Metastasis of Prostate Cancer

Cancer Metastasis – Biology and Treatment

VOLUME 10

Series Editors

Richard J. Ablin, *Ph.D., University of Arizona, College of Medicine and The Arizona Cancer Center, AZ, U.S.A.*
Wen G. Jiang, *M.D., Wales College of Medicine, Cardiff University, Cardiff, U.K.*

Advisory Editorial Board

Harold F. Dvorak, *M.D.*
Phil Gold, *M.D., Ph.D.*
Danny Welch *Ph.D.*
Hiroshi Kobayashi, *M.D., Ph.D.*
Robert E. Mansel, *M.S., FRCS.*
Klaus Pantel *Ph.D.*

Recent Volumes in this Series

Volume 4: Proteases and Their Inhibitors in Cancer Metastasis
Editors: Jean-Michel Foidart and Ruth J. Muschel
ISBN 1-4020-0923-2

Volume 5: Micrometastasis
Editor: Klaus Pantel
ISBN 1-4020-1155-5

Volume 6: Bone Metastasis and Molecular Mechanisms
Editors: Gurmit Singh and William Orr
ISBN 1-4020-1984-X

Volume 7: DNA Methylation, Epigenetics and Metastasis
Editor: Manel Esteller
ISBN 1-4020-3641-8

Volume 8: Cell Motility in Cancer Invasion and Metastasis
Editor: Alan Wells
ISBN 1-4020-4008-3

Volume 9: Cell Adhesion and Cytoskeletal Molecules in Metastasis
Editors: Anne E. Cress and Raymond B. Nagle
ISBN: 1-4020-5128-X

Metastasis of Prostate Cancer

Edited by

Richard J. Ablin
University of Arizona College of Medicine, and the Arizona Cancer Center, Tucson, AZ, U.S.A.

and

Malcolm D. Mason
University of Cardiff, U.K.

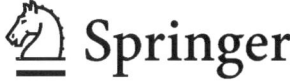

Library of Congress Control Number: 2008920686

ISBN 978-1-4020-5846-2 (HB)
ISBN 978-1-4020-5847-9 (e-book)

Published by Springer,
P.O. Box 17, 3300 AA Dordrecht, The Netherlands.

www.springer.com

Printed on acid-free paper

All Rights Reserved
© 2008 Springer Science+Business Media B.V.
No part of this work may be reproduced, stored in a retrieval system, or transmitted
in any form or by any means, electronic, mechanical, photocopying, microfilming, recording
or otherwise, without written permission from the Publisher, with the exception
of any material supplied specifically for the purpose of being entered
and executed on a computer system, for exclusive use by the purchaser of the work.

TABLE OF CONTENTS

List of Contributors ix

Chapter 1 1
Introduction: Metastasis as a Therapeutic Target
Richard J. Ablin and Malcolm D. Mason

Chapter 2 5
The Natural History of Prostate Cancer
David F. Penson and Peter C. Albertsen

Chapter 3 21
The Search for Genes Which Influence Prostate Cancer Metastasis: A Moving Target?
Norman J. Maitland

Chapter 4 63
Polyunsaturated Fatty Acids and Prostate Cancer Metastasis
Wen G. Jiang

Chapter 5 87
Role of Prostaglandin Synthesis and Cyclooxygenase-2 in Prostate Cancer and Metastasis
Alaa F. Badawi

Chapter 6 111
Cell Cycle Regulation
Ruchi M. Newman and Bruce R. Zetter

Chapter 7 127

Epithelial-Mesenchymal Molecular Interactions in Prostatic Tumor Cell Plasticity

Mary J.C. Hendrix, Jun Luo, Elisabeth A. Seftor, Navesh Sharma, Paul M. Heidger Jr., Michael B. Cohen, Robert Bhatty, Jirapat Chungthapong, Richard E.B. Seftor, and David Lubaroff

Chapter 8 143

Orthotopic Metastatic Mouse Models of Prostate Cancer

Robert M. Hoffman

Chapter 9 171

ß-Catenin, its Binding Partners and Signalling Mechanisms: Implications in Prostate Cancer

Gaynor Davies, Gregory M. Harrison, and Malcolm D. Mason

Chapter 10 197

Hepatocyte Growth Factor/Scatter Factor and Prostate Cancer Metastasis

Gaynor Davies, Wen G. Jiang, and Malcolm D. Mason

Chapter 11 221

Matrix Degradation in Prostate Cancer

Michael J. Wilson and Akhouri A. Sinha

Chapter 12 253

The Biology of Bone Metastases from Prostate Cancer and the Role of Bisphosphonates

Noel W. Clarke and Herbert A. Fleisch

Chapter 13 283

Hormone Therapy for Prostate Cancer

Mike Shelley, Charles Bennett, Derek Nathan, and Oliver Sartor

Chapter 14 309

Strategies for the Implementation of Chemotherapy and Radiotherapy

Paula Scullin, Joe M. O'Sullivan, and Christopher C. Parker

Chapter 15 337
Immuno-Gene Therapy for Metastatic Prostate Cancer
Takefumi Satoh, Terry L. Timme, Yehoshua Gdor, Brian J. Miles, Robert J. Amato, Dov Kadmon, and Timothy C. Thompson

Chapter 16 355
Distilling the Past – Envisioning the Future
Richard J. Ablin and Malcolm D. Mason

Index 399

LIST OF CONTRIBUTORS

Richard J. Ablin, Ph.D.
Department of Immunobiology, University of Arizona College of Medicine and the Arizona Cancer Center, Tucson, AZ, USA

Peter C. Albertsen, M.D.
Division of Urology, Department of Surgery, University of Connecticut, School of Medicine, Farmington, CT, USA

Robert J. Amato, Ph.D.
Scott Department of Urology, Baylor College Of Medicine, Houston, TX, USA

Alaa F. Badawi, Ph.D.
Division of Population Sciences, Fox Chase Cancer Center, Philadelphia, PA, USA

Robert Bhatty, Ph.D.
Department of Anatomy and Cell Biology, University of Iowa, Iowa City, IA, USA

Charles L. Bennett, M.D., Ph.D.
Lakeside Veterans Administration Hospital, Chicago, IL, USA

Noel W. Clarke, M.D.
Christie Hospital, Withington, Manchester, United Kingdom

Jirapat Chunthapong, Ph.D.
Department of Biology, Faculty of Science, Khon Kaen University, Khon Kaen, Thailand

Michael B. Cohen, Ph.D.
Department of Pathology, University of Iowa, Iowa City, IA, USA

Gaynor Davies, Ph.D.
Section of Clinical Oncology, Department of Medicine, Velindre NHS Trust, Cardiff, United Kingdom

Herbert A. Fleisch, M.D.
Department of Pathophysiology, University of Berne, Berne, Switzerland.

Yehoshua Gdor, Ph.D.
Scott Department of Urology, Baylor College of Medicine, Houston, TX, USA

Gregory M. Harrison
Metastasis Research Group, University Department of Surgery, University of Wales College of Medicine, Heath Park, Cardiff, Wales, UK

Paul M. Heidger, Jr., Ph.D.
Department of Anatomy and Cell Biology, University of Iowa, Iowa City, IA, USA

Mary J. C. Hendrix, Ph.D.
Children's Memorial Research Center, Feinberg School of Medicine, Northwestern University, Chicago, IL, USA

Robert M. Hoffman, Ph.D.
Department of Surgery, UCSD Medical Center, Anticancer, Inc., San Diego, CA, USA

Wen G. Jiang, M.B., B.Ch., M.D.
Metastasis and Angiogenesis Research Group, University Department of Surgery, Wales College of Medicine, Cardiff University, Cardiff, United Kingdom

Dov Kadman, Ph.D.
Scott Department of Urology, Baylor College Of Medicine, Houston, TX, USA

David Lubaroff, Ph.D.
Department of Urology, University Of Iowa, Iowa City, IA, USA

Jun Luo, Ph.D.
Brady Urological Institute at Johns Hopkins Medical Institutions, Baltimore, MD, USA

Norman Maitland, M.D.
Department of Biology, Cancer Research Unit, University of York, York, United Kingdom

Malcolm D. Mason, M.D.
Section of Clinical Oncology, Department of Medicine, Velindre NHS Trust, Cardiff, United Kingdom

Brian J. Miles, Ph.D.
Scott Department of Urology, Baylor College of Medicine, Houston, TX, USA

Derek Nathan, B.A.
Lakeside Veterans Administration Hospital, Chicago, IL, USA

Ruchi M. Newman, Ph.D.
The Burnham Institute, La Jolla, CA, USA

Joe M. O'Sullivan, M.D.
Unit of Academic Urology, Institute of Cancer Research, The Royal Marsden NHS Trust, Sutton, Surrey, United Kingdom

Christopher C. Parker, M.D.
Academic Unit of Radiotherapy and Oncology, The Royal Marsden NHS Trust, Sutton, Surrey , United Kingdom

David F. Penson, M.D., M.P.H.
Norris Comprehensive Cancer Center, Department of Urology, Keck School of Medicine, University of Southern California, Los Angeles, CA, USA

A. Oliver Sartor, M.D.
Lank Center for Genitourinary Oncology, Department of Medical Oncology, Dana-Farber Cancer Institute, Harvard Medical School, Boston, MA, USA

Takefumi Satoh, Ph.D.
Scott Department of Urology, Baylor College of Medicine, Houston, TX, USA

Paula Sculin, M.D.
Northern Ireland Cancer Center and Queen's University Belfast, Belfast, Northern Ireland, UK

Elisabeth A. Seftor, M.S.
Children's Memorial Research Center, Feinberg School of Medicine, Northwestern University, Chicago, IL, USA

Richard E.B. Seftor, Ph.D.
Children's Memorial Research Center, Feinberg School of Medicine, Northwestern University, Chicago, IL, USA

Navesh Sharma, Ph.D.
University of Kansas School of Medicine, Kansas City, KS, USA

Michael D. Shelley, Ph.D.
Cochrane Prostatic Diseases and Urological Cancers Group, Cochrane Unit, Research Department, Velindre NHS Trust, Cardiff, United Kingdom

Akhouri A. Sinha, Ph.D.
Department of Research Services, Veterans Administration Medical Center, Minneapolis, MN, USA

Timothy C. Thompson, Ph.D.
Scott Department of Urology, Baylor College Of Medicine, Houston, TX, USA

Terry L. Timme, Ph.D.
Scott Department of Urology, Baylor College Of Medicine, Houston, TX, USA

Michael J. Wilson, Ph.D.
Department of Research Services, Veterans Administration Medical Center, Minneapolis, MN, USA

Bruce R. Zetter, Ph.D.
Children's Hospital, Harvard Medical School, Boston, MA, USA

Chapter 1

INTRODUCTION: METASTASIS AS A THERAPEUTIC TARGET

Richard J. Ablin[1] and Malcolm D. Mason[2]
[1]*Department of Immunobiology, University of Arizona College of Medicine and the Arizona Cancer Center, Tucson, AZ USA and*
[2]*Section of Oncology and Palliative Medicine, University of Wales College of Medicine, Velindre Hospital, Cardiff, Wales, UK*

The National Cancer Act (NCA) of 1971 (1) sounded a clarion call for a critical increase in the interest and activity of the nations endeavours in cancer research and its potential clinical application. Buoyed by the increased enthusiasm and funding for cancer research and specific organ sites, the NCA was followed shortly thereafter by the formation of the National Prostatic Cancer Project. Some 35-years later, we are more often than not reminded that prostate cancer is the most frequently diagnosed cancer in America and the second leading cause of cancer deaths in men after lung cancer. And, although massive, yet to be justified, prostate-specific antigen (PSA) screening, has witnessed a stage migration in the incidence of metastatic to regionally localized disease on initial diagnosis, the mortality from metastatic prostate cancer has changed little and remains the principle cause of prostate cancer related death in man.

In concert with the foregoing and recognizing the continuing insipid sequelae of the progression of prostate cancer to the invasive and metastatic state, we have, challenging as it may be, set "metastasis as a therapeutic target."

Metastasis as a process is the most "central," and yet at the same time the most problematic of all the processes to target as cancer therapy. "Central," because metastasis is the key-defining feature of malignancy, and problematic because of the many patients who present when this process has already taken place, or at least has been started. Upwards of 90% of deaths from cancer are due to metastases (2). It is often argued that success in targeting metastasis *per se* is closely dependent on being able to identify tumors at a pre-metastatic phase, itself a formidable challenge.

However, in the case of prostate cancer, there are other reasons to anticipate targeting metastasis may yield clinical benefits. One of the hallmarks of prostate cancer, with a latent period of ≥ 30 years, is its slow rate of progression. This is particularly true of the time window between first presentation with localized disease, and development of hormone refractory metastatic disease, which, if it occurs, may do so over a time span of many years. It is entirely reasonable, therefore, to hypothesize that if one could effect some reduction in proliferation rate, even in patients with established, but occult metastatic disease, this might translate into a situation where a patient's prostate cancer becomes "irrelevant" in the sense it can be prevented from progressing during their lifetime.

There is another reason for studying the underlying biological basis of the metastasis of prostate cancer. That is, that one of the formidable challenges, if not the most, facing the clinician is being able to distinguish early prostate cancer that may be indolent from one that is aggressive, clinically significant and that should be treated. Currently it is not possible to definitively identify the aggressive tumor. Therefore, many men undergo unnecessary therapy with its attendant morbidities, while other possibly dangerously conservative treatment. And, as the very appropriate, and most often quoted statement by the late, Willet F. Whitmore, Jr., asks: "Is cure possible? Is cure necessary? Is cure possible only when it is not necessary?" (3). It seems an almost inescapable conclusion that insight toward understanding the processes which lead to metastasis of prostate cancer will greatly aid in this critical clinical distinction.

In the 25-years since one of us (RJA) edited one of the early treatises on prostate cancer in 1981 (4), the introduction of the use of the PSA test has revolutionized the practice of urology and changed the face of prostate cancer. In spite of the increased awareness and interest in prostate cancer, the myriad molecular biological investigations, clinical studies and significant decrease in the incidence of metastatic disease on diagnosis, the mortality from metastatic prostate cancer has changed little. What's more, 25–35% of patients with organ-confined disease who undergo radical prostatectomy have a recurrence within 5 years of which a significant number go on to develop metastatic disease and die.

Given the foregoing, it was thought appropriate to take a step back and asses the current state of the reality in setting metastasis of prostate cancer as a "therapeutic target." Toward this end, we have been privileged to assemble international experts to cover the gamut from the fundamentals of molecular biology of metastasis to the patient in the clinic. Last, but not least, in the final Chapter –"Distilling the Past, Envisioning the Future," the endeavor is made to comment and expand on the topics covered within limits, knowing we cannot be all encompassing.

REFERENCES

1. *National Cancer Act*, P.L. No. 99–158, 1971.
2. Hananhan D, Weinberg RA. The hallmarks of cancer. Cell 2000, 100:57–70.
3. Montie JE, JAS Jr. Whitemoreism: Memorable quotes from Willet F.Whitmore, Jr., M.D. Urology 2004, 63:207–09.
4. Ablin RJ. *Prostatic Cancer*. New York: Marcel Dekker, Inc, 1981, pp. 321.

Chapter 2

THE NATURAL HISTORY OF PROSTATE CANCER

David F. Penson[1] and Peter C. Albertsen[2]
[1] University of Washington, Seattle, WA, USA
[2] University of Connecticut Health Center, Farmington, CT, USA

Abstract: Although prostate cancer is the most common solid tumor among American men, it is not a leading cause of cancer death. In fact, the majority of men diagnosed with this malignancy do not ultimately die of their disease. While this may be due in part to effective therapies, it is also likely due to the fact that many prostate cancers are indolent in nature, taking many years to present with clinical manifestations, if at all. The goal of this chapter is to review the literature on the natural history of untreated prostate cancer and to identify factors predictive of clinical significant disease. We begin by reviewing the influence of pathologic differentiation, clinical stage and tumor volume on the natural history of prostate cancer. We then discuss how underlying patients characteristics, such as age and co-morbidity influence outcomes in this disease. By reviewing the effect of these factors on the natural history of prostate cancer, the reader will obtain a better understanding of this malignancy and will be able to improve outcomes in men affected by this common condition.

Key words: prostate cancer, natural history, epidemiology

In 2004, 230,000 new cases of prostate cancer were identified in the United States making this disease the most common solid tumor of men. Despite the high incidence of disease in the U.S., only 30,000 men will die of prostate cancer this year (1). While this may be due, at least in part, to effective management of early prostate cancer, there is little doubt that many newly diagnosed cases are indolent in nature and require no treatment. Many patients are likely to die with, rather than of, prostate cancer. This is particularly true of older men who present with localized disease that can often take decades to metastasize (2).

Once prostate cancer metastasizes, the natural history of the disease is ominous. Patients presenting with symptomatic metastases to bone respond to hormone ablation therapy for an average of only 2 years (3). The disease then progresses to its hormone-insensitive stage with most patients surviving only a matter of months (4). Clearly, one of the great challenges facing both clinicians and researchers is to identify which patients with prostate cancer have aggressive, clinically significant prostate cancer with metastatic potential and which patients have indolent tumors which are unlikely to become problematic during the patient's lifetime.

In contemporary practice, a majority of patients with prostate cancer present with localized disease (5). Understanding which of these malignancies will ultimately become "clinically significant" permits more selective application of aggressive therapy, with a subsequent reduction in morbidity experienced by prostate cancer patients and an improved quality of life. To appreciate which tumors will impact clinical outcomes, known biologic characteristics of the tumor, including tumor volume (as evidenced by baseline prostate-specific antigen (PSA) levels), pathologic differentiation (as measured by Gleason score) and stage at presentation, must be balanced against underlying host factors (such as age and co-morbid conditions.) The goal of this chapter is to review the existing literature on the natural history of untreated prostate cancer and to identify which factors are predictive of clinically significant disease. By providing the reader with a better understanding of the relationship between tumor characteristics, underlying host factors and clinical outcomes, clinicians and researchers alike will understand better the natural history of prostate cancer, which hopefully will lead to improved clinical care and properly constructed, risk-adjusted research.

1. TUMOR CHARACTERISTICS THAT AFFECT THE NATURAL HISTORY OF PROSTATE CANCER

1.1 Influence of Histologic Differentiation on Natural History

Clearly, not all prostate cancers are "equal". Some tumors have considerably greater biologic potential for local and/or distant progression than others. The degree of histologic differentiation, or pathologic grade, is an important variable that is clearly associated with the malignant potential of the tumor. Prior to the publication of the Gleason grading system as part of the Veterans Administration Cooperative Urological Research Group's

(VACURG) clinical trials of the 1960's and 70's, many pathologists found it difficult to classify pathologic differentiation in adenocarcinoma of the prostate. As part of the VACURG trials, Dr. Gleason classified prostate cancer specimens from 270 men enrolled in VA cooperative trials. After reviewing the pathology of each of these tumors, he developed a relatively simple scoring system for grading pathologic differentiation (6). Not surprisingly, patients with higher grade prostate cancer were more likely to present with advanced disease (7). However, patients with higher primary Gleason score (more poorly differentiated prostate cancers) were also more likely to die of prostate cancer at both 6 and 30 months following diagnosis (see Table 1). This finding underscores the fact that histological differentiation of the tumor impacts natural history in men with prostate cancer.

Gleason updated his grading system in 1974 using the 1032 cases enrolled in the VACURG trials nationally that had prostate tissue available for review (8). When considering the results of this study, readers should remember that the trials included men who were randomized to various treatments for prostate cancer according to one of four protocols. They included: 1) radical prostatectomy vs. radical prostatectomy and 5 mg of diethylstilbesterol (DES) per day for localized disease; 2) radical prostatectomy versus no therapy for men with localized disease; 3) placebo vs. 5 mg DES/day vs. orchiectomy alone vs. orchiectomy and 5 mg of DES/day for regional or

Table 1. The relationship of Gleason pathologic score and survival in 270 men diagnosed with prostate cancer in the pre-PSA era. Results from Bailer et al. (7)

Pathologic pattern	6 month outcome			30 month outcome		
	N	Total deaths (%)	Prostate-cancer specific deaths (%)	N	Total deaths (%)	Prostate-cancer specific deaths (%)
Primary						
1	30	1 (3)	0 (0)	16	1 (6)	0 (0)
2	89	4 (4)	0 (0)	57	10 (18)	2 (4)
3	121	8 (7)	4 (3)	71	17 (24)	9 (13)
4	10	1 (10)	1 (10)	6	2 (33)	2 (33)
5	20	5 (25)	2 (10)	12	9 (75)	6 (50)
Secondary						
1	9	0 (0)	0 (0)	4	0 (0)	0 (0)
2	57	1 (2)	0 (0)	36	3 (8)	1 (3)
3	152	11 (7)	3 (2)	89	24 (27)	10 (11)
4	20	3 (15)	0 (0)	12	3 (25)	1 (8)
5	32	4 (13)	4 (13)	21	9 (43)	7 (33)

metastatic disease or; 4) 1 mg DES/day vs. 2.5 mg of estrogen/day vs. 30 mg of progesterone/day alone vs. 30 mg progesterone and 5 mg DES/day for regional or metastatic disease. Despite the differing treatments, one can draw reasonable conclusions regarding the impact of histological differentiation on the natural history of prostate cancer in these patients. The VACURG investigators did this by calculating number of deaths per patient-year of follow-up. This variable was derived by taking the number of deaths and dividing by the sum of follow-up times for all patients for whom tissue was available. The results are presented in Figure 1. Unlike Gleason's prior work, where he had identified both primary and secondary pathologic patterns within a tumor, in this report he combined two scores into a single sum on a scale from 2 to 10, with higher scores being more poorly differentiated disease. As the data indicate, men with more poorly differentiated prostate cancer (Gleason sum 8–10) are more likely to die of their disease than men with well-differentiated disease (Gleason sum 2–5).

Others have also noted the strong influence of histology on the natural history of prostate cancer. In particular, Johansson et al. (9–11) have studied both 10 and 15 year survival rates in a population-based cohort of men with early, untreated localized prostate cancer. From a group of 648 consecutive men who were diagnosed with prostate cancer at Orebro Medical Center from March 1977 through February 1984, they identified 223 with localized disease who did not receive any initial treatment. Overall ten and fifteen year survival was 41% and 21%, respectively. Importantly, 10 and 15 year prostate cancer-specific survival (corrected for causes of death other than prostate cancer) was much higher, 86 and 81% respectively. When

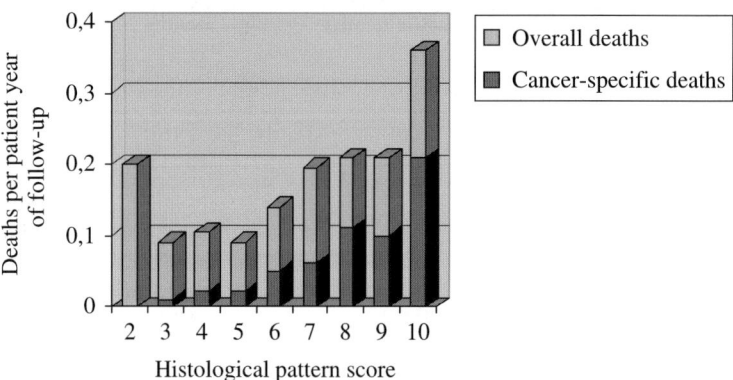

Figure 1. Deaths per patient year follow-up in the VACURG trials stratified by Gleason pathologic sum. Data from Gleason et al. (8).

stratified by histologic grade, men with poorly differentiated prostate cancer were more likely to develop metastases and to die from prostate cancer, as demonstrated in Table 2.

While the results from this study illustrated the relationship between histology and the natural history of localized prostate cancer, the authors' final conclusion that "patients with localized prostate cancer have a favorable outlook following watchful waiting, and that the number of deaths potentially avoidable by radical initial treatment is limited"(11) generated considerable controversy. In particular, critics noted that the study cohort was primarily comprised of men with well-differentiated prostate cancer (148 out of 223, presumably with Gleason grade 2–5/6 disease). This does not reflect current diagnostic trends in the United States, where most men present with moderately differentiated (Gleason 5–7) prostate cancer(12). Furthermore, critics of the Johansson studies note that the advanced age of patients at diagnosis (62% were over the age of 70) limits the number of years they are at risk for disease progression or prostate cancer-specific death. In other words, the patients never had a chance to experience problems from their prostate cancer because they had such a short life expectancy at entry into the cohort. In support of this, Aus et al. (13) from Goteborg, Sweden, used the Swedish Cancer Registry to identify all men with prostate cancer who died in Goteborg of any cause between 1988 and 1990. A cohort of 536 men, selected for younger, healthier men with higher grade disease, was initially identified, from which 14 cases were excluded because they were diagnosed at autopsy, 6 because they were treated with curative intent and 2 because they were lost to follow-up. Of the remaining 514 patients, 301 (59%) had non-metastatic disease at the time of presentation. In this group of patients, the longer a subject survived after diagnosis, the more likely he was to die of prostate cancer. For men who survived 0–5 years

Table 2. Fifteen year local and metastatic progression rates and prostate-cancer specific deaths in 223 men with localized prostate cancer treated expectantly in Orebro, Sweden. Data from Johansson et al. (11)

Pathologic differentiation	Total number of patients	Number with local progression (%)	Number with metastatic progression (%)	Number who died from prostate cancer (%)
Highly (grade I)	148	37 (25)	2 (8)	9 (6)
Moderately (grade II)	66	33 (50)	2 (18)	11 (17)
Poorly (grade III)	9	3 (33)	6 (67)	5 (56)

after diagnosis, the risk of prostate cancer death was 39%. This increased to 54% for men who survived 5–10 years after diagnosis, 57% for those who survived 10–15 years, 71% for those who survived 15–20 years and 71% for those who survived more than 20 years. The Aus study calls into question the generalizability of the Johansson data to younger and healthier men diagnosed with localized prostate cancer. In addition, it supports the observation that histology impacts natural history, as men with poorly differentiated prostate cancer were still more likely to die of their disease (risk of prostate cancer-related death was 43% for men with well-differentiated disease, 48% with moderately differentiated disease and 60% for men with poorly differentiated disease.)

More recently, Lu-Yao and Yao (14) studied a group of 59,876 American men aged 50–79 years diagnosed with localized prostate cancer from 1983 through 1992. This population-based cohort was identified using the Surveillance, Epidemiology and End Results (SEER) dataset maintained by the National Cancer Institute (NCI). In this cohort, 19,898 (33.2%) initially received conservative management. Within the group of watchful waiting patients, 9804 (49%) had histologically well-differentiated disease, 6198 (31%) had moderately differentiated disease, 2236 (11%) had poorly differentiated disease, and 9% had cancer of unknown pathologic grade. Patients initially managed with watchful waiting tended to be older than men receiving radical prostatectomy (mean age at diagnosis: 70.7 vs. 65.8 years respectively). Mean follow-up was 44.5 months with 10% of patients followed for 92 months or longer. An intention-to-treat analysis was performed and 10-year overall and disease-specific survival rates were calculated utilizing annual mortality rates. Ten-year prostate cancer-specific survival in all 19,898 men with localized prostate cancer electing conservative management was 82%. However, stratifying the results by pathologic grade illustrates the importance of this variable in predicting the natural history of this disease. In men with well-differentiated disease, 10 year prostate cancer-specific survival was 93%; in moderately differentiated disease, it was 77%; and in poorly differentiated disease, it dropped to 45%. Lu-Yao and Yao (14) clearly demonstrate that pathologic grade is an important predictor of the natural history of localized prostate cancer.

1.2   Influence of Stage on Natural History

While there is little debate that men who present with metastatic disease have a worse prognosis than those who present with localized disease, the impact of tumor volume in localized prostate cancer patients is less clear. In a controversial meta-analysis of 6 non-randomized studies examining survival in men with localized prostate cancer who elected conservative management, Chodak et al. (15) used proportional hazards analysis to examine the independent effect of grade, stage and age on disease-specific survival. Like the prior studies (one of which (10) was included in the meta-analysis), higher pathologic grade was a strong predictor of worse survival in the multivariable analysis. Ten-year disease specific survival was 87% for both men with well-differentiated (Grade 1) and moderately differentiated (Grade 2) prostate cancer, while men with poorly differentiated (Grade 3) disease had a ten-year survival of only 34%. In the Cox regression, which controlled for age, study cohort and stage at presentation, men with Grade 2 disease were 1.64 times more likely to die of prostate cancer than men with grade 1 disease, although this did not quite reach statistical significance ($p = 0.08$). However, men with Grade 3 disease were 10 times more likely to die of prostate cancer than men with Grade 1 disease and this relationship was highly statistically significant ($p < 0.001$).

While the results from the Chodak meta-analysis concerning pathologic grade are fairly conclusive, the data regarding stage at presentation are considerably less clear. The cohorts included in the study were all accrued prior to the introduction and use of prostate-specific antigen as a screening test. Therefore, most of the patients were detected either at the time of transurethral resection of the prostate (TURP) or by palpable disease on digital rectal exam. Stage at presentation was categorized using a combination of the 1992 AJCC TNM Staging System,(16) the Jewitt-Whitmore system(17) and the Chisholm system.(18) Of the 828 subjects in the meta-analysis, 19% had Stage A1 disease, 26% had A2 disease, 12% had B1 disease, 42% had B2 or B3 disease, while stage was unknown in the remaining 1%. In the Cox regression analysis, Stage A1 was chosen as the referent category. When controlling for age, grade and study cohort, there was a trend towards higher stage cancer being associated with increased prostate cancer-specific mortality, but this did not reach statistical significance (risk ratios: $A2 = 1.38$, $B1 = 1.77$, and $B2/3 = 2.38$ when compared to men with A1 disease). The unreliability of digital rectal examination or transurethral resection of the prostate as staging tests that adequately quantify overall tumor volume may explain why tumor stage is not a more powerful predictor of overall mortality.

1.3   Influence of Tumor Volume, as Evidenced by Serum PSA Levels, on Natural History

Prior studies have shown that serum PSA levels can serve as reasonable proxies for tumor volume, at least in the aggregate. Catalona et al. (19)

collected data on 10,251 men aged 50 years or older who participated in a community screening program for prostate cancer. In patients with PSA levels above 10 ng/ml, only 45% had disease localized to the prostate, indicating that PSA may be a proxy marker for tumor volume. If tumor volume reflects the natural history of prostate cancer, it follows that PSA at the time of diagnosis may also reflect the natural history of this disease. Although there are no studies looking specifically at this issue in men treated with expectant management, there are a number of reports that document this relationship in men treated with aggressive therapy. For example, Kupelian et al. (20) studied a cohort of 423 patients treated with radical prostatectomy for presumably localized prostate cancer at a single institution. Five year biochemical recurrence-free survival was 88% in men with a preoperative PSA of less than or equal to 4 ng/ml, 62% in men who presented with a PSA from 4–10 ng/ml, 48% for men who presented with a PSA between 10–20 ng/ml and 31% for those who presented with a PSA greater than 20 ng/ml. In fact, in the multivariable analysis of the same dataset, baseline PSA was the strongest predictor of 5-year recurrence-free survival, although baseline Gleason score and surgical margin status were also found to be significant predictors of outcomes. D'Amico and colleagues (21) also found baseline PSA to be an important predictor of biochemical recurrence in a proportional hazards analysis of 688 men undergoing radical prostatectomy at a single institution. They later confirmed these findings in a larger group of patients that included 468 men undergoing radiotherapy for localized disease, demonstrating that baseline PSA is a predictor of outcomes in localized prostate cancer (22).

Researchers have also suggested that longitudinal changes in PSA may be useful in identifying men who have occult prostate cancer. Carter et al. (23) performed a case-control study using serum from men participating in the Baltimore Longitudinal Study of Aging. The study consisted of 16 men with no prostate cancer (controls), 20 men with a histological diagnosis of benign prostatic hyperplasia (BPH) and 18 men over age 60 with pathologically confirmed prostate cancer who had participated in the study for at least 7 years prior to diagnosis. Patients were classified as having local, regional or distant disease on the basis of clinical examination, prostatic acid phosphatase levels, bone scan results and information from the treating physician's medical records. While there was serum available from subjects on several occasions, this was not collected at each visit and, therefore, the number and interval of PSA measurements was not standardized. A mixed-effects regression model was used to test the hypothesis that, after controlling for the effect of age at diagnosis, PSA values increase faster in subjects with prostate cancer compared with controls. Mean PSA levels

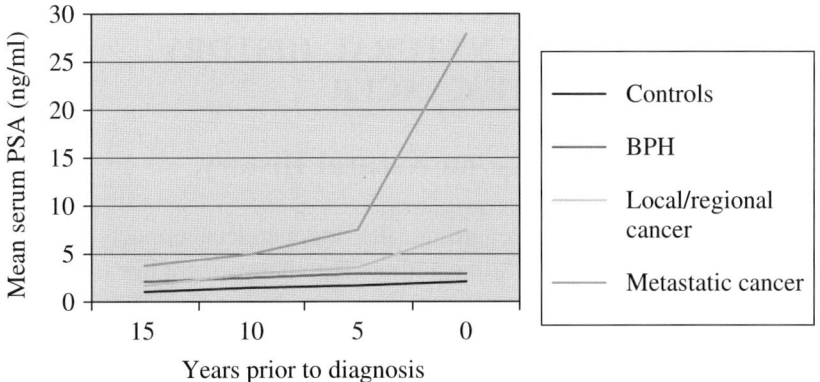

Figure 2. Mean prostate-specific antigen levels of 44 men from the Baltimore Longitudinal Study of Aging with either no prostate cancer, benign prostatic hyperplasia or prostate cancer at 5 year interval prior to diagnosis. (Data from Carter et al. (23)).

for the various groups of patients in the study are presented graphically in Figure 2. Patients with prostate cancer had significantly higher rates of change of PSA than those without prostate cancer up to 10 years prior to diagnosis. Rates of change in serum PSA also helped distinguish between men with localized and metastatic prostate cancer, as shown in Figure 2. Although the study did not provide information regarding Gleason score, it does demonstrate that patients with prostate cancer have elevated serum PSA levels well before the diagnosis of prostate cancer and that the rate of change of PSA may be helpful in identifying men with more advanced disease.

The studies described above summarize the available evidence on the influence of various tumor characteristics, such as pathologic differentiation, clinical stage at presentation and tumor volume on the natural history of localized prostate cancer. There is little doubt that as our comprehension of the genetic mechanisms involved in prostate cancer development and growth improves, we will identify additional markers of more aggressive disease that will be useful in understanding the natural history of prostate cancer. Any advances in our understanding of prostate cancer tumor biology, however, must be framed against the underlying host characteristics of the patient. As life expectancies of men with the most aggressive prostate cancers are often still measured in years, as opposed to months, other factors, such as age at diagnosis and co-morbid conditions must be considered when counseling patients on the natural history of their disease.

2. HOST CHARACTERISTICS THAT AFFECT THE NATURAL HISTORY OF PROSTATE CANCER

2.1 Influence of Age on Natural History

There is some debate regarding the independent impact of age on outcomes in prostate cancer. Some authors feel that younger age is associated with more aggressive disease (24), while others do not (25). When assessing non-randomized cohort studies of men with localized prostate cancer who elect conservative management, age is often an important predictor of survival, due at least in part to the selected nature of observational cohorts of men choosing watchful waiting. In particular, selection bias may be present in two forms: first, elderly men (>75 years) with short life expectancies (less then 10 years) are often counseled by their providers to choose conservative management, as many providers feel aggressive therapy should be reserved for men with longer life expectancies. Alternatively, younger men (<60 years) who elect watchful waiting tend to have significant co-morbid disease which makes them more likely to die of other conditions and impacts any analysis of the natural history of localized disease in this population. This observation underscores the importance of controlling for both age and co-morbid conditions when assessing the impact of treatment on outcomes in prostate cancer.

To address this issue, Albertsen et al. (2) studied 767 men diagnosed with clinically localized prostate cancer between 1971 and 1984 who were managed expectantly. Using the Connecticut Tumor Registry to identify patients eligible for inclusion in this population-base study, the authors limited their analysis to men aged 55 to 74 years at the time of diagnosis. They obtained original histology specimens and reanalyzed these slides using contemporary Gleason grading criteria. They then stratified their cohort by both age at diagnosis and Gleason grade. Using both the Connecticut tumor registry and the vital statistics bureau of the Department of Public Health, long-term disease-specific and overall survival information was collected. The mean follow-up of the cohort from diagnosis to death was 8.6 years. Of the 157 patients lost to follow-up or known to be alive as of March 1, 1997, the mean follow-up was 15.4 years. Cause of death was determined using death certificate data according to accepted algorithms for assessing this outcome from these data.

The results of the stratified survival analysis are shown in Figure 3. These data underscore the importance of considering both tumor factors

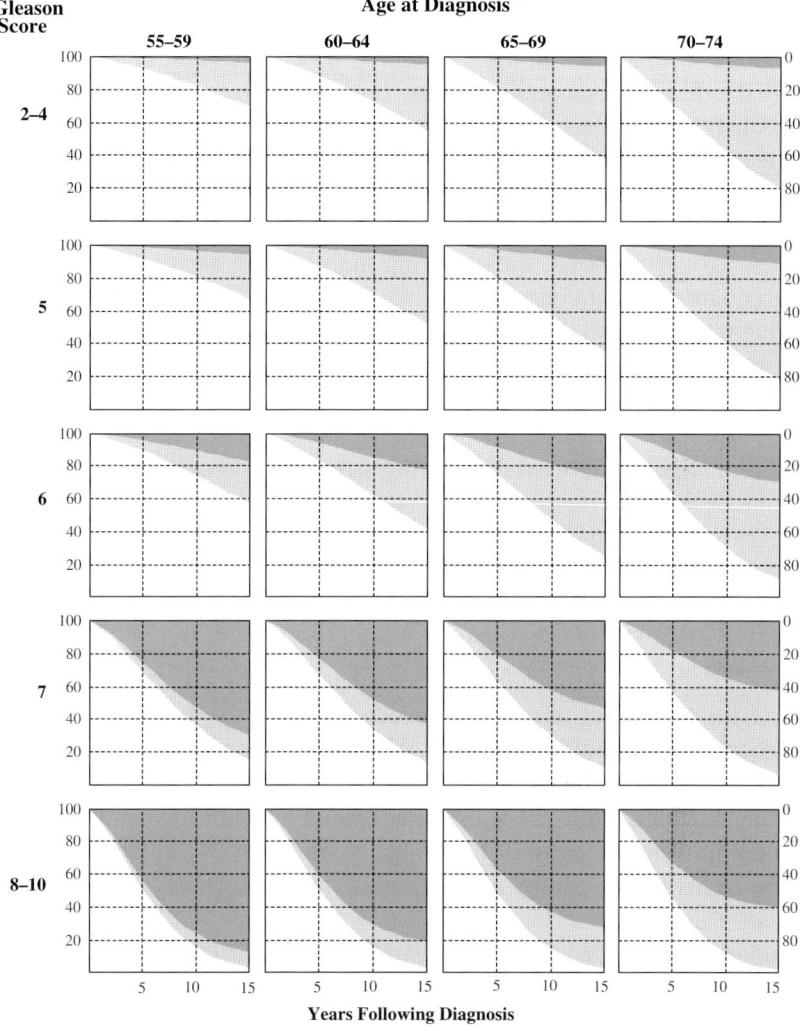

Figure 3. Survival (white lower band) and cumulative mortality from prostate cancer (dark gray upper band) and all other causes (light gray middle band) up to 15 years following diagnosis stratified by age at diagnosis and Gleason score. The percentage of men alive can be read from y-axis on the left, and the percentage of men who have died of prostate cancer or other causes can be read from the y-axis on the right. (From Albertsen et al. (2) with permission. Copyrighted 1998, American Medical Association).

(histological grade) and host characteristics (age at diagnosis) when studying the natural history of localized prostate cancer.

Patients with low-grade disease (Gleason 2–4) were unlikely to die of prostate cancer within 15 years of diagnosis. Older men (age 70–75) with low-grade disease had an approximately 20% overall survival at 15 years due to deaths from competing causes. If one is to counsel a patient regarding his probability of dying from localized prostate cancer, these data underscore that both the Gleason score of the tumor and the age of the patient must be considered. Men with high grade disease (Gleason 8–10) experienced high prostate-cancer specific mortality within 15 years of diagnosis, regardless of their age at diagnosis, underscoring the very aggressive nature of poorly differentiated prostate cancer.

The results from Albertsen and colleagues' research are remarkably consistent with the studies mentioned earlier (10, 14, 15). After 15 years, men diagnosed with low-grade disease (Gleason 2–4) have a small risk of dying from prostate cancer. Men with moderate-grade disease (Gleason 5–6) have a slightly higher risk of dying from their disease, while those with high-grade disease (Gleason 7–10) have a substantial risk of dying from prostate cancer if managed conservatively.

2.2　　Influence of Co-Morbid Conditions on Outcomes

The number of co-morbid conditions a patient has at the time of diagnosis also affects outcomes in prostate cancer. Patients may be more likely to die of a competing condition than die of prostate cancer. It follows that, if a patient has another illness that significantly limits his life expectancy, he may be a better candidate for expectant management. The natural history of indolent prostate cancer will be clinically irrelevant. To this end, a number of researchers have examined the impact of co-morbidity on outcomes in prostate cancer.

Albertsen et al. (26) studied the impact of co-morbidity on life expectancy in men with prostate cancer using three well-known, validated co-morbidity indexes. They used the Connecticut tumor registry to identify men aged 65 to 75 years old diagnosed with prostate cancer between 1971 and 1976 at one of the 39 hospitals in the state. Four hundred and fifty-one men were included in the cohort with a mean age of 70.9 years and mean follow-up of 15.5 years. Information on Gleason score, clinical stage at presentation, current vital status and cause of death was obtained from hospital medical records and from the Connecticut Tumor Registry. In the univariate analysis, Gleason score was still the best single independent predictor of age-adjusted survival. However, all three co-morbidity indexes were also predictive of survival in this cohort. In a multivariate analysis, the combination of Gleason score and co-morbidity index score was more predictive than Gleason score, age or clinical stage alone, demonstrating the importance of assessing co-morbid conditions when considering the natural history of prostate cancer.

Given the fact that host factors, such as age and co-morbid condition, can affect outcomes in prostate cancer as much as tumor characteristics, researchers must develop methods of incorporating this information into prognostic systems to help clinicians understand the clinical significance of newly diagnosed disease. Although there are many nomograms available that predict proxy outcomes, such as biochemical-free survival (27, 28) or pathological outcomes following surgery (29), there are few that prognosticate overall or disease-specific survival. Clemens et al. (30) developed such a system in 1986, prior to the introduction of PSA. Using a cohort of 230 men diagnosed with prostate cancer at a single institution in the late 1970's, they employed a statistical method called conjunctive consolidation to develop a staging system that stratified patients using conventional anatomic staging (Jewitt/VACURG score), age, urinary and systemic symptoms and co-morbidity. Although the system did not incorporate Gleason score, it was still able to identify patients who were more likely to survive at least 5 years following diagnosis of prostate cancer. The staging system calculated a score from 0-10 with worse scores predicting poorer prognosis. Men with scores from 0–2, 3–5, 6, and 7–10, had a five-year survival of 91%, 61%, 31% and 9% respectively. Although this "clinical-anatomic" staging system is now somewhat outdated, given the introduction of PSA testing and the importance of Gleason score as a predictor of outcomes, it still demonstrates the importance of using information regarding both the tumor and the host to improve our understanding of the natural history of prostate cancer.

3. SUMMARY

Prostate cancer is a heterogeneous disease that is influenced by a number of variables. Clearly, the best predictor of its natural history is histological differentiation, commonly measured using the Gleason scoring system. However, this is not sufficient when counseling patients with newly diagnosed disease. Stage at presentation and serum PSA must also be considered when assessing the metastatic potential of any prostate tumor. Given the fact that all prostate cancers will eventually progress to systemic disease and death if given sufficient time, it is important to consider host factors when treating men with newly diagnosed prostate cancer or conducting epidemiological studies. The impact of age at diagnosis and concurrent illnesses should not be underestimated. Only by incorporating information on all of these variables will we obtain a better understanding of the natural history of prostate cancer and improve outcomes in men affected by this common disease.

REFERENCES

1. Jemal A, Tiwari RC, Murray T, Ghafoor A, Samuels A, Ward E et al. Cancer statistics, 2004. Cancer J Clin 2004, 54:8–29.
2. Albertsen PC, Hanley JA, Gleason DF, Barry MJ. Competing risk analysis of men aged 55 to 74 years at diagnosis managed conservatively for clinically localized prostate cancer. J Am Med Assoc 1998, 280:975–80.
3. Jacobi GH. LH-RH agonist monotherapy in patients with carcinoma of the prostate and reflections on the so-called total androgen blockade. Recent results. Cancer Res 1990, 118:174–85.
4. Beynon LL, Chisholm GD. The stable state is not an objective response in hormone-escaped carcinoma of prostate. Br J Urol 1984, 56:702–5.
5. Stephenson RF. Population-based prostate cancer trends in the PSA era: Data from the SEER program. Monogr Urol 1998, 91:1–19.
6. Gleason DF. Classification of prostatic carcinomas. Cancer Chemother Rep 1966, 50:125–8.
7. Bailar JC, 3rd, Mellinger GT, Gleason DF. Survival rates of patients with prostatic cancer, tumor stage, and differentiation–preliminary report. Cancer Chemother Rep 1966, 50:129–36.
8. Gleason DF, Mellinger GT. Prediction of prognosis for prostatic adenocarcinoma by combined histological grading and clinical staging. J Urol 1974, 111:58–64.
9. Johansson JE, Adami HO, Andersson SO, Bergstrom R, Krusemo UB, Kraaz W. Natural history of localised prostatic cancer. A population-based study in 223 untreated patients. Lancet 1989, 1:799–803.
10. Johansson JE, Adami HO, Andersson SO, Bergstrom R, Holmberg L, Krusemo UB. High 10-year survival rate in patients with early, untreated prostatic cancer. J Am Med Assoc 1992, 267:2191–6.
11. Johansson JE, Holmberg L, Johansson S, Bergstrom R, Adami HO. Fifteen-year survival in prostate cancer. A prospective, population-based study in sweden. J Am Med Assoc 1997, 277:467–71.
12. Stephenson RA, Stanford JL. Population-based prostate cancer trends in the united states: Patterns of change in the era of prostate-specific antigen. World J Urol 1997, 15:331–5.
13. Aus G, Hugosson J, Norlen L. Long-term survival and mortality in prostate cancer treated with noncurative intent. J Urol 1995, 154:460–5.
14. Lu-Yao GL, Yao SL. Population-based study of long-term survival in patients with clinically localised prostate cancer [see comments]. Lancet 1997, 349:906–10.
15. Chodak GW, Thisted RA, Gerber GS, Johansson JE, Adolfsson J, Jones GW et al. Results of conservative management of clinically localized prostate cancer. N Engl J Med 1994, 330:242–8.
16. Schroder FH, Hermanek P, Denis L, Fair WR, Gospodarowicz MK, Pavone-Macaluso M. The TNM classification of prostate cancer. Prostate Suppl 1992, 4:129–38.

17. Whitmore WF Jr. Natural history and staging of prostate cancer. Urol Clin North Am 1984, 11:205–20.
18. Chisholm GD. Treatment of advanced cancer of the prostate. Semin Surg Oncol 1985, 1:38–55.
19. Catalona WJ, Smith DS, Ratliff TL, Basler JW. Detection of organ-confined prostate cancer is increased through prostate-specific antigen-based screening. J Am Med Assoc 1993, 270:948–54.
20. Kupelian PA, Katcher J, Levin HS, Klein EA. Stage T1-2 prostate cancer: A multivariate analysis of factors affecting biochemical and clinical failures after radical prostatectomy. Int J Radiat Oncol Biol Phys 1997, 37:1043–52.
21. AV DA, Whittington R, Schultz D, Malkowicz SB, Tomaszewski JE, Wein A. Outcome based staging for clinically localized adenocarcinoma of the prostate. J Urol 1997, 158:1422–6.
22. AV DA, Desjardin A, Chung A, Chen MH, Schultz D, Whittington R et al. Assessment of outcome prediction models for patients with localized prostate carcinoma managed with radical prostatectomy or external beam radiation therapy. Cancer 1998, 82:1887–96.
23. Carter HB, Pearson JD, Metter EJ, Brant LJ, Chan DW, Andres R et al. Longitudinal evaluation of prostate-specific antigen levels in men with and without prostate disease [see comments]. J Am Med Assoc 1992, 267:2215–0.
24. Gronberg H, Damber JE, Jonsson H, Lenner P. Patient age as a prognostic factor in prostate cancer. J Urol 1994, 152:892–5.
25. Neulander EZ, Duncan RC, Tiguert R, Posey JT, Soloway MS. Deferred treatment of localized prostate cancer in the elderly: The impact of the age and stage at the time of diagnosis on the treatment decision. BJU Int 2000, 85:699–704.
26. Albertsen PC, Fryback DG, Storer BE, Kolon TF, Fine J. The impact of co-morbidity on life expectancy among men with localized prostate cancer [see comments]. J Urol 1996, 156:127–32.
27. Kattan MW, Eastham JA, Stapleton AM, Wheeler TM, Scardino PT. A preoperative nomogram for disease recurrence following radical prostatectomy for prostate cancer. J Natl Cancer Inst 1998, 90:766–71.
28. Kattan MW, Wheeler TM, Scardino PT. Postoperative nomogram for disease recurrence after radical prostatectomy for prostate cancer. J Clin Oncol 1999, 17:1499–507.
29. Partin AW, Kattan MW, Subong EN, Walsh PC, Wojno KJ, Oesterling JE et al. Combination of prostate-specific antigen, clinical stage, and gleason score to predict pathological stage of localized prostate cancer. A multi-institutional update [see comments] [published erratum appears in J Am Med Assoc 1997 9;278:118]. J Am Med Assoc 1997, 277:1445–51.
30. Clemens JD, Feinstein AR, Holabird N, Cartwright S. A new clinical-anatomic staging system for evaluating prognosis and treatment of prostatic cancer. J Chronic Dis 1986, 39:913–28.

Chapter 3

THE SEARCH FOR GENES WHICH INFLUENCE PROSTATE CANCER METASTASIS: A MOVING TARGET?

Norman J. Maitland

YCR Cancer Research Unit, Department of Biology (Area 13), University of York, York, UK

Abstract: The process of cancer and prostate cancer metastasis is complex and requires fundamental changes to the behaviour of the parent cell. While the stage at which essential mutations for prostate cancer metastasis occur remains controversial, it is likely, based on current evidence, that an accumulation of genetic damage is required. However, the study of cancer metastasis is clearly dependent on the availability of suitable *in vitro* and *in vivo* models. Not every model represents the full *in vivo* situation in man, but a combination of these models is now becoming available in prostate cancer and should allow a more detailed assessment of the specific genes involved in metastasis and the preferential adhesion in bone. Identification of specific genes associated with particular pathology has also taken tremendous steps forward in the last few years. Differential expression analysis, of both the RNA and also protein levels are providing new targets for therapy, specifically directed against metastatic disease. However, for longer term prospects the ability to detect metastasis in a simple blood sample would offer the most hope of permanent treatment or indeed cure. Based on serum profiling, such methods should soon be available to the oncologist in the clinic. On-line catalogues of genes whose expression is perturbed in metastatic processes offer the first clues to the key events in this complex biological process. It is perhaps from these catalogues improved animal models and indeed the more global analysis of patient samples from bio-banks that the key events and a genetic basis will be identified.

Key words: prostate cancer metastasis, genomics, proteomics, *in vitro* tests

1. INTRODUCTION

Without metastasis, prostate cancer would be both tolerable and treatable. The high incidence of indolent and organ confined disease is testament to this sweeping generalisation. Equally, if molecular markers of metastatic spread can be identified, then the choice of treatment for many patients would be easier and more radical, even curative. However, should prevention and treatment of the primary tumors prove difficult or impossible, then a knowledge of the phenotype of advanced metastatic tumors should allow us to target these lesions for destruction by conventional (drug based) or more innovative means such as gene and/or immunotherapy (1).

The process of metastasis has been reviewed many times (e.g., 2) and has been subdivided for ease of analysis into a number of discrete stages (see Figure 1). It has been suggested that at least 10 separate genetic

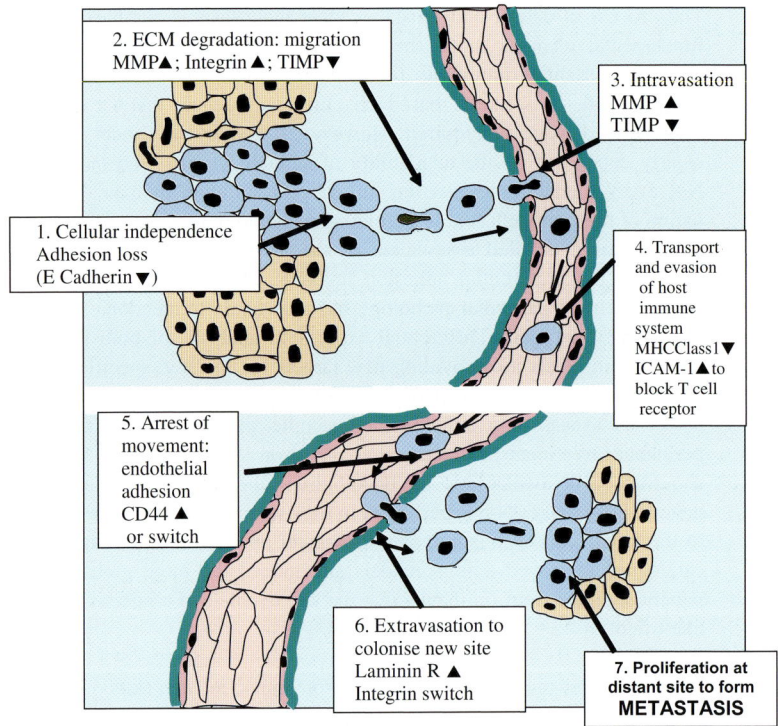

Figure 1. Stages in prostate cancer metastasis. Basic processes in tumor metastases are indicated in the boxes with some key changes in gene expression indicated at each stage by the solid arrows.

alterations and/or genetic selections could be required to permit establishment of a tumor at an extra-prostatic site (3), and many investigations have concentrated on defining a role for genes of known function within the metastatic process. Thus demarcations in the stages of metastasis development as shown in Figure 1, and the primary consequences of the changes at each stage have dominated thinking on the types of genes investigated. Perhaps the complexity of the phenomenon demands a more even-handed and unbiased investigation, now possible in the days of whole genome analysis, and mass proteomics. To provide an alternative approach, I have adopted a technology-based approach to prostate cancer, and will seek to justify the inevitable preferences and prejudices about the significance of the many metastatic markers, more on the basis of genetic preference (4) rather than a seed and soil (5) approach. As metastasis is a basic property of most tumor types, at an advanced stage, then it is likely that many of the basic parameters will be shared (as outlined in Figure 1), but the behaviour of prostate tumors is sufficiently different even from breast cancer at the metastatic site, for example in its osteoblastic nature, compared to the osteolytic properties of breast carcinoma (reviewed in 6) to suggest the existence of certain unique features. For this reason, I have also deliberately eliminated a detailed discussion of angiogenesis, as one of the most basic necessary and important steps in metastatic escape. The subject has been reviewed in great detail, and I would direct the interested reader to reviews on this topic such as Folkman (7).

2. GENETIC ALTERATIONS: A MATTER OF PERMANENCE

Cancer is normally associated with a loss of genetic information i.e., a dominant recessive disease, and it has long been supposed that metastasis occurs as a result of removal or suppression of "metastasis suppressors". However, there is also good evidence for metastasis activators or enhancers, where a gene is expressed either aberrantly or at higher levels than normal. Genome wide expression screens have identified candidates of both positively and negatively acting gene groups (see below).

What is perhaps more important however, are the mechanisms by which the altered levels of expression of the two types of gene are ultimately obtained. These are outlined in diagrammatic form in Figure 2. Firstly, for autosomal *suppressor* genes, one or both copies can be inactivated by deletion or mutation in the classical tumor suppressor gene mechanism, as shown in Figure 2a. Most frequently one of the two

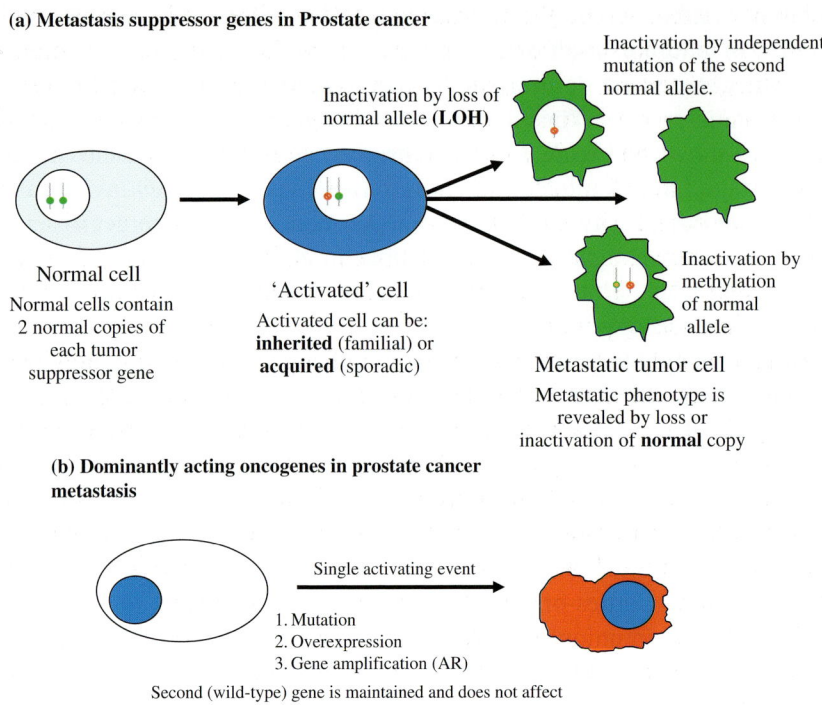
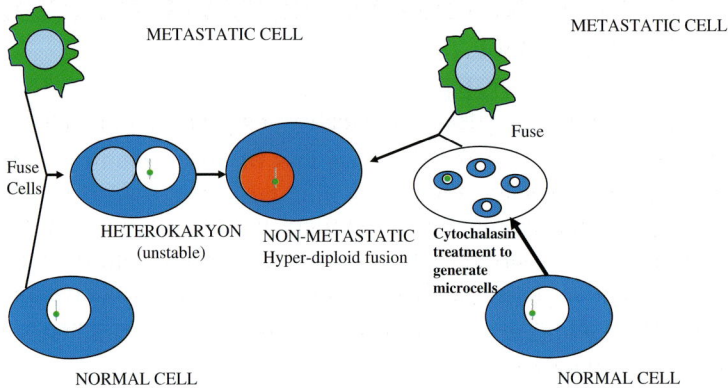

Figure 2. Human metastasis genes. **A:** The principles behind metastasis suppressor genes. The three methods of inactivation of a normal suppressor allele are illustrated. **B:** Dominantly acting metastasis enhancers, a subset of known oncogenes act by direct over expression, either in a wild-type or constitutively active mutant form to promote tumor spread. **C:** Identification of metastasis suppressor gene loci by cell fusion or direct chromosomal introduction into indicator metastatic cells.

alleles is deleted, whilst the remaining allele is silenced by epigenetic or mutational mechanisms. For a sex-linked gene in males, the situation is more straightforward, with a single gene inactivation required to abolish expression. A good example of this is the gene for androgen receptor, which is located on the X chromosome. Chromosomal alterations leading to over-expression of a metastasis *activator* are easier to explain, with both intra-chromosomal tandem duplications and minute chromosomes observed containing amplicons of both the metastasis activator and closely linked genes (Figure 2b). This latter co-amplification can result in false identification of implicated genes.

An increasingly common mechanism of changing gene expression levels is epigenetic alteration. A full description of the various intra-nuclear modifications, which lead to activation or silencing can be found elsewhere (8). The most commonly recognised and observed mechanism for selective gene silencing is CpG methylation in promoter and enhancer regions associated with the gene in question. The great advantage in changes of this type is their reversibility. For a (cancer) cell to survive *adaptability* must be a major advantage, and the permanent changes in gene expression produced by the various chromosomal alterations would be a poor strategy in a hostile environment, for example when establishing residence in an extra-prostatic site.

3. BIOLOGICAL ASSAY SYSTEMS TO STUDY GENE FUNCTION IN PROSTATE CANCER METASTASIS

In order to carry out detailed genetic analysis of the genes, which are activated in *metastasis* of prostate cancer, quite distinctly from genes activated in prostate cancer, the choice of biological material is paramount. The old adage about the quality of the input matching the output is particularly true here. The source of the material has ranged from rodent models through to material dissected from clinical material. All have produced candidate genes, but in the case of rodent models, their relevance to human disease has in some cases yet to be confirmed.

3.1 *In vitro* Approaches

Considerable experimental work has been conducted on the standard prostate cancer cell lines as an attempt to analyse metastasis. The PC3 cell line was originally isolated from a bone marrow metastasis, LNCaP is derived from a lymph node metastasis and DU145 from a brain metastasis (an extremely rare occurrence for prostate cancer) (reviewed in 9). Comparisons between these cell lines have been made, in attempts to define both site-specific changes, and androgen sensitivity of genes up-regulated in metastasis. There are considerable shortcomings in this approach, particularly as the different cell types and cultures derived from normal tissue, such as the PNT series (9), are all from different patients, and were established in culture using different methods. After many years in culture, they have become grossly aneuploid and also heterogeneous. Unless cross-related to the tissue arrays (or similar) as discussed later, these simple models only offer a small fragment of the metastasis story.

A better approach would be to use malignant variants of the same cell type. Most cell lines do throw off variants in both culture and *in vivo* selection (for example the multiple xenograft variants reviewed in van Weerden and Romijn, 10). Comparisons of non-malignant cells "progressed" by treatment with chemical and viral carcinogens offer the controlled baseline for comprehensive analysis of metastatic changes. One such comparison was reported by Hukku et al. (11) who analysed the multiple genetic changes that occurred when a non-malignant HPV18-immortalised cell line, progressed to malignancy as judged by the ability to form tumors in severe combined immunodeficient (SCID) mice. However, no analysis of metastasis was presented, although the model should lend itself to such studies.

3.2 Cell Fusion/Single Chromosome Transfer

As long ago as 1969, Harris et al. (12) showed that fusion of malignant cells with non-malignant cells would result in a non-malignant phenotype. Further experiments by Sidebottom and Clark (13) extended this "suppressor gene" hypothesis to metastasis (in the chosen cell type at least) implying that metastasis is a recessive disease. The assay was taken forward by Stanbridge, who used the dominance of the murine karyotype over human chromosomes in murine:human cell hybrids to produce stable murine cell lines with relatively few human chromosomes. Suppression of the malignancy of the murine parent in the hybrid indicated that the retained human chromosome contained one or more suppressor gene (14). To further improve the technology, a series of murine cell lines, each containing a single human chromosome (and a drug selection marker to permit primary selection) were developed. These systems have been successfully employed to map senescence genes and other tumor suppressor, and formed the basis of metastasis suppressor identification in the Dunning model (e.g., Mashimo et al., 15) which is described in more detail below. The principles of cell fusion mediated suppression of metastasis are illustrated in Figure 2c.

The resources of the Human Genome Program, now offer bacterial artificial chromosomes and cosmid clones which span the entire genome in manageable segments, to permit more precise "biological" mapping. While these whole chromosome methods may seem crude, they have the major advantage of transferring gene clusters and associated genes, while overcoming single gene silencing (often observed in integrative gene transfers) by transfer of a large genomic segment.

However, the biological assays all require a means of quantifying metastasis (e.g., 16). Perhaps the simplest approach is to measure the ability of cells to form viable colonies in semi-solid support medium; this is a strong indicator of independence from normal cellular controls, and interdependence between stromal and epithelial cells for example. A more precise measure of invasion in metastasis is the long established chamber assay, where the tumor cells are layered on top of a matrix (frequently collagen or matrigel for example), prepared in a cylindrical insert for a tissue culture chamber. By comparison with a known metastatic cell, the rate at which the test cell migrates through the matrix is measured by crystal violet staining of the distal surface of the membrane after various time points. Most cells will eventually penetrate such matrices, but truly metastatic cells will appear within 24 hours, at the distal surface, having penetrated and frequently digested the matrix. There are variants on this procedure:

(i) Embedding of stromal cells in the matrix can provide both positive and negative stimuli to invasion and

(ii) Introduction of a layer of endothelial cells can simulate the essential penetration of microvasculature as a first step in migration out of a tissue such as prostate.

3.3 Motility Assays in Two Dimensions

In vitro analysis of metastatic tumor cells, have provided good evidence that the most metastatic cells display greatly altered motility and cellular organisation. The original model for this was the 3T3, 3T6 and 3T12 embryonic mouse cells. The highly tumorigenic 3T12 cells displaying all of the properties of a true tumor, while 3T3 cells remained 'normal' with elements of growth control and special regulation. Quantification of *motility* remains problematical. Some guidelines were provided by Mohler et al. (17) studying the Rat Dunning system (see above), and this can be translated into studies on prostate epithelium, either in mono-culture or in tissue recombinations (16). Since different tumor cells exhibit different sets of properties almost certainly defined by genetic changes, a combination of scores for ruffling, pseudopodial movement, translative movement results in an overall motility index, which correlates well in most (but not all) cell lines with metastatic ability (Table 1) (18). In combination experiments, prostatic stroma positively regulated motility, while in most cases not affecting growth rates (16).

The significance of this reductionist approach to metastasis has recently been given extra credibility by microarray studies on metastatic human and mouse melanoma cells (19, 20). Using the mouse techniques described above, metastatic variants were selected and screened by 7k cDNA microarray. This biologically sound approach, which reduced the extreme "noise" often seen in such experiments, resulted in over-expression of fewer than 20 genes, but no significant fingerprint for metastasis in melanoma. As shown by Kozlowski et al. (21), there are independent routes to and origins for a metastatic phenotype, and the gene profiling simply provided sound evidence for this 20 year old hypothesis. However, the expression of 3 genes: RhoC, 1fibronectin and thymosin β4 was elevated in all of the mouse and human metastases (19). Fibronectin has been linked to cell migration, as it is a component of the extracellular matrix and was a common upregulation product in both recent studies on melanoma. Thymosin β4, like other thymosins, binds to monomeric actin, sequestering it and preventing polymerisation into fibres, and as a result reduces cellular motility via lamellipodial extension (22). Here there is a clear relationship to prostate cancer, where earlier studies on the Rat Dunning model revealed Thymosin β15 as an over expression product in metastatic cells, while anti-sense inhibition of Thymosin β15 in metastatic cells prevented metastasis (23).

Table 1. Quantification of prostate epithelial cell motility as a determinant of invasiveness

Motile property				Scoring system			
Ruffling Pseudopodia	**Score:**	**0** None	**1** None/little 1–49%	**2** Average 50%	**3** High 51–99%	**4** 100%	
Translation	**Score:**	**0** None	**1** Little movement as a tight colony	**2** High movement as a tight colony	**3** Movement as a scattered colony	**+1*** <50% of cells show individual translation	**+2*** >50% of cells show individual translation

*The extra scores for individual translation are added to the basic scores of 0–3 for translation

Finally, overexpression of RhoC (a GTP-hydrolysing protein like ras) has also been shown to affect cell migration (24). However the microarray analysis failed to detect changes in Rho A and B, and only re-introduction and overexpression of RhoC was able to convert non-metastatic melanoma to a metastatic phenotype. No direct involvement of RhoC in prostate cancer invasion has been reported in a recent comprehensive review (25), although Rho kinase inhibitors appear to suppress malignancy in experimental PC3 models of carcinoma of the prostats (CaP) (26).

4. SYNGENEIC MODELS OF PROSTATE CANCER

4.1 Rat Dunning Model

Amongst the first models to be exploited was the Rat Dunning carcinoma, which exists as metastatic and non-metastatic variants (e.g., AT2.1 and AT3.1). Cell fusion experiments between the variants resulted in a non-metastatic heterokaryon (27). The Dunning metastatic cells were therefore used as an indicator system for similar metastasis suppressor genes, leading to the identification of firstly loci at 8p, 10q and 11p 17p and later positive identification of the metastasis suppressor genes KAI1 at 11p12 and a role for CD44 (at 11p13) and MAPK kinase 4 (at 17p11.2)

4.2 Mouse Prostate Reconstitution Model

The ability to derive differentiated prostate tissue from reconstitution of individual cell types has provided powerful tools for the study of glandular development for more than 30 years (28). More recently Thompson and co-workers were able to use a similar model to investigate carcinogenesis in the mouse prostate by transfections of dominantly acting oncogenes into the epithelial component of the reconstitution (29). The model has been further refined by the use of p53 knockout mice as the recipient of the myc and ras oncogenes, which resulted in development of micro-metastases in bone and other tissue (30), implying a critical role for p53 in metastatic development in this system, paralleling the demonstration of p53 mutants in metastatic human prostate cancer (31). The model has therefore generated the correct, genetically matched background, from which genetic lesions can be assessed (reviewed in Thompson et al., 32). Using primary tumor and lung metastases for example, and differential display (see below) a role for overexpression of Caveolin 1, which is present in membrane invaginations responsible for small molecule transport, urokinase signalling and with integrin mediated signalling has been postulated (reviewed by Bangma et al., 33). Caveolin expression is undetectable in normal human prostatic epithelium, but appears to be upregulated in human metastatic tumors (34).

4.3 Transgenic Mouse Models

Considerable investment has been made in murine models of human cancers (35). For gene isolation and functional characterisation, the mouse is closely related to man, and is clearly a better experimental model for investigation of molecular therapies, in particular immune therapy for metastatic disease. However, the relatively short lifespan of the mouse probably prevents the accumulation of necessary mutations to spontaneously develop prostate cancer. Indeed the mouse is more likely to die of other tumor types. There are a number of other significant biological differences, which promote some caution in the extrapolation of the mouse situation to humans:

Firstly, the murine prostate atrophies with age, in contrast to human prostate, in which hypertrophy is observed. Secondly, the mouse prostate has 3 lobes, in direct contrast to the alobular human prostate, which is a single gland composed of transitional, peripheral and central zones.

To produce prostate cancer in mice requires tissue specific expression of a strong oncogene from a tissue-specific promoter (36). Not all of the models however produce metastatic disease. The TRAMP model (probasin promoter driven SV40 T antigen, (37)), results in tumors in the dorsolateral lobe (murine equivalent of the peripheral zone) which metastasise to lymph node, lung and (in the correct genetic background) to bone. However, the probasin promoter is active in luminal cells of the murine prostate, and most human prostate cancers probably arise from the basal epithelium. The genetic changes observed are however similar if not identical to human disease, including the loss of E-cadherin expression. The TRAMP model also allows derivation of individual cell lines, which behave in a predictable and similar manner to the original Tag –induced tumors when transplanted into syngeneic hosts (38) and should also form the ideal raw material for gene identification. For example, expression of the murine homologues of a number of human prostate carcinogenesis-associated genes is frequently observed (39). TRAMP C2 metastatic lesions can be induced by abrogation of transforming growth factor beta (TGF-β) responses in bone marrow (40) and re-expression of maspin (one of the most common negatively regulated genes found in human CaP by microarray) also leads to reduced metastatic potential (41).

Other models using dominant oncogenes, which are capable of producing metastases include (i) the C3(1) driven T antigen (42) and (ii) the murine cryptdin (CR2) driven T antigen model (43), which differs from the other in that it targets the neuroendocrine cell component of prostate.

As our knowledge of the genes deleted during prostatic carcinogenesis increases, the specific deletions in tumor suppressors can be modelled in transgenic knockout mice. Two good examples of such tumor suppressor genes, where loss of heterozygosity is frequently observed in human carcinoma are PTEN (chromosome 10q23) and Nkx3.1 (chromosome 8p21). Single knockout mice in Nkx3.1 develop lesions perhaps akin to prostatic intraepithelial neoplasia (PIN) (44), whereas PTEN knockout mice develop adenocarcinomas in multiple tissues (45). The addition of a p27 KIP1 cyclin dependent kinase inhibitor knockout on the PTEN background results in prostate carcinogenesis. The triple knockout results in true carcinogenesis, which should further progress to metastasis in the absence of the viral oncogenes used in the TRAMP and similar models. Development of these systems should allow functional characterisation of metastasis candidate genes, and development of therapies, in a prostate-specific manner.

4.4   Xenograft in Nude/SCID Mice

The nude (athymic) and now the severe combined immunodeficient mouse systems, offer the ability to culture a range of human tumor types, both by inoculation of established tumor cell lines (21) and direct graft of tumor tissues such as CWR22 (46). The range of systems available was reviewed recently by van Weerden and Romijn (10).

Again the system makes compromises, as the lack of a functional immune system can affect both location and take rate of the grafted tumors. One solution to this was described by Nemeth et al. (47), who engrafted human tumor cells located within macroscopic human bone fragments into SCID mice, to study the metastatic lesion in its ultimate environment. In this model, only PC3 (originally from a bone metastasis) was able to colonise bone fragments after intravenous injection, whereas *all* of the tumor cells injected showed an ability to grow when grafted in human but not murine bone. Significantly, evidence of intense stromal:epithelial interaction was observed in the human:human grafts. In contrast to the majority of natural human tumors which are osteoblastic, the grafted cell lines produced ostolytic growth.

The PC3 cell is much favoured in studies of this type, as sub-lines with particular metastatic abilities can be readily generated (48, 49) by orthotopic inoculation. However, the LNCaP (androgen responsive) cell line, derived originally from a lymph node metastasis, can also be used to generate androgen independent and specifically metastatic sublines (50). These cell variants provide homogeneous sources of material for gene isolation and functional analysis, although in all cases the ability of the cells to colonise the metastatic sites can be modulated by the presence of human stroma (51).

Most recently new sublines have been developed which express fluorescent markers such as GFP (52) and luciferase (53), which offer the added advantage of real time monitoring of the metastatic process.

To identify metastasis associated genes, sublines of the CWR22 xenograft have been employed. Multiple variants are now available, including androgen independent (54) and highly metastatic cells (55) which have been directly employed in microarray analyses to identify implicated genes such as S100P, whose role in prostate tumorigenesis has been suggested in other studies (56). Although the S100P gene is androgen regulated, linkage of over-expression to both androgen independent and recurrent, metastatic disease was observed by Mousses et al. (55). Other members of the calcium and magnesium binding protein family of S100 proteins such as S100A4 have been linked directly to metastatic disease ((57, 58) and I Bronstein, unpublished results), which suggests that the metastatic role could predominate.

Lastly, and possibly of relevance to the metastatic process in prostate, is a study of skin carcinogenesis in the mouse. Detailed study of the changes in signalling pathways in clonally derived skin carcinoma cell lines (59) confirmed that, after initiation by H-ras activation, over-expression or gene amplification (only rarely seen in human prostate cancers) TGF-β signalling induces an epithelial/mesenchymal transition (overexpression observed in metastatic human prostate cancers). Phosphatidylinositol-3 kinase activation, which is observed as a result of PTEN inactivation in CaP ((60) and M Sharrard, personal communication), can also co-operate to inhibit TGF-β induced apoptosis. The key downstream event for TGF-β signalling is now the activation state of the SMAD 2 and 3 proteins: ie whether they are phosphorylated and nuclear in location, resulting in upregulation of SMAD transcription control targets (61). Such activation has been observed in CaP (62), and is a key player in the increased migratory capacity (via structural changes to the cellular cytoskeleton), rather than the proliferative capacity (via abrogation of cell cycle controls) of the tumor cells. This data, and its obvious application to carcinoma of the prostate provides further strong *in vivo* and *in vitro* evidence for the importance of the epithelial:mesenchymal transition in the development of metastatic potential (63).

4.5 Primary Tissue Comparisons: Tissue Microarrays

The data reported by Mousses et al. (55), see previous section) was given added relevance to native disease by validation using in situ hybridization and immuno-histochemistry on tissue microarrays, in which 60% of metastatic tumor samples over-expressed S100P. In contrast to many of the earlier studies, where statistical relevance was always hampered by the need for multiple immuno-staining, or in situ hybridization to many individual sections of tissue. The advent of a tissue microarray, in which many different types of pathological disorder are represented on a single slide from multiple patients (64) can produce significant data in a single reproducible experiment, which also can take account of the heterogeneity of the prostate cancer phenotype. It is useful not only for determining intracellular location of proteins whose expression is changed in metastasis, for example in the DNA micro-array study of Dhanasekaran et al. (65), who confirmed hepsin and the serine-threonine kinase pim-1 over expression, but also in the analysis of gene copy number. Interphase cytogenetics, to detect amplified and translocated genes in prostate cancers have been instrumental in confirming the amplification of the AR and c-myc genes in a single survey of 371 specimens (66) and have now become an essential tool in providing clinical relevance for candidate genes. The various chromosomal loci and specific metastasis genes, which have been identified by direct application of cellular and animal models are listed in Table 2 and illustrated on an ideogram of the normal human karyotype in Figure 3a.

5. IDENTIFICATION OF GENES

In order to study metastasis genes the *techniques* remain the most critical decision. Perhaps the easiest approach taken is to simply test the deletion/amplification status and expression patterns of genes implicated in the metastasis of other more easily studied tumor types. This is not the most imaginative approach, but given the ubiquitous nature of most of the processes involved in metastasis it has been very popular, although the choice of biological material is variable. As I shall demonstrate, the most recent exploitation of the database provided by the human genome mapping program is a fingerprint of metastasis that is tumor type independent, but may have significant consequences for tumor diagnosis and therapy.

Table 2. Chromosomal changes implicated in Human prostate Cancer Metastasis: Cell and Animal models

Source of metastases	Gene	Chromosomal locus	Activator (+) or suppressor (−)	Method(s) of isolation	Reference(s)
PC3M	?	1q21-22,	(+)	CGH	(67)
	PTEN	10q23-ter,	(−)		
	?	18q12-21	(−)		
LNCaP	BRCA2 ?	13q12-13	(+)	CGH	(67)
	?	16q23-ter	(−)		
	?	16q21	(−)		
Dunning Model	KAI 1(CD82)	11p11.2	(−)	Microcell Fusion	(109)
	CD44	11p13	(−)		(110)
	MAPK kinase	17p11.2	(−)		
	4	2p22-25	(−)		
	?	7q21-27/7q31.2-32	(−)		
	?	8p21	(−)		
	?	10cen-q23	(−)		
	?	12cen-q13/12q24-ter	(−)		
	?	16q24.2	(−)		
	?	20p11.23	(−)		
	?	Yq11.1/	(+)		
	Thymosin β15				
Mouse prostate reconstitution	Caveolin	7q31.1	(+)	DD	(34)
(myc/ras/p53)	p53	17p13.1	(−)		(32)

Table 2. (Continued)

Melanoma 'fingerprints'	Rho A/C	3p21/1p31.1	(+)	Microarray	(19)
	Fibronectin	2q34	(+)		
	Thymosinβ4	Xq21	(+)		
TRAMP	TGF-β	19q13.1	(+)	Various	(40)
	E-cadherin	18q21.3	(−)		(41)
		16q	(−)		(39)
					(45)
					(44)
Compound Knockout mice	PTEN	10q23	(−)		(35)
	Nkx3.1	8p21	(−)		
	P27KIP1	12p13.1	(−)		
CWR22 (orthotopic mouse)	S100P	4p16	(+)	Microarray	(55)

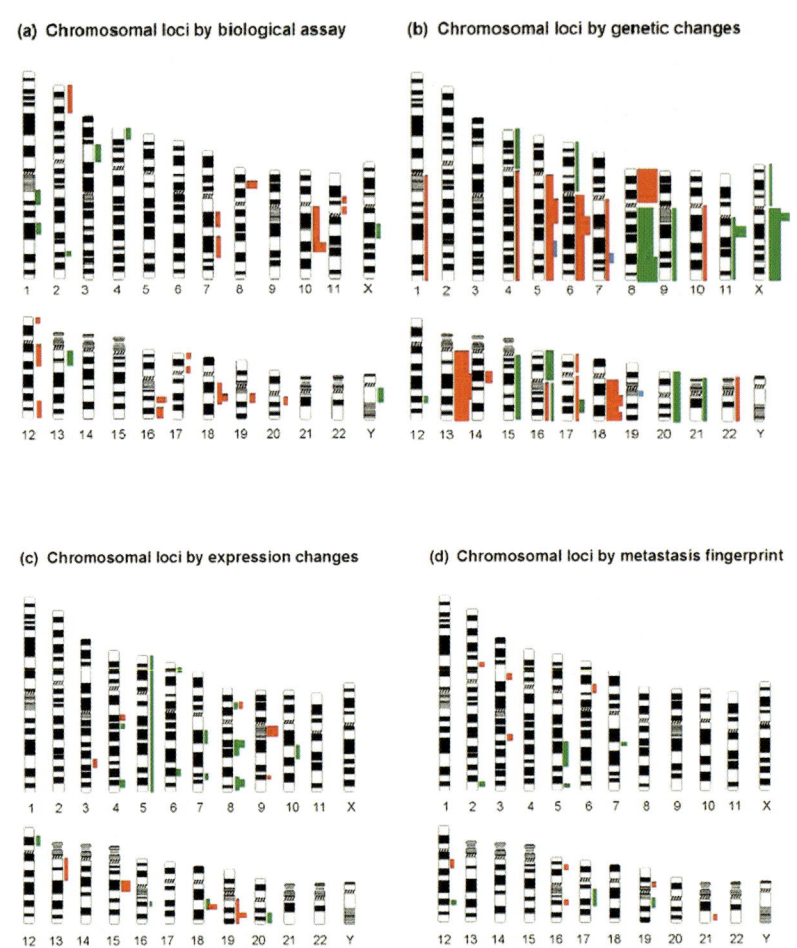

Figure 3. Chromosomal locations of genetic changes observed in prostate cancer metastases. Data is detailed in the text and in Tables 2–5. Gains (gene amplifications) are indicated by green bars and losses by red bars. The frequency of changes are denoted by the thickness of the bars.

6. TECHNIQUES TO IDENTIFY GENE LOSS AND AMPLIFICATION

6.1 Cytogenetics/Comparative Genomic Hybridization

Numerous cytogenetic abnormalities have been shown in prostate cancers, although consistent data has been elusive. Most tumors appear on

Table 3. Chromosomal changes implicated in Prostate Cancer Metastasis: Genetic Analyses of Human Tissues

Source of metastases	Gene	Chromosomal locus	Activator (+) or suppressor(−)	Method(s) of isolation	Reference(s)
Human metastatic tissue relative to intraprostatic disease		18q21 18q22-23	(−) (−)	LOH	(111)
Human lymph node and bone metastases		8q 8p	(+) (−)	CGH / Cytogenetics/ Interphase *in situ* hybridization	(112)
Linkage analysis in brothers with CaP		5q31-33 7q32 19q12	?	Linkage analysis	(71)
Human tissue microarrays	Androgen receptor c-myc	X 8q	(+) (+)	FISH/tissue microarrays	(66)
Human Tissues		*5q(1), 6q(1), 7q(1), 8p(4), 10q(1), 13q(1) 16q(1), 17p(1), 17q(2) 18q(3)	(−)	LOH	Reviewed in 113

Table 3. (Continued)

Source of metastases	Gene	Chromosomal locus	Activator (+) or suppressor(−)	Method(s) of isolation	Reference(s)
Human bone marrow metastatic deposits		8p, 13q, 18q 8q, 9q, 20, X	(−) (+)	M-FISH and CGH	(114)
"Advanced" prostate cancer		1q, 4q, 5q14-21, 6q16.1-21, 13q21.3-22, 14q21, 22 4p, 6p, 8q24.1-24.3, 11q, 12q23, 15q, 16p, 17q23-24, 20,21	(−) (+)	FISH and CGH	(115)
"Advanced" prostate cancer	AR c-myc cyclin D1	8p, 13q, 6q, 18q, 5q (2q, 4q, 16q) 8q, Xq, Xp Amplifications at Xq12, 8q24 11q13	(−) (+)	CGH	(116)
Microdissected human lymph node metastases		13q 9q, 16	(−) (+)	CGH	(117)

Table 4. (Continued)

Gene	Function	Positive or negative effector	In vitro (V) or in vivo activity (T)	Chromosomal location	Reference(s)
DAB-2 interacting protein (DAB2IP)		−	V	9q33.1-33.3	(134)
Annexin I	Calcium binding adhesion, membrane trafficking, cell signaling	−	T&V	9q12	(135, 136)
Annexin II				15q21	
Parathyroid hormone-related protein (PRHrP)	Peptide hormone	−	T	12p12	(137)
PRHrP receptor	Hormone receptor	+			
C13	Nuclear, glutamine and alpha helix rich	−	T(DD)	13q12-14	(138)
Autocrine motility factor (AMF)	Cytokine	+	V	16q21	(139)
Progastrin-releasing peptide (ProGRP)	Cytokine	+		18q21	(140)
Maspin	Serine protease inhibitor (adhesion to ECM)	−	V&T	18q21.3	(41)
TGF-β family	Cytokine	−	V	19q13	(40)
CLAR1	Proline-rich with SH3 binding domains	+	T (DD)	19q13.3	(141)
Bone morphogenetic proteins (e.g., 6 & 7)	Cytokine (osteoblast differentiation)	+	T	6p24	(142, 143)
Matrix metalloproteinases	Proteases (tissue and vascular escape)	+	T	20q13 Multiple	Reviewed in (144)
Connexins	Intracellular communication	+/−	T	Multiple	Reviewed in (145, 146)

Table 4. Multiple Gene Expression changes implicated in prostate cancer metastasis

Gene	Function	Positive or negative effector	In vitro (V) or in vivo activity (T)	Chromosomal location	Reference(s)
Tazarotene-induced gene 1 (TIG1)	Retinoic acid responder gene	−	T&V(DD)	3q25.32	(118)
Hevin	Extracellular matrix, antiadhesive acidic cysteine-rich glycoprotein	−	T&V (DD)	4q22.1	(119)
NF-κB	Transcription factor	+	V	4q24	(120)
VEGFC	Cytokine(angiogenesis)	+	T	4q34	(121)
Type XXIII Collagen	Transmembrane (type 11)collagen	+	V (rat) (DD)	5	(122)
Endothelin	Cytokine	+	T	6p24	(123)
Src-suppressed C Kinase substrate (SSeCKS/Gravin)	Tumor suppressor	−	V&T	6q24-25.2	(124)
Hepatocyte growth factor	Multiple growth factor-like activities	+	V&T	7q21	(125, 126)
CAT-like	Re-absorption of Ca++	+	V&T(?)	7q33-34	(127)
c-erbB2/neu	Cytokine	−	T&V	8p21	(128)
Nkx3.1	Transcription factor	+	T&V	8p21	(129)
Elongin C	Multifunctional	+	T&V	8q21	(130)
Urokinase-type plasminogen activator	Protease	+	V (DD)	10q22	
Cutaneous fatty acid binding protein	Fatty acid binding	+		8q21.1	(131)
Osteoprotegerin	Cytokine (Osteoblastic)	+	T	8q24	(132)
Prostate stem cell antigen	GPI anchored cell surface antigen	+	T	8q24.2	(133)

(*Continued*)

Table 5. Genes expression changes included in the 'Metastasis Signature' (all tumors), (Taken from Ramaswamy et al., (76))

Overexpressed genes	Chromosomal location
Elongation factor 4E-like 3 (EIF-4EL3)	2q37.1
Lamin B1 (LMNB1)	5q23-31
Securin (PTTG1)	5q35.1
Heterogeneous nuclear ribonucleoprotein A/B (HNRPAB)	5q35.3
Type 1 collagen a2 (COL1A2)	7q22.1
Small Nuclear Ribonucleoprotein F (SNRPF)	12q23.1
Type 1 collagen a1 (COL1A1)	17q21-22
Deoxyhypusin synthase (DHPS)	19p13.1
Underexpressed genes	
Actin g2 (ACTG2)	2p13.1
RNA binding motif 5 (RBM5)	3p21.3
Myosin light chain kinase (MYLK)	3q21
MHC Class II, DPb1 (HLA-DPB1)	6p21.3
Nuclear Hormone receptor TR3 (NR4A1)	12q13
Myosin heavy chain 11 (MYH11)	16p13.1
Metallothionein 3 (MT3)	16q13
Calponin 1 (CNN1)	19p13.1
Runt- related transcription factor 1 (RINX1)	21q22.3

culture to have a normal karyotype, which could reflect difficulties in culture technology. A more precise estimate can be gained by *comparative genomic hybridization* (68), which employs metastatic tumor DNA labelled with one fluorochrome (test DNA) and normal (male) diploid DNA, preferably but not essentially from the same patient, labelled with a different fluorochrome. The DNA's are denatured and allowed to anneal to form double strands, in the presence of a repetitive unlabelled DNA sample (Cot-1), to eliminate noise. After extensive annealing, the mixture is further hybridised to spreads of normal human karyotypes. Since any gains in the test DNA relative to the normal DNA will be over represented as labelled single strands in the hybridization mixture, the regions on the chromosomes homologous to these sequences will be labelled. By convention these are coloured green. The converse is true for losses in the metastatic cell DNA relative to the normal, when excess labelled, unhybridized normal DNA will be present in the hybridization mixture, and can anneal to its homologous location on the human chromosome (red label). Detailed cytogenetic analysis under ultra-violet illumination, and computer-assisted visualisation identifies the altered chromosomal loci. The technique is more suited to cell line analysis than extracted tissues, as it requires up to 1 microgram of pure DNA, and data obtained with PC3 and LNCaP metastatic variants confirms the presence of a number of known metastasis associated loci in prostate tumors as summarised in Tables 2 and 3 (e.g., 67).

6.2 Allelic Linkage/Loss of Heterozygosity

Numerous studies of allelic losses and gains in prostate cancer have been published over the last 10 years. Analysis is based on microsatellites in the human genome, which consist of multiple polymorphic repeats of simple di tri or tetra nucleotides. Some of these repeats are associated with pathology, such as the CAG (polyglutamine encoding) repeat in the human androgen receptor. Mostly they lie outwith coding sequences, and inheritance of different unit repeats at the same locus from an individual's mother and father generates a heterozygote. If a section of chromosome or locus (i.e. containing a tumor/metastasis suppressor) is lost from on chromosome relative to normal DNA from the same patient, then loss of heterozygosity (LOH) has occurred (69). High density microsatellite collections are now available for the entire human genome, and have now been supplanted by even more widely and evenly distributed Single Nucleotide Polymorphisms (SNP's) (70). Precise location of genes can be accomplished in this way, but both fragile chromosomal sites and the inherent genomic instability in tumors can generate "noise" in the analysis.

Most LOH studies have focussed on differentiating either normal tissue from tumors or low Gleason grade tumors from high Gleason grade tumors. Whilst the higher Gleason grades have greater *potential* to metastasise, the data do not differentiate advanced, poorly differentiated tumors with multiple genetic changes from truly metastatic lesions. The data are variable, probably as metastatic lesions are both heterogeneous and difficult to obtain. Any conclusions about metastatic genes from LOH analysis are therefore less reliable than with some other technologies (see Table 3). The various gene loci identified by these techniques (Table 3) are also illustrated in Figure 3b.

A different and complementary approach was taken by (71) who exploited the large number of families in their population study for familial tumors. By comparing the 'aggressiveness' of cancers from 513 brothers where the Gleason score of their tumors was known and wide differences were observed, they carried out a traditional linkage analysis with 364 equally spaced polymorphic microsatellites. The results indicated the presence of an additional 3 'markers' of aggressiveness, which could be equated to malignancy at 5q31-33, 7q32 and 19q12 (indicated in blue on Figure 3b).

The sample size was sufficiently large to achieve high statistical significance in the analysis, and at least 2 of these loci correspond to gene loss hotspots.

7. TECHNIQUES TO IDENTIFY DIFFERENTIALLY EXPRESSED GENES

The search for novel metastasis genes in prostate carcinoma is more difficult. As with other studies, in prostate cancer, the lack of effective models precludes decisive results. Many of the results are technology dependent, providing interesting new candidates from *in vitro* studies, which are infrequently confirmed in larger scale studies of human tumor material.

The ability to detect differences between populations of nucleic acids from metastatic and non-metastatic cellular populations has been exploited over many years. However many of the differences are subtle, and technology was unable to resolve these from background until the power of gene amplification was combined with the subtractive hybridization technologies. Also, most of the techniques require rather large starting quantities of RNA, which poses problems in heterogeneous metastatic lesions.

7.1 Subtractive Hybridization

The easiest way to compare two nucleic acid populations is to selectively hybridise them together, to leave an under and over represented population in an unpaired state, where imbalances have occurred. The basic procedure is illustrated in Figure 4, but the enduring problem with a sound methodology has always been the yield of unpaired molecules, which restricted the changes detected to those of great magnitude, or aberrant hybrid formation (72). However, by combination with gene amplification, the technology is able to analyse much smaller differences in expression levels. When combined with use of cDNA micro-arrays (73, 74) and SAGE tagging an even greater sensitivity and identification of multiple new target genes as described later.

7.2 DNA Microarray

Recent advances in mass gene analysis such as printed oligonucleotide gene tissue arrays have resulted in the definition of sets of candidate carcinogenesis and metastasis genes. A meta analysis of the major studies was recently published (75), but like most studies of this type in prostate

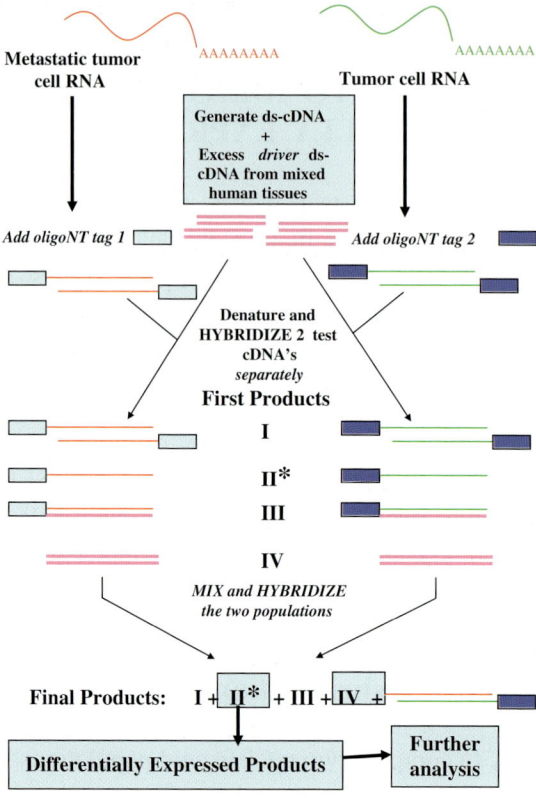

Figure 4. Suppression subtractive hybridization. Comparisons between different nucleic acid populations are compromised by abundant base sequences which can mask significant differences. The suppression subtraction technology, illustrated here for an mRNA comparison, can be extended to DNA by initiating the comparison after the RT step. The suppression step with excess ''driver' cDNA reduces background from abundant mRNA's. Population II (indicated by *) represents the unique species from the subtraction, to be used either as templates for PCR amplification (employing the tag for example) or for direct labelling and hybridization to microarrays. The final analysis step can be by either comparative genomic hybridization to metaphase chromosomal spreads or to DNA microarrays (the 5' oligonucleotide tagging (OligoNT) step is not necessary for microarray).

cancer, obtaining sufficient material from genuine metastatic lesions to carry our the analysis remains a problem. However in the study by Dhanasekaran et al. (65) 20 metastatic samples were included in the analysis, with an equivalent number of benign (19) and localised samples (14). Even allowing for the heterogeneity of prostate tumors, this population of metastases can provide clues as to the key over-expression products, which could be linked to genetic deletions and amplifications. Aside from some previously determined over- and under-expression products such as e-cadherin (−), PTEN (−) fatty acid synthetase (+) and c-myc (+) the major products which emerged as diagnostic aids were hepsin (+), maspin (−) and AMACR (+), although their mechanistic relevance to the metastatic process remains questionable.

For a definitive analysis of genes over-expressed in metastasis, the best measurement has currently been obtained from 64 primary and 12 metastatic adenocarcinomas originating from prostate, lung, colon, breast, ovary and uterus (76). The initial screen produced a set of 128 genes, which could distinguish the metastatic lesions from primary tumors. However, some primary tumors also showed altered expression of genes from the distinguishing set. The authors raised the possibility that these organ-confined tumors already contained cells pre-programmed to metastasise, particularly with lung tumors. This could equally apply in those "difficult" prostate tumors with a Gleason score of 5–7 where prognosis is a major diagnostic problem. Further refinement of the data set resulted in a minimal signature of genes over and under-expressed in metastases. Without further confirmation by RT-PCR or northern blotting, the minimal set of 17 genes was applied to sets of test tumors, including 21 prostate tumors, where the prediction had a p value of 0.022 (77). The genes included in the 'metastasis signature' are listed in Table 5 and mapped on to the human karyotype in Figure 3d. The predictive power applied to a range of tumors, indicating that the genes whose expression must be altered in order for a tumor to metastasise is probably a basic biological function, independent of the tissue of origin, although tissue-specific functions do probably exist.

Finally, the power of microarray analysis may not be exploited to its fullest extent, or in an extreme case, be providing misleading data. Most analyses reduce the differential expression to a ratio, relative to 'normal' tissues. There are good statistical reasons to be cautious with this approach, and the distinct possibility remains that these analyses are detecting over-expression epiphenomena; a result of signal amplification from a critical upstream event, which may be more subtle (78).

7.3 Differential Display

One of the earliest methods of comparative gene expression, differential display (DD) has been used to analyse differences in gene expression between normal and tumor cell from prostate (79), but the required amounts of RNA for the analysis are relatively large, which precludes use with small metastatic lesions. By selection and cloning of individual products, the DD technology can isolate individual genes based on different sequence and biological criteria, but the procedure can be time consuming. To accelerate gene discovery, it can be combined with cDNA microarrays (80) to reveal multiple expression alterations between metastatic and non-metastatic cell lines. These candidates remain to be confirmed on tissues however. A number of candidate genes have emerged from DD analysis. Some of these are listed in Table 4 (indicated by DD).

7.4 Serial Analysis of Gene Expression (SAGE)

This technology was devised to overcome the laborious nature of differential display, by amplifying differentially expressed sequence tags of 10 base pairs as concatamers with defined ends. The small sequence tags are finally used to screen sequence databases to identify specific products, whose expression changes are confirmed by other technologies in the target tissue (81). It is considerably faster than expressed sequence tag (EST) analysis, from which it is derived, and with the human genome map now complete (April 2003) final analyses and gene identification will be more rapid.

With prostate cancer, SAGE analysis has identified a number of expression changes such as E2F4 and Daxx (82) from a total of 156 detected changes. Links to metastasis have still to be confirmed. In a separate study genes implicated in the evasion of cellular senescence in prostate cancer were analysed by SAGE. In this case 273 changes were observed, which could be related to both phenotype and senescent stage. The data has to be extended to tissues however (83).

In summary therefore, the listing of 'metastasis associated' gene expression changes in Table 4 is unlikely to be complete, or *universally* applicable, given the technique (and clinical material) dependency of the analyses carried out. Most likely the sheer number of changes observed reflects gross perturbations in gene expression required by the metastatic cell to survive in its new extra-prostatic environment. The most common genes, whose expression changes are recorded in Table 4, have been mapped on to the human genome in Figure 3c.

7.5 Proteomics: Analysis of Gene Products in Metastasis

All of the previously discussed genetic changes will provide either a chromosomal or an expression fingerprint for metastatic cancer, although it is obvious from the preceding that considerable refinement is still required. As far as mechanistic genetics are concerned, translation of the DNA and RNA studies into altered protein levels is necessary. The main aims of the 'post-genomic'era are to develop the proteome, and its application to the genetics of metastasis in prostate cancer are still relatively primitive, compared to the nucleic acid studies. Again however, the quality of the results obtained will be determined by the strength of the biological systems. To permit proteomic analysis, new technologies for the precise analysis of the many protein forms within cells have been developed (see review by Nelson et al. (84)). The sheer complexity of protein expression patterns can be simply explained as follows: In the human genome there are about 40,000 genes. Many of these produce multiply spliced mRNA, which results in translation into different polypeptide chains. These polypeptides are further modified by proteolysis, glycosylation, phosphorylation etc, to produce protein with often radically different biological activities.

The application of proteomics to the study of prostate cancer metastasis can be divided into several enabling technologies as follows:

7.5.1 Analysis of the Proteome of Extracted Prostatic Tissues and Cells

To assist in the analysis of the total proteome, databases from multiple prostate tumors are being assembled (e.g., Nelson et al. (85)). To achieve cellular homogeneity, microdissection has to be carried out. However the technique does not always produce reliable results on traditional formalin fixed tissue, and frozen or ethanol fixed tissues must be used. A minimum of 10^5 cells is required for the 2D polyacylamide gel electrophoretic analysis, followed by spot picking and conventional protein mapping by mass spectrometry, which could restrict its use in multiple metastatic lesions. To date there is no information on the proteome of bone metastasis for example, although the difficulty in applying the technology was recently confirmed by Ahram et al. (86), who compared 12 matched normal prostate samples with corresponding high grade tumors (presumably with metastatic potential). The results confirmed the heterogeneity of prostate cancers at this level of analysis, since despite detecting forty changes in protein constitution, none were conserved between all of the tumors. No really new candidate metastasis associated genes were identified, although genes previously expressed in tumors such as lactate dehydrogenase, laminin receptor and tropomyosin-β were upregulated.

SELDI analysis, which has been developed for the analysis of small volumes of serum (see below), can equally be applied to the analysis of the protein complement and differences between microdissected cell populations (87). The problem remains the assignment of the peaks from the MS analysis to specific protein for which complex algorithms are only now being developed (88, 89).

7.5.2 Tissue and Antibody 'Chips' to Facilitate Large Scale Marker Screening

The external surface presented by metastatic tumors to its environment is important for interaction with other cell types, matrix and of course the immune system. Many studies have analysed the distribution of individual cell surface proteins on prostate cancer cells, with a resulting heterogeneity frequently observed. Liu (90) adopted a more general approach, using a forerunner of commercially available antibody arrays to produce 'macroarrays' each containing 16 immobilised antibodies to screen the expression of 119 different CD antigens in the common prostate cancer cell lines. Unsurprisingly, all were different and also displayed heterogeneity of staining intensity *within* populations of the same cell culture type, for example for CD44 antigen. While the paper speculated about this heterogeneity, it could simply be a result of genetic instability in the established tumor cell cultures. Similar analysis of metastatic lesions should produce important data about immune targeting, for example, although the disaggregation methods to be used will have to be carefully controlled to avoid antigen degradation.

There are now commercial antibody microarrays, to enable the researcher to probe multiple components of intracellular signalling pathways, activated in cancer and apoptosis, for example.

7.5.3 Analysis of Serum Markers of Metastasis

A serum protein to enable early and error free detection of metastatic prostate cancer is the ultimate goal of many marker studies (see review by Bok and Small, (91)). There already exist 2 examples of genes detected by this method. Both have been known for more than 10 years! The first, and still a reliable marker of metastatic disease was prostatic acid phosphatase (92). A better marker, of course is PSA, whose serum levels have been exploited extensively (93). The major drawback in using these two secreted proteins is their lack of specificity for metastatic disease. Elevated levels can be the result of a number of non-malignant conditions, and a search for new markers using proteomics has been under way for several years. The problem here is of course the source of material. Variously, blood (serum) ejaculate and prostatic fluid expressed after massage have been used as a source of material. The problem of course remains the complex nature of all of these fluids. Prostate cancer cells have been detected in serum by a variety of means, including RT-PCR for tumor-specific markers such as PSA and PSMA (94). However, the protein content to be analysed is sufficiently complex to confound visual or even computer assisted analysis. The increasing database of known proteins should facilitate such analyses.

In a recent antibody microarray study (95), a comparison of the protein profiles in serum from 33 prostate cancer and 20 normal serum samples using a 183 antibody microarray detected significant differences between the two populations in the expression of five proteins: von Willebrand factor, immunoglobulins G and M, alpha-1 antichymotrypsin, and villin. These could form the basis of new tests for early metastasis detection.

The choice of technology for this type of analysis (96) lies between the conventional 2D gel separation followed by mass-spectrometry assisted sequencing and confirmation of protein identity (97). A simpler technique, now employed routinely for serum analysis is direct separation of protein components by Surface Enhanced Laser Desorption Ionisation (SELDI)-Time of Flight Mass Spectroscopy (TOF-MS) (98). The Ciphergen SELDI has been used to advantage to separate unknown serum proteins to provide a further fingerprint, by making use of the multiple affinity spots on the proteinchip arrays. These act as successive protein fractionation steps to remove abundant serum proteins such as albumin and gamma globulin, to allow more detailed analysis of minor species (normally masked in 2D gel analysis) which could provide the key to better and earlier diagnosis of metastasis, for example PSMA (99). By applying 'reverse genetics' the peptides recovered from the time of flight mass spectrometer can be used to isolate the genes involved. It is interesting to speculate, given the diversity of genes and loci in Tables 2–5 and in Figure 3, whether alternative methodology simply provides a further layer of complexity.

7.6   In Silico Searching: Genes at Your Fingertips

The availability of public databases associated with or produced as a result of the human genome mapping program, allows basic research results to be put into a wider context. For example, most enzyme activity has down and upstream consequences. Therefore perturbation of one stage of a pathway has measurable effects on the connected steps in signal transduction or metabolism (for example). However, the situation is complicated by salvage, branched and alternative pathways, which are also activated when a particular reaction is inhibited or over-stimulated. The capacity to measure all of these effects is beyond the capacity of the human intellect, and computer algorithms come into their own.

For prostate, specific gene expression and structural changes have been collected into a series of such databases: the Prostate Expression database (85) at http://www.pedb.org. This allows rapid screening for the normal and malignant expression patters of more than 20,000 human genes, and is linked to a similar murine database for use with animal models. Such databases have been used to mine for prostate-specific products, and by combination with specific libraries from different cell and tissue types to electronically derive candidate genes for further study as markers of malignancy (84, 100). This type of analysis can even be carried out completely electronically using the Binary Indexing Search Algorithm (101). However the approach does have some limitations, and of course all results must be confirmed experimentally. The technique has identified two new cancer associated expression differences, in cysteine-rich secretory protein 3 (CRISP3, upregulated by more than 50 fold) and de-adenylating nuclease (DAN, downregulated by more than 80%). Linkage to *metastatic* disease was not reported however.

7.7 Metastasis Genes: How Many Activation Events Are Required or... Making Sense of the Data

The information which we are being deluged with as a result of both genome wide scans, analysis of the total proteome and microarray for both DNA and mRNA expression changes seems to suggest that an almost infinite number of changes in gene structure and expression are required for the development of prostate cancer metastasis. Recent estimates of around ten independent events (3) seem extremely wide of the mark if the number of gene loci in Figure 3 a–d are summed. What should be considered are the critical genetic changes. Many of the changes above, although seemingly important in prostate, could easily represent epi-phenomena, or downstream reactions to the changes in environment at the metastatic site. The key changes included in Figure 1 are often represented in prostate, allowing escape, survival and re-establishment of the tumor cells outside of the prostatic capsule. Some are clearly bone specific, allowing the prostate tumor cells to proliferate and/or survive.

The most telling results are those from the general survey of Ramaswamy et al. (76) which does reveal a general 'fingerprint' of metastasis, independent of tumor type. Are these gene expression changes fundamental? More probably not; given the nature of the genes, they probably represent further downstream effects.

Perhaps a significant feature of the genes in Table 5 is that at least some of the over-expressed products are normally expressed in *stromal* cells, while four of the downregulated genes are *smooth muscle* and two are *haematopoetic* cell genes. Does this expression pattern represent at least part of the epithelial: mesenchymal transition which is a frequent property of malignant tumors (see review by Thiery, 63). Two of the major mediators of this transition, TGF-β and HGF are both upregulated genes in prostate cancers, and the intracellular responses to such signalling in terms of apoptosis induction are short-circuited in metastatic lesions. Indeed one of the most reliable stromal markers: vimentin: is frequently over-expressed in malignant prostate tumors and can provide a good indication of metastatic potential in the primary tumor (102). A similar situation is found for cyclo-oxygenase 2 (COX2), which is expressed in prostate stromal cells in the premalignant state but over-expressed in the epithelium in the malignant state (103, 104). There are numerous other examples in prostate to suggest that the malignant cell has compensated for the lack of stromal contribution by establishing autocrine signalling loops to replace the paracrine signalling in the normal state. The signals probably have very little to do with growth, but rather cellular survival and motility. There also exists a clear role for reactive stroma, and bone stroma for the survival of the metastatic prostatic carcinoma cells (105, 106). Several studies, for example Macintosh et al. (107) have suggested that the changes in the stroma may extend from expression reprogramming to permanent genetic changes.

8. CONCLUSIONS

The data summarised above are neither comprehensive nor conclusive. There are many more anecdotal reports of phenotypic changes in metastatic prostate cancers not included, and more candidate genes are being identified almost monthly. However all of these are the result of genetic changes, and the various levels of control of gene expression discussed earlier. Some of these genetic changes are transient, some are of fundamental importance, while others may be unimportant to the development of the metastasis, but remain as reliable markers of extra-prostatic disease. As the knowledge base increases, it is likely that "metastatic prostate cancer" will be subdivided into a number of tumor types with a sound scientific basis, and an accurate set of prognostic indicators.

A meta-analysis of Figures 3a–d serves to underline this conclusion. On the surface there is little in common between the multiple loci identified by different technologies, although losses at 8p, 10q and 18q are consistently observed, being detected by all 4 technical approaches. A number of loci are identified by 2 approaches, but given that there is no requirement for downregulation of expression to be reflected in gene loss (although the gene loss is related to expression changes), whereas gene amplification can be directly related to overexpression (for example amplification/overexpression of the c-myc oncogene on chromosome 8q), this type of analysis is probably too premature, until the gene loss/amplification studies are further refined to more precise locations. This can readily be achieved by further exploitation of microarray technology (108).

The biggest danger for the future is to confuse a genetic change with diagnostic potential, with a fundamental change, which could be exploited in therapy. The ideal therapeutic target should be tumor restricted, and essential for the survival of the tumor in the metastatic site. The same is true for immunological targets. Prostate metastases have a capacity both to hide from the immune system, and to vary protein/antigen production, either as a population or a fraction of a tumor mass. By attacking the wrong targets, we would simply be producing new classes of recurrent tumors, as observed in the changes within androgen receptor signalling pathways (both androgen and growth factor mediated) after use of anti-androgen therapies. The current status of prostate cancer genetics is akin to an unedited electronic manuscript: most of the information is out there, some of it is in the wrong place (although some *is* misleading because of imperfect biology), but it must be referenced, annotated and assembled into a coherent whole for the benefit of more than 20,000 new patients diagnosed every year with CaP in the UK.

ACKNOWLEDGEMENTS

I wish to thank Michelle Mounter for her invaluable assistance in preparing the manuscript and particularly Dr Karen Woodward, University of Sheffield whose PhD thesis provided the basis for Figure 1. Research in this area is supported in York by a program grant from Yorkshire Cancer Research and a center of Excellence grant (Northern Collaborative) from the UK National Cancer Research Institute.

REFERENCES

1. Maitland NJ, Stanbridge LJ, Dussupt V. Targeting gene therapy for prostate cancer. Curr Pharm Des 2004, 10:531–55.
2. Fidler IJ. Critical determinants of cancer metastasis; rationale for therapy. Cancer Chemother Pharmacol 1991, 43:S3–S10.

3. Bernards R, Weinberg RA. A progession puzzle. Nature 2002, 418:823.
4. Greaves M. *Cancer: the Evolutionary Legacy*. Oxford, New York: Oxford Univ Press, 2000, pp. 57–61.
5. Paget S. The distribution of secondary growths in cancer of the breast. Lancet 1889, 1:99–101.
6. Mundy GR. Metastasis to bone: Causes, consequences and therapeutic opportunities. Nat Rev Cancer 2002, 2:584–93.
7. Folkman J. Role of angiogenesis in tumor growth and metastasis. Semin Oncol 2002, 29:15–18.
8. Ng H-H, Bird A. DNA methylation and chromatin modification. Curr Opin Genet Dev 1999, 9:158–63.
9. Maitland NJ, Macintosh CA, Hall J, Sharrard M, Quinn G, Lang S. *In vitro* models to study cellular differentiation and function in human prostate cancers. Radiat Res 2001, 155:133–42.
10. Van Weerden WM, Romijn JC. Use of nude mouse xenograft models in prostate cancer research. Prostate 2000, 43:263–71.
11. Hukku B, Mally M, Cher ML, Peehl DM, Kung HF, Rhim JS. Stepwise genetic changes associated with progression of nontumorigenic HPV-18 immortalized human prostate cancer-derived cell line to a malignant phenotype. Cancer Genet Cytogenet 2000, 120:117–26.
12. Harris H, Miller OJ, Klein G, Worst P, Tachebana T. Suppression of malignancy by cell fusion. Nature 1969, 223:363–8.
13. Sidebottom E, Clark SR. Cell fusion regulated progressive growth from metastasis. Br J Cancer 1983, 47:399–406.
14. Anderson MJ, Stanbridge EJ. Tumor suppressor genes studied by cell hybridization and chromosome transfer. FASEB J 1993, 7:826–33.
15. Mashimo T, Watabe M, Cuthbert AP, Newbold RF, Rinker-Schaeffer CW, Helfer E, Watabe K. Human chromosome 16 suppresses metastasis but not tumorigenesis in rat prostatic tumor cells. Cancer Res 1998, 58:4572–6.
16. Lang SH, Stower M, Maitland NJ. In vitro modelling of epithelial and stromal interactions in non-malignant and malignant prostates. Br J Cancer 2000, 82:990–7.
17. Mohler JL, Partin AW, Isaacs JT, Coffey DS. Metastatic potential prediction by a visual grading system of cell motility: Prospective validation in the dunning R-3327 prostatic adenocarcinoma model. Cancer Res 1988, 48:4312–17.
18. Partin AW, Isaacs JT, Treiger B, Coffey DS. Early cell motility changes associated with an increase in metastatic ability in rat prostatic cancer cells transfected with the v-harvey-*ras* oncogene. Cancer Res 1988, 48:6050–3.
19. Clark EA, Golub TR, Lander ES, Hynes RO. Genomic analysis of metastasis reveals an essential role for rhoc. Nature 2000, 406:532–5.
20. Khan J, Saal LH, Bittner ML, Chen YD, Trent JM, Meltzer PS. Expression profiling in cancer using cDNA microarrays. Electrophoresis 1999, 20:223–9.
21. Kozlowski JM, Fidler IJ, Campbell D, Xu ZL, Kaighn ME, Hart IR. Metastatic behavior of human tumor cell lines grown in the nude mouse. Cancer Res 1984, 44:3522–9.
22. Chen YH, Lu Q, Schneeberger EE, Goodenough DA. Restoration of tight junction structure and barrier function by down-regulation of the mitogen-activated protein kinase pathway in ras-transformed madin-darby canine kidney cells. Mol Biol Cell 2000, 11:849–62.

23. Bao LR, Loda M, Janmey PA, Stewart R, Anand-Apte B, Zetter BR. Thymosin (15: A novel regulator of tumor cell motility upregulated in metastatic prostate cancer. Nat Med 1996, 2:1322–8.
24. Hall A. Rho gtpase and the actin cytoskeleton. Science 1998, 279:509–14.
25. Sahai E, Marshall CJ. RHO-gtpases and cancer. Nat Rev Cancer 2002, 2:133–42.
26. Somlyo AV, Bradshaw D, Ramos S, Murphy C, Myers CE, Somlyo AP. Rho-kinase inhibitor retards migration and *in vivo* dissemination of human prostate cancer cells. Biochem Biophys Res Commun 2000, 269:652–9.
27. Ichikawa T, Ichikawa Y, Isaacs JT. Genetic factors and suppression of metastatic ability of prostatic cancer. Cancer Res 1991, 51:3788–92.
28. Cunha GR. Epithelio-mesenchymal interaction in primodial gland structures will become responsive to androgenic stimulation. Anat Rec 1973, 172:179–96.
29. Thompson TC, Kadmon D, Timme TL, Merz VW, Egawa S, Krebs T *et al*. Experimental oncogene induced prostate cancer. Cancer Surv 1991, 11:55–71.
30. Thompson TC, Park SH, Timme TL, Ren C, Eastham JA, Donehower LA *et al*. Loss of P53 function leads to metastasis n ras+ myc-initiated mouse prostate cancer. Oncogene 1995, 10:869–79.
31. Bookstein R, MacGrogan D, Hilsenbeck SG, Sharkey F, Allred DC. P53 is mutated in a subset of advanced-stage prostate cancers. Cancer Res 1993, 53:3369–73.
32. Thompson TC, Timme TL, Park SH, Yang G, Ren CZ. Mouse prostate reconstitution model system: A series of in vivo and in vitro models for benign and malignant prostatic disease. Prostate 2000, 43:248–54.
33. Bangma CH, Nasu Y, Ren CZ, Thompson TC. Metastasis-related genes in prostate cancer. Semin Oncol 1999, 26:422–7.
34. Yang G, Truong LD, Wheeler TM, Thompson TC. Caveolin-l expression in clinically confined human prostate cancer: A novel prognostic marker. Cancer Res 1999, 59:5719–23.
35. Abate-Shen C, Shen MM. Mouse models of prostate carcinogenesis. Trends Genet 2002,S1–5.
36. Sharma P, Schreiber-Agus N. Mouse models of prostate cancer. Oncogene 1999, 18:5349–55.
37. Gingrich JR, Barrios RJ, Morton RA, Boyce BF, DeMayo FJ, Finegold MJ *et al*. Metastatic prostate cancer in a transgenic mouse. Cancer Res 1996, 56:4096–102.
38. Voeks DJ, Martiniello-Wilks R, Russell PJ. Derivation of MPR and TRAMP models of prostate cancer and prostate cancer metastasis for evaluation of therapeutic strategies. Urol Oncol 2002, 7:111–18.
39. Yang D, Holt GE, Velders MP, Kwon ED, Kast WM. Murine six membrane epithelial antigen of the prostate, prostate stem cell antigen and prostate-specific membrane antigen: Prostate-specific cell surface antigens highly expressed in prostate cancer of transgenic adenocarcinoma mouse prostate mice. Cancer Res 2001, 61:5857–60.
40. Shah AH, Tabayoyong WB, Kundu SD, Kim SJ, Van Parijs L, Liu VC *et al*. Suppression of tumor metastasis by blockade of transforming growth factor beta signaling in bone marrow cells through a retroviral-mediated gene therapy in mice. Cancer Res 2002, 62:7135–8.
41. Abraham S, Zhang W, Greenberg N, Zhang M. Maspin functions as tumor suppressor by increasing cell adhesion to extracellular matrix in prostate tumor cells. J Urol 2003, 169:1157–61.

42. Maroulakou IG, Anver M, Garrett L, Green JE. Prostate and mammary adenocarcinoma in transgenic mice carrying a rat C3(1) simian virus 40 large tumor antigen fusion gene. Proc Natl Acad Sci USA 1994, 91:11236–40.
43. Garabedian EM, Humphrey PA, Gordon JI. A transgenic mouse model of metastatic prostate cancer originating from neuroendocrine cells. Proc Natl Acad Sci USA 1998, 95:15382–7.
44. Bhatia-Gaur R, Donjacour AA, Sciavolino PJ, Kim M, Desai N, Young P et al. Roles for NKX3.1 In prostate development and cancer. Genes Dev 1999, 13:966–77.
45. Podsypanina K, Ellenson LH, Nemes A, Gu JG, Tamura M, Yamada KM et al. Mutation of *Pten*/MMAC1 in mice causes neoplasia in multiple organ systems. Proc Natl Acad Sci USA 1999, 96:1563–8.
46. Wainstein MA, He F, Robinson D, Kung H-J, Schwartz S, Giaconia JM et al. CWR22: Androgen-dependent xenograft model derived from a primary human prostatic carcinoma. Cancer Res 1994, 54:6049–52.
47. Nemeth JA, Harb JF, Barroso U Jr, Grignon DJ, Cher ML. Severe combined immunodeficient-hu model of human prostate cancer metastasis to human bone. Cancer Res 1999, 59:1987–93.
48. Pettaway CA, Pathak S, Greene G, Ramirez E, Wilson MR, Killion JJ, Fidler IJ. Selection of highly metastatic variants of different human prostatic carcinomas using orthotopic implantation in nude mice. Clin Cancer Res 1996, 2:1627–36.
49. Kocheril SV, Grignon DJ, Wang CY, Maughan RL, Montecillo EJ, Talati B et al. Responsiveness of human prostate carcinoma bone tumors to interleukin-2 therapy in a mouse xenograft tumor model. Cancer Detect Prev 1999, 23:408–16.
50. Thalmann GN, Sikes RA, Wu TT, Degeorges A, Chang SM, Ozen M et al. LNCap progression model of human prostate cancer: Androgen-independence and osseous metastasis. Prostate 2000, 44:91–103.
51. Gleave M, Hsieh J-T, Gao C, Von Eschenbach AC, Chung LWK. Acceleration of human prostate cancer growth *in vivo* by factors produced by prostate and bone fibroblasts. Cancer Res 1991, 51:3753–61.
52. Patel BJ, Pantuck AJ, Zisman A, Tsui KH, Paik SH, Caliliw R et al. CL1-GFP: An androgen independent metastatic tumor model for prostate cancer. J Urol 2000, 164:1420–5.
53. Adams JY, Johnson M, Sato M, Berger F, Gambhir SS, Carey M et al. Visualization of advanced human prostate cancer lesions in living mice by a targeted gene transfer vector and optical imaging. Nat Med 2002, 8:891–897.
54. Chen CT, Gan YB, Au JLS, Wientjes MG. Androgen-dependent and -independent human prostate xenograft tumors as models for drug activity evaluation. Cancer Res 1998, 58:2777–83.
55. Mousses S, Bubendorf L, Wagner U, Hostetter G, Kononen J, Cornelison R et al. Clinical validation of candidate genes associated with prostate cancer progression in the CWR22 model system using tissue microarrays. Cancer Res 2002, 62: 1256–60.
56. Averboukh L, Liang P, Kantoff PW, Pardee AB. Regulation of S100P expression by androgen. Prostate 1996, 29:350–5.
57. Takenaga K, Nakamura Y, Sakiyama S. Expression of antisense RNA to S100A4 gene encoding an S100-related calcium-binding protein suppresses metastatic potential of high-metastatic lewis lung carcinoma cells. Oncogene 1997, 14:331–7.

58. Tarabykina S, Scott DJ, Herzyk P, Hill TJ, Tame JR, Kriajevska M et al. The dimerization interface of the metastasis-associated protein S100A4 (MTS1): In vivo and in vitro studies. J Biol Chem 2001, 276:24212–22.
59. Oft M, Akhurst RJ, Balmain A. Metastasis is driven by sequential elevation of H-ras and SMAD2 levels. Nat Cell Biol 2002, 4:487–94.
60. Chu LW, Pettaway CA, Liang JC. Genetic abnormalities specifically associated with varying metastatis potential of prostate cancer cell lines as detected by comparative genomic hybridization. Cancer Genet Cytogenet 2001, 127:161–7.
61. Sharrard RM, Maitland NJ. Phenotypic effects of overexpression of the MMAC1 gene in prostate epithelial cells. Br J Cancer 2000, 83:1102–9.
62. Schuster N, Krieglstein K. Mechanisms of TGF-(-mediated apoptosis. Cell Tissue Res 2002, 307:1–14.
63. Blanchère M, Mestayer C, Saunier E, Broshuis M, Mowszowicz I. Transforming growth factor in the human prostate: Its role in stromal-epithelial interactions in non-cancerous cell culture. Prostate 2001, 46:311–18.
64. Thiery JP. Epithelial-mesenchymal transitions in tumor progression. Nat Rev Cancer 2002, 2:442–54.
65. Kononen J, Budendorf L, Kallioniemi A, Barlund M, Schraml P, Leighton S et al. Tissue microarrays for high-throughput molecular profiling of tumor specimens. Nat Med 1998, 4:844–7.
66. Dhanasekaran SM, Barrette TR, Ghosh D, Shah R, Varambally S, Kurachi K et al. Delineation of prognostic biomarkers in prostate cancer. Nature 2001, 412:822–6.
67. Bubendorf L, Kononen J, Koivisto P, Schraml P, Moch H, Gasser TC et al. Survey of gene amplifications during prostate cancer progression by high throughput fluorescence in situ hybridization on tissue microarrays. Cancer Res 1999, 59:803–6.
68. Forozan F, Karhu R, Kononen J, Kallioniemi A, Kallioniemi O-P. Genome screening by comparative genomic hybridization. Trends Genet 1997, 13:405–9.
69. Macintosh CA, Murant S, Hopwood L, Anderson M, Phillips S, Stower M, Maitland NJ. Analysis of chromosomal instability in prostatic carcinoma using fluorescent microsatellites to map preferentially altered loci. Urol Res 1994, 23:P61.
70. Dumur CI, Dechsukhum C, Ware JL, Cofield SS, Best AM, Wilkinson DS et al. Genome-wide detection of LOH in prostate cancer using human SNP microarray technology. Genomics 2003, 81:260–9.
71. Witte JS, Goddard KAB, Conti DV, Elston RC, Lin J, Suarez BK et al. Genomewide scan for prostate cancer-aggressiveness loci. Am J Hum Genet 2000, 67:92–9.
72. Diatchenko L, Lau YF, Campbell AP, Chenchik A, Moqadam F, Huang B et al. Suppression subtractive hybridization: A method for generating differentially regulated or tissue-specific cDNA probes and libraries. Proc Natl Acad Sci USA 1996, 93:6025–30.
73. Xu JC, Stolk JA, Zhang XQ, Silva SJ, Houghton RL, Matsumura M et al. Identification of differentially expressed genes in human prostate cancer using subtraction and microarray. Cancer Res 2000, 60:1677–82.
74. Porkka KP, Visakorpi T. Detection of differentially expressed genes in prostate cancer by combining suppression subtractive hybridization and cDNA library array. J Pathol 2001, 193:73–9.
75. Rhodes DR, Barrette TR, Rubin MA, Ghosh D, Chinnaiyan AM. Meta-analysis of microarrays: Interstudy validation of gene expression profiles reveals pathway dysregulation in prostate cancer. Cancer Res 2002, 62:4427–33.

76. Ramaswamy S, Ross KN, Lander ES, Golub TR. A molecular signature of metastasis in primary solid tumors. Nat Genet 2003, 33:49–54.
77. Singh D, Febbo PG, Ross K, Jackson DG, Manola J, Ladd C *et al.* Gene expression correlates of clinical prostate cancer behavior. Cancer Cell 2002, 1:203–9.
78. Newton D, Kendziorski CM, Richmond CS, Blattner FR, Tsui KW. On differerential variability of expression ratios: Improving statistical inference about gene expression changes from microarray data. Comput Biol 2001, 8:37–52.
79. Scheurle D, DeYoung MP, Binninger DM, Page H, Jahanzeb M, Narayanan R. Cancer gene discovery using digital differential display. Cancer Res 2000, 60:4037–43.
80. Chakrabarti R, Robles LD, Gibson J, Muroski M. Profiling of differential expression of messenger RNA in normal, benign, and metastatic prostate cell lines. Cancer Genet Cytogenet 2002, 139:115–25.
81. Velculescu VE, Zhang L, Vogelstein B, Kinzler KW. Serial analysis of gene expression. Science 1995, 270:484–7.
82. Waghray A, Schober M, Feroze F, Yao F, Virgin J, Chen YQ. Identification of differentially expressed genes by serial analysis of gene expression in human prostate cancer. Cancer Res 2001, 61:4283–6.
83. Untergasser G, Koch KB, Menssen A, Hermeking H. Characterization of epithelial senescence by serial analysis of gene expression: Identification of genes potentially involved in prostate cancer. Cancer Res 2002, 62:6255–62.
84. Nelson PS, Han D, Rochon Y, Corthals GL, Lin BY, Monson A *et al.* Comprehensive analyses of prostate gene expression: Convergence of expressed sequence tag databases, transcript profiling and proteomics. Electrophoresis 2000, 21:1823–31.
85. Nelson PS, Pritchard C, Abbott D, Clegg N. The human (PEDB) and mouse (mPEDB) prostate expression databases. Nucleic Acids Res 2002, 30:218–20.
86. Ahram M, Best CJM, Flaig MJ, Gillespie JW, Leiva IM, Chuaqui RF *et al.* Proteomic analysis of human prostate cancer. Mol Carcinog 2002, 33:9–15.
87. Wellmann A, Wollscheid V, Lu H, Ma ZL, Albers P, Schutze K *et al.* Analysis of microdissected prostate tissue with PROTEINCHIP arrays–a way to new insights into carcinogenesis and to diagnostic tools. Int J Mol Med 2002, 9:341–7.
88. Qu Y, Adam BL, Yasui Y, Ward MD, Cazares LH, Schellhammer PF *et al.* Boosted decision tree analysis of surface-enhanced laser desorption/ionization mass spectral serum profiles discriminates prostate cancer from noncancer patients. Clin Chem 2002, 48:1835–43.
89. Ball G, Mian S, Holding F, Allibone RO, Lowe J, Ali S *et al.* An integrated approach utilizing artificial neural networks and SELDI mass spectrometry for the classification of human tumor and rapid identification of potential biomarkers. Bioinformatics 2002, 18:395–404.
90. Liu AY. Differential expression of cell surface molecules in prostate cancer cells. Cancer Res 2000, 60:3429–34.
91. Bok RA, Small EJ. Bloodborne biomolecular markers in prostate cancer development and progression. Nat Rev Cancer 2002, 2:918–26.
92. Kontturi M. Is acid phosphatase (PAP) still justified in the management of prostatic cancer. Acta Oncol 1991, 30:169–70.
93. Howanitz JH. Prostate specific antigen (PSA). Dis Markers 1993, 11:3–10.
94. Corey E, Arfman EW, Oswin MM, Melchior SW, Tindall DJ, Young CYF *et al.* Detection of circulating prostate cells by reverse transcriptase polymerase chain

reaction of human glandular kallikrein (hK2) and prostate-specific antigen (PSA) messages. Urology 1997, 50:184–8.
95. Miller JC, Zhou H, Kwekel J, Cavallo R, Burke J, Butler EB *et al*. Antibody microarray profiling of human prostate cancer sera: Antibody screening and identification of potential biomarkers. Proteomics 2003, 3:56–63.
96. Diamandis EP. Serum proteomic patterns for detection of prostate cancer. J Natl Cancer Inst 2003, 95:489–90.
97. Petricoin EFIII, Ornstein DK, Paweletz CP, Ardekani A, Hackett PS, Hitt BA *et al*. Serum proteomic patterns for detection of prostate cancer. J Natl Cancer Inst 2002, 94:1576–8.
98. Issaq JH, Veenstra TD, Contads TP, Felshow D. The seldi-tof ms approach to proteomics: Protein profiling and biomarker identification. Biochem Biophys Res Commun 2002, 292:587–92.
99. Wang S, Diamond DL, Hass GM, Sokoloff R, Vessella RL. Identification of prostate specific memvrane antigen (PSMA) as the target of monoclonal antibody 107-1A4 by proteinchip®; array, surface-enhanced laser desorption/ionization (SELDI) technology. Int J Cancer 2001, 92:871–6.
100. Huang GM, Ng WL, Farkas J, He L, Liang HA, Gordon D *et al*. Prostate cancer expression profiling by cDNA sequencing analysis. Genomics 1999, 59:178–86.
101. Asmann YW, Kosari F, Wang K, Cheville JC, Vasmatzis G. Identification of differentially expressed genes in normal and malignant prostate by electronic profiling of expressed sequence tags. Cancer Res 2002, 62:3308–14.
102. Lang SH, Hyde C, Reid IN, Hitchcock IS, Hart CA, Bryden AAG *et al*. Enhanced expression of vimentin in motile prostate cell lines and in poorly differentiated and metastatic prostate cancer. Prostate 2002, 52:253–63.
103. Yoshimura R, Sano H, Masuda C, Kawamura M, Tsubouchi Y, Chargui J *et al*. Expression of cyclooxygenase-2 in prostate carcinoma. Cancer 2000, 89:589–96.
104. Kirschenbaum A, Liu XH, Yao S, Levine AC. The role of cyclooxygenase-2 in prostate cancer. Urology 2001, 58:127–31.
105. Tuxhorn JA, Ayala GE, Rowley DR. Reactive stroma in prostate cancer progression. J Urol 2001, 166:2472–83.
106. Cunha GR, Hayward SW, Wang YZ. Role of stroma in carcinogenesis of the prostate. Differentiation 2002, 70:473–85.
107. Macintosh CA, Stower M, Reid N, Maitland NJ. Precise microdissection of human prostate cancers reveals genotypic heterogeneity. Cancer Res 1998, 58:23–8.
108. Clark J, Edwards S, Feber A, Flohr P, John M, Giddings I *et al*. Genome-wide screening for complete genetic loss in prostate cancer by comparative hybridization onto cDNA microarrays. Oncogene 2003, 22:1247–52.
109. Ichikawa T, Nihei N, Kuramochi J, Kawana Y, Killary AM, Rinker-Schaeffer CW *et al*. Metastasis suppressor genes for prostate cancer. Prostate 1996,:31–5.
110. Kauffman EC, Robinson VL, Stadler WM, Sokoloff MH, Rinker-Schaeffer CW. Metastasis suppression: The evolving role of metastasis supressor genes for regulating cancer cell growth at the secondary site. J Urol 2003, 169:1122–33.
111. Padalecki SS, Troyer DA, Hansen MF, Saric T, Schneider BG, O'Connell P, Leach RJ. Identification of two distinct regions of allelic imbalance on chromosome 18q in metastatic prostate cancer. Int J Cancer 2000, 85:654–8.

112. Alers JC, Krijtenburg PJ, Rosenberg C, Hop WCJ, Verkerk AM, Schröder FH et al. Interphase cytogenetics of prostatic tumor progression: Specific chromosomal abnormalities are involved in metastasis to the bone. Lab Invest 1997, 77:437–48.
113. Karan D, Lin MF, Johansson SL, Batra SK. Current status of the molecular genetics of human prostatic adenocarcinomas. Int J Cancer 2003, 103:285–93.
114. Kraus J, Pantel K, Pinkel D, Albertson DG, Speicher MR. High-resolution genomic profiling of occult micrometastatic tumor cells. Genes Chromosomes. Cancer 2003, 36:159–66.
115. Kasahara K, Taguchi T, Yamasaki I, Kamada M, Yuri K, Shuin T. Detection of genetic alterations in advanced prostate cancer by comparative genomic hybridization. Cancer Genet Cytogenet 2002, 137:59–63.
116. El Gedaily A, Bubendorf L, Willi N, Fu W, Richter J, Moch H et al. Discovery of new DNA amplification loci in prostate cancer by comparative genomic hybridization. Prostate 2001, 46:184–90.
117. Zitzelsberger H, Engert D, Walch A, Kulka U, Aubele M, Höfler H et al. Chromosomal changes during development and progression of prostate adenocarcinomas. Br J Cancer 2001, 84:202–8.
118. Jing C, El Ghany MA, Beesley C, Foster CS, Rudland PS, Smith P, Ke Y. Tazarotene-induced gene 1 (TIG1) expression in prostate carcinomas and its relationship to tumorigenicity. J Natl Cancer Inst 2002, 94:482–90.
119. Nelson PS, Plymate SR, Wang K, True LD, Ware JL, Gan L et al. Hevin, an antiadhesive extracellular matrix protein, is down- regulated in metastatic prostate adenocarcinoma. Cancer Res 1998, 58:232–6.
120. Huang SY, Pettaway CA, Uehara H, Bucana CD, Fidler IJ. Blockade of NF-kappab activity in human prostate cancer cells is associated with suppression of angiogenesis, invasion, and metastasis. Oncogene 2001, 20:4188–97.
121. Tsurusaki T, Kanda S, Sakai H, Kanetake H, Saito Y, Alitalo K, Koji T. Vascular endothelial growth factor-C expression in human prostatic carcinoma and its relationship to lymph node metastasis. Br J Cancer 1999, 80:309–13.
122. Banyard J, Bao L, Zetter BR. Type XXIII collagen: A new transmembrane collagen identified in metastatic tumor cells. J Biol Chem 2003, 18:20989–20994.
123. Nelson JB, Hedican SP, George DJ, Reddi AH, Piantadosi S, Eisenberger MA, Simons JW. Identification of endothelin-1 in the pathophysiology of metastatic adenocarcinoma of the prostate. Nat Med 1995, 1:944–9.
124. Xia W, Unger P, Miller L, Nelson J, Gelman IH. The *Src*-suppressed C kinase substrate, ssecks, is a potential metastasis inhibitor in prostate cancer. Cancer Res 2001, 61:5644–51.
125. Humphrey PA, Zhu X, Zarnegar R, Swanson PE, Ratliff TL, Vollmer RT, Day ML. Hepatocyte growth factor and its receptor (c-MET) in prostatic carcinoma. Am J Pathol 1995, 147:386–96.
126. Naughton M, Picus J, Zhu XP, Catalona WJ, Vollmer RT, Humphrey PA. Scatter factor-hepatocyte growth factor elevation in the serum of patients with prostate cancer. J Urol 2001, 165:1325–8.
127. Wissenbach U, Niemeyer BA, Fixemer T, Schneidewind A, Trost C, Cavalié A et al. Expression of cat-like, a novel calcium-selective channel, correlates with the malignancy of prostate cancer. J Biol Chem 2001, 276:19461–8.

128. Zhau HYE, Zhou JX, Symmans WF, Chen BQ, Chang SM, Sikes RA, Chung LWK. Transfected neu oncogene induces human prostate cancer metastasis. Prostate 1996, 28:73–83.
129. Bowen C, Bubendorf L, Voeller HJ, Slack R, Willi N, Sauter G et al. Loss of NKX3.1 Expression in human prostate cancers correlates with tumor progression. Cancer Res 2000, 60:6111–15.
130. Porkka K, Saramäki O, Tanner M, Visakorpi T. Amplification and overexpression of elongin C gene discovered in prostate cancer by cDNA microarrays. Lab Invest 2002, 82:629–37.
131. Jing C, Beesley C, Foster CS, Rudland PS, Fujii H, Ono T et al. Identification of the messenger RNA for human cutaneous fatty acid-binding protein as a metastasis inducer. Cancer Res 2000, 60:2390–8.
132. Zhang J, Dai J, Qi Y, Lin DL, Smith P, Strayhorn C et al. Osteoprotegerin inhibits prostate cancer-induced osteoclastogenesis and prevents prostate tumor growth in the bone. J Clin Invest 2001, 107:1235–44.
133. Gu Z, Thomas G, Yamashiro J, Shintaku IP, Dorey F, Raitano A et al. Prostate stem cell antigen (PSCA) expression increases with high gleason score, advanced stage and bone metastasis in prostate cancer. Oncogene 2000, 19:1288–96.
134. Chen H, Pong RC, Wang Z, Hsieh JT. Differential regulation of the human gene DAB2IP in normal and malignant prostatic epithelia: Cloning and characterization. Genomics 2002, 79:573–81.
135. Xin W, Rhodes DR, Ingold C, Chinnaiyan AM, Rubin MA. Dysregulation of the annexin family protein family is associated with prostate cancer progression. Am J Pathol 2003, 162:255–61.
136. Liu JW, Shen JJ, Tanzillo-Swarts A, Bhatia B, Maldonado CM, Person MD et al. Annexin II expression is reduced or lost in prostate cancer cells and its re-expression inhibits prostate cancer cell migration. Oncogene 2003, 22:1475–85.
137. Iddon J, Bundred NJ, Hoyland J, Downey SE, Baird P, Salter D et al. Expression of parathyroid hormone-related protein and its receptor in bone metastases from prostate cancer. J Pathol 2000, 191:170–4.
138. Schmidt U, Fiedler U, Pilarsky CP, Ehlers W, Füssel S, Haase M et al. Identification of a novel gene on chromosome 13 between BRCA-2 and RB-1. Prostate 2001, 47:91–101.
139. Silletti S, Yao JP, Pienta KJ, Raz A. Loss of cell-contact regulation and altered responses to autocrine motility factor correlate with increased malignancy in prostate cancer cells. Int J Cancer 1995, 63:100–5.
140. Yashi M, Muraishi O, Kobayashi Y, Tokue A, Nanjo H. Elevated serum progastrin-releasing peptide (31–98) in metastatic and androgen-independent prostate cancer patients. Prostate 2002, 51:84–97.
141. Rondinelli RH, Tricoli JV. CLAR1, a novel gene that exhibits enhanced expression in advanced human prostate cancer. Clin Cancer Res 1999, 5:1595–602.
142. Thomas BG, Hamdy FC. Bone morphogenetic protein-6: Potential mediator of osteoblastic metastases in prostate cancer. Prostate Cancer Prostatic Dis 2000, 3:283–5.
143. Masuda H, Fukabori Y, Nakano K, Takezawa Y, Suzuki T, Yamanaka H. Increased expression of bone morphogenetic protein-7 in bone metastatic prostate cancer. Prostate 2003, 54:268–74.
144. Westermarck J, Kähäri V-M. Regulation of a matrix metalloproteinase expression in tumor invasion. FASEB J 1999, 13:781–92.

145. Kelsell DP, Dunlop J, Hodgins MB. Hum diseases: Clues to cracking the connexin code. Trends Cell Biol 2001, 11:2–6.
146. Govindarajan R, Zhao S, Song XH, Guo RJ, Wheelock M, Johnson KR, Mehta PP. Impaired trafficking of connexins in androgen-independent human prostate cancer cell lines and its mitigation by alpha-catenin. J Biol Chem 2002, 277:50087–97.

Chapter 4

POLYUNSATURATED FATTY ACIDS AND PROSTATE CANCER METASTASIS

Wen G. Jiang
Metastasis Research Group, University Department of Surgery, University of Wales College of Medicine, Heath Park, Cardiff, Wales, UK

Abstract: Polyunsaturated fatty acids have been demonstrated to have anticancer activities, on a number of tumor types including prostate cancer. There is evidence that these fatty acids may also influence the metastatic process of cancer. The anti-metastasis function is probably via the effects on more than one aspect of the metastatic process, including angiogenesis, cell adhesion and communication, matrix degradation and invasion, as well as the growth and death of prostate cancer cells. Clinical and epidemiological evidence has also pointed to the involvement of various fatty acids in the development and progression of prostate cancer. Some of the fatty acids have been evaluated for the possible anticancer effects *in vivo* and in limited clinical studies. This chapter summarises the recent development in scientific and clinical research into the possible impact of polyunsaturated fatty acids on prostate cancer.

Key words: prostate cancer, polyunsaturated fatty acids, essential fatty acids, metastasis, angiogenesis

Fatty acids and their impact on the incidence of cancer has been an ongoing debate for the past decades (1, 2, 3, 4). While evidence exists that certain fatty acids may be involved in the development certain type cancers, recent studies have also revealed that some fatty acids, primarily selected polyunsaturated fatty acids of ω-3 and ω-6 series, are important regulators in cancer development and metastasis. This chapter will discuss firstly the scientific evidence of the impact of fatty acids on cancer, and then the epidemiological and clinical studies of the role of fatty acids in the development and metastasis of prostate cancer.

1. POLYUNSATURATED FATTY ACIDS

There are 4 series of unsaturated fatty acids (ω-3, ω-6, ω-7, and ω-9), named so because of the position of the first double bond from the methyl end of the molecules (Figure 1 and Figure 2). Two of these series, the ω-3 and ω-6 are known to be essential fatty acid (EFA) series (Figure 1). This is due to the fact that the first fatty acids linoleic acid (LA) (ω-6) and alpha-linolenic acid (ALA) (ω-3) in the respective series has to be obtained from diets, as our body is unable to synthesise these fatty acids. These two fatty acids are therefore referred to as being essential.

Parent forms of fatty acids (LA and ALA) are converted to its down stream highly unsaturated fatty acids (referred to HUFAs in some cases) by way of elongation and desaturation. The elongation step involves adding

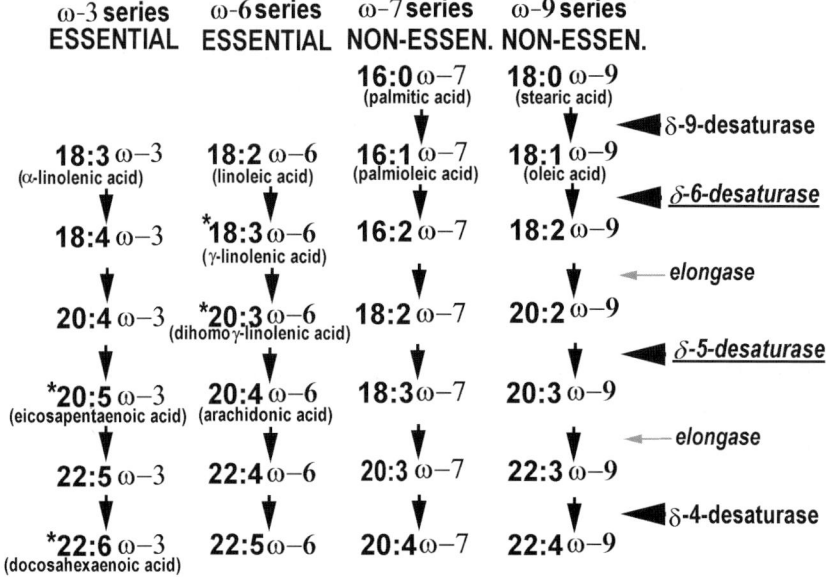

Figure 1. Unsaturated fatty acids. ω-3 and ω-6 are essential series as the parent fatty acids in the series, α-linolenic acid and linoleic acid have to be obtained from diets. ω-7 and ω-9 series are non-essential fatty series as our body can synthesised all the fatty acids in the series. Parent fatty acids are becoming more saturated with addition of more double bonds to their carbon chain, by desaturases. The length of the carbon chain is increased with addition of new carbon atom to the backbone of the lipid by elongase. δ-6, and δ-5 desaturases are thought to be deficient in cancer cells and cancer tissues. Fatty acids marked by a star sign are those known to be highly unsaturared and usually highly toxic to cancer cells.

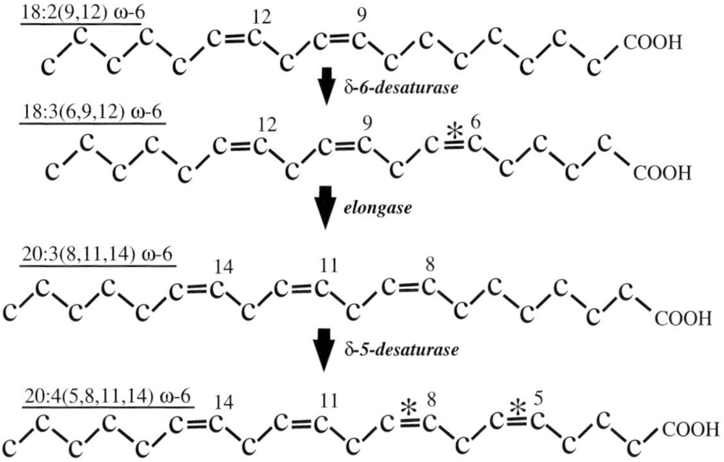

Figure 2. Desaturation and elongation of ω-6 series essential fatty acids. The essential fatty acid, 18:2 (9, 12) ω-6 (linoleic acid) which has two unsaturated double bonds at position 9 and 12, is desaturated by δ-6-desaturase, with the addition of the double bond at position 6 (marked with a star). The product thus produced has three unsaturated double bonds and is known as γ-linolenic acid. This is followed by addition of two carbon atoms to the backbone of the fatty acids by elongase, forming a product which now has a chain of 20 carbon atoms and 3 unsaturated bond and is known as dihomo-γ-linolenic acid. dihomo-γ-linolenic acid is further desaturated by δ-5-desaturase, to form arachidonic acid which has 4 unsaturated double bonds.

additional carbon atoms and the desaturation step adding unsaturated double bond (Figure 2). It is those highly unsaturated fatty acids, notably eicosapentaenoic acid (EPA) and docosahexaenoic acid (DHA) of the ω-3 series (Figure 1) and gamma linolenic acid (GLA) and dihomogamma linolenic acid (DGLA) of the ω-6 series (Figure 2) are generally known to have anti-cancer effects and will be discussed in later parts.

One of the important features of the unsaturated fatty acids is that they can be swiftly converted to downstream metabolites, such as prostaglandins, leukotrienes, etc., collectively known as eicosanoids, via different pathways. Figure 3 is an example of the pathways, by which fatty acids of the ω-6 series are converted into large number of different eicosanoids. Most of the eicosanoids are unstable, and have not been well studies in the context of cancer. However, some of them have been shown to have direct effect on cancer cells, such as 12-HETE and 13-HODE. The role of these eicosanoids in cancer is beyond the scope of this chapter.

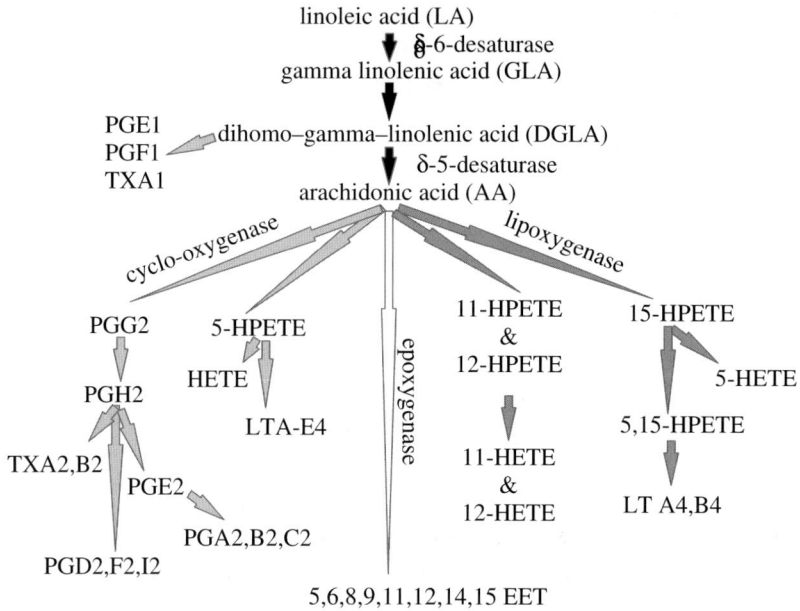

Figure 3. Production of eicosanoids from ω-6 polyunsaturated fatty acids. Polyunsaturated fatty acids can be converted into a large of number of eicosanoids by different enzyme pathways. Many of the eicosanods are bioactive and exert functions on cancer cells.

2. FATTY ACIDS AND CANCER

Although the direct scientific support for a role of fatty acids in the development and metastasis of cancer has only become evident in recent years, many of the early observations have already indicated that lack of essential fatty acids, in clinical situations such as essential fatty acid deficiency (EFAD) (5, 6), often results in damage to cell/tissue functions in the body that closely resemble that seen in cancer. During essential fatty acid deficiency, a rare condition in modern societies, it was frequently observed that there was a significant increase widening of the intercellular space, loss or reduction of desmosomes, and increased vascular permeability (7, 8, 9, 10, 11, 12, 13, 14). These changes are well known to occur during cancer development and in particular during cancer metastasis (for a review (see 15, 16)). Recent evidence suggests fatty acids do, indeed, regulate cell functions that are corresponding to some of the changes seen in EFAD (17), aspects of these new discoveries will be discussed in later part of the chapter.

2.1 Fatty Acids, Cell Growth and Cell Death

Perhaps one of the most studied areas in the relationship between cancer and fatty acid is the cytotoxic effects of unsaturated fatty acid in cancer cells (for a review see 4 and 18). After early reports showing a toxic effect of polyunsaturated fatty acid on some cancer cell lines (19, 20, 21), a large number of human and non-human cancer cell lines have since been tested. These cells cover almost all the solid tumor types as well as leukemic cells. As one would probably expect, the responses of these cells to fatty acids are various and are largely divided into: no response, response with decrease cell growth or increase of cell death, and response with an increase in cell growth. A summary of these changes can be seen in a recent review (22). While it is difficult to draw a clear conclusion as to which fatty acids are more toxic to cancer cell, it is generally recognised that that highly unsaturated fatty acids with more than three double bonds in both ω-3 and ω-6 series are generally toxic to cancer cells, including eicosapentaenoic acid, docosahaexanoic acid, gamma linenic acid and dihomogamma linolenic acid (Figure 1). Linolenic acid of the ω-6 series and in some cases (i.e. prostate cancer) alpha linolenic acid of the ω-3 series have been reported to increase the growth of various cancer cells. It is evident from these studies that to simply conclude that any particular series of fatty acids are pro- or against cancer is unfair, as fatty acids from both essential series can be toxic to cancer cells, whereas others in the same series can enhance the growth of the cells. For obvious reasons as discussed in later part, comparison should be perhaps be best made between individual fatty acid.

Fatty acids, under appropriate conditions and concentrations, are also reported to induce apoptosis in cancer cells (23, 24). This is probably via the direct or indirect effect of fatty acids on intracellular mediators, such as p53, bcl family, cell cycle regulators, and MAPK that modulate apoptotic events (24, 25).

2.2 Cytoxic Effects of Fatty Acids are Partly Dependent on Lipid Peroxidation, the Role of Fatty Acids Desaturases

It has been recognised for some years that the toxic effects of fatty acids on cancer cells are, at least in part, mediated by the peroxides and superoxides generated from lipid peroxidation (4, 18). The free radicals thus generated inside cancer cells results in damage to DNA and vital functions in cancer cells, which in turn leads to the death of cancer cells.

The reason why cancer cells are particularly sensitive to highly unsaturated fatty acids has been a focus of interest in cancer research. It was suggested that one of the possibilities is the abnormality of fatty acid metabolism in cancer cells and tumor tissues (4, 26, 27, 28, 29), including prostate cancer tissues (30, 31). As shown in Figures 1 and 2, parent fatty acid alpha linolenic acid of ω-3 and linoleic acid of ω-6 series have to be converted by enzymes to have more unsaturated bonds. This is achieved by fatty acid desaturates (FAD). Notable ones are δ-6-desaturase and δ-5-desaturase. These two desaturases enable the parent fatty acids, which must be obtained from the diet (and hence essential), to be converted to highly unsaturated forms. Early studies have indicated that in both cancer cells and cancer tissues, the activities of these enzymes are either lower or absent when compared with normal cells and tissues (31, 32, 33, 34). These abnormalities were demonstrated by using cell/tissue extracts as source of the enzymes and radioisotope labelled parent fatty acid as substrate. A few studies have demonstrated the deficiency of both δ-6-desaturase and δ-5-desaturase activities in cancer.

However, it was not until recently that human δ-6-desaturase and δ-5-desaturase have been cloned and sequenced by Clarke's group. The human δ-6 desaturase gene encode a 444-amino acid peptide, and was predicts to contains two membrane-spanning domains as well as a cytochrome b(5)-like domain that is characteristic of nonmammalian δ-6-desaturases. Expression of the enzyme increases the production of the downstream unsaturated products (35). Interestingly, the tissue with the highest level of the enzyme is brain. The human δ-5 desaturase gene encodes a 444-amino acid peptide, and contains two membrane-spanning domains, three histidine-rich regions, and a cytochrome b(5) domain (36). δ-5 desaturase is highly homologous to δ-6 desaturase. Many tissues express δ-5 desaturase mRNA, but highest levels are seen in the liver, brain and heart.

The cloning of these enzymes would have some profound impact on the understanding of the biology of unsaturated fatty acids in cancer. However, the expression of these enzymes is yet to be fully investigated in cancer. Furthermore, it may be essential to evaluate if restoring δ-6-desaturase and δ-5-desaturase in cancer cells may increase their sensitivity to fatty acid such as alpha-linolenic and linoleic acids. Inhibition of the activities of δ-6-desaturase using specific inhibitors such as SC-26196, has been shown reduce the metablsm of linoleic acid in vivo, and result in the increase of tumorigenesis in animal models (37). We may expect some more progress of the impact of manipulating these specific desaturases in the regulation of cancer cells functions and if these offer some possible therapeutic potentials in cancer.

2.3 Peroxisome-Proliferator Activated Receptors (PPAR) in the Action of Fatty Acids

Peroxisome proliferator activator receptors (PPARs) belong to a nuclear hormone receptor superfamily that regulates gene expressions (38, 39, 40, 45). A typical PPAR contains a DNA binding domain that recognises response elements in the promoters of its target genes (41). PPARs have been shown to control retinoic acid (RA) regulated genes and also to control lipid metabolism in peroxisomes (42). They can be activated by anti-cancer agents and indomethacin (43, 44). PPARs occur in three main forms, α–, β- and γ-. PPARs are also known to transduce external signals to the nucleus. The receptor ligands are lipophilic compounds and include retinoids, peroxisome proliferators and certain fatty acids and prostaglandins (PG J2) (45, 46, 47). These receptors also directly interact with PUFAs, including linoleic acid, arachidonic acid, linolenic acid and certain eicosanoids (PGJ2) (46, 47, 48). PPARs control gene expression in a number of circumstances. PPARγ modulates the inflammatory process by affecting the inflammatory cytokine production from macrophages (49, 50). PPARα may also regulate the inflammatory process, but more likely through the mediation of leukotriene B4 (LTB4) (51, 52). PPARα, however, does not participate in polyunsaturated fatty acid regulation of enzyme synthesis (53). Certain cancer cells have been shown to express PPAR, such as breast cancer MCF-7 and T45D cells (54).

Recent studies showed that these receptors also directly interact with PUFAs, including LA, AA, linolenic and certain eicosanoids (PGJ) and served as their receptor (45, 52, 53, 54). Clearly, more efforts are required to identify the genes that are regulated by the PPAR response elements and those that are responsible for PUFA induced expressions. Our recent study has demonstrated that a number of the effects exerted by highly unsaturated fatty acids can be partly attributed to the action of PPARγ in cancer cells (45, 55).

2.4 Fatty Acids and the Metastatic Process of Cancer

Metastatic spread of cancers is the single most important event that affects the clinical outcome of patients with cancer. The process of formation of tumor metastases can be referred to as the metastatic cascade (16, 56). The success of establishing a secondary tumor by a cancer cells requires the completion of a good number of separate but essential steps, including the loss of cell-cell adhesion at the primary site, adhesion to and invasion of the basement membrane and extracellular matrix (ECM), intravasation, travel in the host blood circulation and survival of host immune responses, adhesion to the endothelium and departure from the blood stream (extravasation), and finally establishment of secondary foci assisted by the formation of neovasculature and angiogenesis. Experimental evidence suggests that fatty acids may affect a number of these events.

2.4.1   Fatty Acids and Cell-Cell Adhesion Mechanisms in Cancer

Cell-cell adhesion mechanism plays a key role in the maintenance of tissue/organ integrity and almost all the physiological functions in the body. A range of cell adhesion molecules have been identified and can be grouped into four superfamilies: cadherins, integrins, the immunoglobulin superfamily and others (16, 56). Amongst these adhesion structures, E-cadherin complex and desmosomal cadherin complex are known to be suppressors of tumor metastasis.

As discussed previously, studies in the fifties and sixties have indicated a possible damage to what is now known as cell-cell adhesion mechanisms, during essential fatty acid deficiency (EFAD) (5, 6, 7, 8, 9, 10, 11). Recently experimental evidence has suggested that certain polyunsaturated fatty acid can up-regulate the expression of E-cadherin and desomosomal cadherin, desmoglein in cancer cells, thus reducing the invasive and metastatic potential of cancer cells.

2.4.2   Fatty Acids and Cell-Matrix Adhesion

The adhesion of tumor cells to the extracellular matrix is a crucial event that facilitates matrix degradation and invasion, cell survival and migration of tumor cells (60, 61, 62). Tumor cell-matrix attachment is mediated by integrin molecules on the cell surface. Expression of selected integrin, in combination of matrix protein, are known to be a key part in the early phase of cancer cell invasion and dissociation. There have been some compelling evidence to show that polyunsaturated fatty acids, such as GLA, EPA, and DHA are able to reduce tumor adhesion to a range of matrix components, including collagen type IV, fibronectin, laminin, vitronectin, and the basement membrane (57, 58, 59, 60). The inhibition was also associated with a reduction in the number of tumor cells lodging in blood vessels in animal studies (64, 65, 66). Although a precise mechanism is yet to be sought for the action of PUFAs on tumor cell-matrix adhesion, a recent study (67) indicated that this was at least partly via the inhibition of the tyrosine phosphorylation of FAK and paxillin, key regulatory mediators in cell-matrix adhesion signalling.

2.4.3 Fatty Acids and Extracellular Matrix Degradation by Cancer Cells

It has been demonstrated that fatty acids, such as EPA and GLA are able to inhibit both tissue type and urokinase type plasminogen activators (tPA and uPA) in cancer cells (68, 69). It has also been shown that the level of plasminogen activator inhibitor I, a member of the serpin class of protease inhibitors, was enhanced by DGLA and DHA (70). Although linoleic acid has been shown to stimulate 92-kDa type IV collagenase production in vitro; GLA however inhibited invasion and did not induce activity of the proteolytic enzyme (64, 71, 59, 72). Interestingly, this appeared to be the response of another recently identified tumor suppressor and member of the serpin family, maspin (73, 74, 75). GLA and EPA selectively increased the protein and mRNA level of maspin in a range of cancer cells (76).

2.4.4 Tumor-Endothelial Interaction Can Be Regulated by Fatty Acids

The adhesion of tumor cells to endothelium and subsequent invasion of the endothelium, the extravasation process, is a key part in the metastatic process. Short-term culture of endothelial cells with fatty acid such as GLA would result in a marked reduction of tumor cell adhesion to the endothelium (77). DHA has been reported to inhibit cytokine-induced expression of adhesion molecules in endothelial cells, including VCAM-1, ICAM-1 and E-selectin (78, 79, 80). Similar inhibition has been reported with metabolites of linoleic acid. The phenomenon may be the result of regulation of adhesion molecules both in cancer cells and in endothelial cells. It may also involve regulation of intercellular communication amongst endothelial cells as well as between endothelial cells and cancer cells.

2.4.5 Regulation of Cellular Motility and Migration by Unsaturated Fatty Acids

Fatty acids are known to regulate the motile and migratory behaviour of cancer cells, a cell function primary required during the metastatic process. Fatty acids such as GLA and EPA can reduce the migration of cancer cells on plastic culture ware as well as over ECM. Part of this reduction may be attributed to by the effects of fatty acids on tumor-matrix adhesion, and partly due to the alteration of intracellular events that govern cell migration, such as the cytoskeleton and cytoskeletal associated protein, including the ezrin-ridixin-moesin family (81).

2.4.6 Polyunsaturated Fatty Acids are Anti-Angiogenic

The central role of angiogenesis in the metastatic spread of cancer has been well established. The therapeutic value of anti-angiogenesis approaches has also been recognised. Fatty acids including EPA and GLA are known to be anti-angiogenic both *in vitro* and *in vivo*, as seen by a reduction of tubule forming from endothelial cells and reduction of angiogenesis in the corneal model (82, 83, 84, 85, 86). The possible mechanisms underlying this action is perhaps at the followingfolds: first the reduction of endothelial motility by fatty acid; this is an established function of polyunsaturated fatty acid; second inhibition of endothelial morphogenesis; and third modulation of other events involved in angiogenesis, including the alteration of adhesion mechanism specific to endothelial cell and angiogenesis such as vascular endothelial (VE)-cadherin in vascular endothelial cells (87, 88).

3. EPIDEMIOLOGICAL EVIDENCE THE DIFFERENT FATTY ACIDS HAVE A DIFFERENT IMPACT ON PROSTATE CANCER

In a prospective study of over 47 thousands participants by Giovannucci et al. (89), the risk of having advanced prostate cancer was directly related with the consumption of total fat of the diet, particularly that of animal fat. Interestingly, saturated, monosaturated fat, and alpha linolenic acid were associated with advanced prostate cancer (89). The study did not find a correlation between prostate cancer and linoleic acid. The same group has also analysed the plasma level of fatty acids from 14916 U.S. male physicians (90). It was revealed that the levels of alpha-linolenic acid, but not linoleic acid was correlated with the risk of prostate cancer. The recent study from the group investigated over 51,000 men amongst whom 1897 prostate cancer and 249 metastatic prostate cancers were identified (91). Consumption of red meat and levels of alpha linolenic acid were found to associate with the incidence of metastatic prostate cancer. These studies have shown a strong link between alpha-linolenic acid in the development of prostate cancer and metastatic prostate cancer, but not linoleic acid as demonstrated in *in vitro* and certain animal studies, which will be discussed in later sections. The same conclusion was not drawn in Godley's studies (92, 93), when use erythrocyte membrane fatty acid as biomarkers. This study also shows a correlation between lenoleic acid and the risk of prostate cancer.

In a study that involves 8 European countries and Israel, it has been shown that n-6 fatty acid including linoleic acid, are not associated with the incidence of cancer, including prostate cancer. While the cis-monounsaturated fatty acids are negatively associated with cancer, trans fatty acids are positively associated with the incidence (94).

In an epidemiological study, it was found that an increasing risk for prostate cancer was associated with increasing quartiles of palmitoleic, palmitic and alpha-linolenic acid, and an inverse risk association was found with increasing levels of tetracosanoic acid and with the ratios of linoleic to alpha-linolenic acid and arachidonic to eicosapentaenoic acid. There was no clear association between the risk effect of total ω-3 and total ω -6 fatty acids. There were no indications of a relationship between fatty acids and more aggressive cancers, thus suggesting a possible positive association between alpha-linolenic acid and a negative association between the ratio of linoleic to alpha-linolenic acid and the risk of prostate cancer (95).

The epidemiological data is further confused by other studies shown a complex correlation between dietary fatty acid and cancer incidence (96). In a small scale study which compared the serum levels of fatty acid in normal controls (n = 21), benign prostate hyperplasia (n = 24) and prostate cancer (n = 19), a positive correlation between n-6 fatty acid with prostate cancer and negative correlation between n-3 fatty acid was claimed (97). Another study comparing the levels of erythrocyte membrane fatty acids in 317 patients with prostate cancer and 480 matched control has shown a reduced risk of prostate cancer with high level of phophatidylchline of eicosapentaenoic acid (EPA) and docosapentaenoic acid (DHA) (Norrish et al., 1999).

4. EXPERIMENTAL EVIDENCE THE DIFFERENT FATTY ACIDS HAVE A DIFFERENT IMPACT ON PROSTATE CANCER

4.1 Growth and Death of Prostate Cancer Cells are Affected by Fatty Acids

Prostate cancer cells respond differently to ω-3 and ω-6 polyunsatured fatty acids. Rose and Connolly (99) demonstrated that the growth of PC-3, but not DU-145, prostate cancer cells were enhanced by linoleic acid (LA) of ω-6 series over a wide range of concentrations (5-750 ng/ml). This insensitivity of DU145 appears to have a link with the EGF dependency, as the growth DU145M variant which has different EGF receptor profile can be increased by LA (100). In contrast, eicosapentaenoic acid (EPA) and docosahexaenoic acid (DHA) of ω-3 series strongly inhibited the growth of both prostate cancer cell lines. In separate studies, using both human and animal prostate cancer cell lines, it was shown that at low level, linoleic acid of ω-6, linolenic acid and eicosapentaenoic acid of ω-3 all enhanced the growth of prostate cancer cells (18).

It has been shown that oleic acid (OA) and eicosapentaenoic acid (EPA) enhanced proliferation of DU-145 cells at 0.004 and 0.04 mM for up to 4 days. However, alpha-linolenic acid (ALA), linoleic acid (LA), gamma linolenic acid (GLA) and arachidonic acid (AA) suppressed cell proliferation under the same condition, possibly as a result of inhibition of DNA and protein synthesis as measured using labelled thymidine and glycine incorporation. In contrast to the cell proliferation, uPA production was inhibited by all the unsaturated fatty acids under investigation (68). However, malignant cancer cells and non-neoplastic prostate cells did not exhibited a different response to GLA and LA in cell growth (101).

A number of fatty acids including eicosapentaenoic acid (EPA), gamma-linolenic acid (GLA) and alpha-linolenic acid (ALA) have been shown to be toxic to prostate cancer cells, while others (oleic acid (OA), arachidonic (AA) and linoleic acid (LA) have significant effects (102). Interestingly, combinations of various fatty acids showed either no effects or diverse effects that is hard to interpret. EPA and oleic acid were shown to inhibit the growth of prostate cancer cell PC-3, gamma linolenic and linoleic acid increase the growth (103).

The possible signaling events leading the fatty acid-mediated effects in prostate cancer has recently reported (104). Eicosapentaenoic and linoleic acids LA can increase total protein kinase C (PKC) activity and reduce membrane bound PKCδ. Oleic acid, however, reduced membrane bound PKCδ. EPA appears strongly reduced PKCgamma membrane abundance. Although most fatty acids tested increased cytosolic PKCiota, only EPA and LA increased its membrane fraction.

Both DHA and EPA inhibit androgen-stimulated cell growth and inhibited androgenic induction of prostate-specific antigen (PSA). Furthermore, DHA was found to decrease the mRNA levels of five androgen up-regulated genes, PSA, ornithine decarboxylase, NKX 3.1, immunophilin fkbp 51 and Drg-1, which appears to occur at transcription level. Furthermore, the proto-oncoprotein c-jun was increased by DHA treatment (105).

4.2 Contribution of Fatty Acid Metabolites to the Growth and Death of Prostate Cancer Cells

The relation between fatty acids and prostate cancer has also been demonstrated with the downstream metabolites (eicosanoids) (106, 107). 5-hydroxyeicosatetraenoic acid (5-HETE) is one of the eicosanoids from arachidonic acid by 5-lipoxygenase. 5-HETE has been found to prevent prostate cancer from developing apoptosis. When inhibitors to 5-lipoxygenase is used and formation of 5-HETE is blocked, prostate cancer cells would rapidly develop apoptosis. The product of 15-lipoxygenase-2, 15S-hydroxyeicosatetraenoic acid (HETE), can also activate PPAR-γ and inhibit the proliferation of prostate cancer cells.

Arachidonic acid and its cyclooxygenase-2 (COX-2) metabolites, prostaglandin E2 (PGE2), are known to stimulate the growth of prostate cancer cells (45, 103, 109). AA has not only increase the production of prostaglandin PGE2 and COX2, accompanied by the aberrant expression of low density lipoprotein receptor (LDLr) in prostate cancer which deliver. This suggests that the abnormal level of lipids as well as unregulated over-expression of lipid delivery vehicles (LDLr) to prostate cancer cells is one of the key alterations in prostate cancer.

4.3 The Role of Peroxisome Proliferator Activated Receptor Gamma (PPAR-γ) Prostate Cancer Cells

Peroxisome proliferator activated receptors are members of a nuclear receptor family, which co-ordinated the transcription events. PPAR-γ is of particular interest, as it is also the receptor for polyunsaturated fatty acids including linolenic, linoleic and gamma linolenic acids. Conventional PPAR-γ agonists such as phenylacetates are known to have anti-tumor effect in prostate cancer (110). Although both benign and tumor tissues of the prostate expressed PPAR-γ mRNA, PPAR-γ agonist significantly inhibited the proliferation of prostate cancer cells (111). The product of 15-lipoxygenase-2, 15S-HETE, can also activate PPAR-γ and inhibit the proliferation of prostate cancer cells (111).

In a clear contrast to PPAR-γ, it has been reported that the other PPAR family member, namely PPARα, appears to play an opposite role to that by PPARγ. It has been shown that PPARα was over-expressed in prostate cancer tissues compared with normal prostate epithelial cells. Stimulation of prostate cancer cells with androgen resulted in the reduction of PPARα mRNA (112). Given the role of PPARα as lipid agonists and gene transcription regulator, it is proposed that PPARα may integrate dietary fatty acid and steroid hormone signalling pathways in prostate cancer and may be involved in the progression of prostate cancer.

Thus, PPAR-γ and PPAR-α may play an important role in the regulation of cell growth and gene transcription in prostate tissues and cells. The loss of the balance between these two nuclear receptors, loss of balance of their agonists, loss of the balance between the two pathways, may result in prostate cancer cell in different growth/death status and different invasive/metastatic potential (45).

PPARγ may be expressed at similar or higher level in prostate cancer cells than normal prostate epithelial cells. However, supplementation of gamma linolenic acid results in at least three folds increase in the level of PPARγ in normal prostate epithelial cells, but not in prostate cancer cells (113). This interesting observation may provide some evidence that manipulating fatty acids and its nuclear receptor may be a window of opportunity in the treatment of prostate cancer.

5. CLINICAL EVIDENCE OF THE IMPACT OF FATTY ACID ON PROSTATE CANCER AND ITS INVASION AND METASTATIC SPREAD

Perhaps the most direct clinical evidence between fatty acids and prostate cancer metastasis is from a recent study by Freeman and colleagues (114). Tissues from 49 patients with prostate cancer were collected and analysed for their fatty acid levels. The percentage of polyunsatured fatty acids and the ratio of polyunsaturated to saturated fatty acids were significantly lower in tumors with perineural invasion, late stage tumor and seminal vesical involvement. It was also interesting to note that alpha-linolenic acid was low in tumors that already extended over surgical margins or other tissues. Both ω–3 and ω-3/ω-6 ratio were also found to be low in invasive prostate cancer.

A similar positive conclusion was seen between alpha-linolenic acid and prostate cancer was reached in a study comparing 217 prostate cancer patients and 431 matched controls (115). The positive correlation between alpha linolenic acid and the risk of prostate cancer has also been demonstrated in a study involving 217 prostate cancer patients and 434 controlled population in Spain (116). Erythrocyte membrane fatty acids profile in 67 prostate cancer and 156 controls showed an increased alpha-linolenic acid levels and −6 fatty acids levels in prostate cancer patients (117).

6. DO FATTY ACIDS HAVE THERAPEUTIC VALUE IN PROSTATE CANCER?

Although experimental evidence for a role of polyunsaturated fatty acids in cancer including prostate cancer is becoming clear, clinical trials using these fatty acids in the treatment of cancer are sparsely reported. Limited studies of using polyunsaturated fatty acids have been reported with pancreatic cancer (118, 119, 120), breast cancer (121), glioma (122, 123), colorectal cancer (124, 125), and other cancers (126, 127, 128). Some of these studies showed a promising effects with very little side effects. However, a study on prostate cancer is yet to be carried out. The limit of the clinical studies is perhaps due to, first the supply of purified fatty acid, and second the difficulties to design a good trial without bias from other dietary factors and third the still confusing conclusion of fatty acid and cancer. As already indicated in earlier section, the use of correct fatty acid, the purity of the lipid, and ability to deliver good dosage may be essential in clinical trials.

Dietary supplementation of low fat and fish oil in patients with prostate cancer results in significant alteration in the the ω–3/ω-6 ratio and importantly it reduces the expression of COX2 in these patients (129).

PPARγ may be expressed at similar or higher level in prostate cancer cells than normal prostate epithelial cells. However, supplementation of gamma linolenic acid results in at least three folds increase in the level of PPARγ in normal prostate epithelial cells, but not in prostate cancer cells (113). This interesting observation may provide some evidence that manipulating fatty acids and its nuclear receptor may be a window of opportunity in the treatment of prostate cancer.

7. CONCLUSION AND PERSPECTIVES

It is evident that polyunsaturated fatty acids participate in the regulation of a number of functions in cancer cells. The effects depend on the type of fatty acids as well as tumor types. Prostate cancer cells appear to be sensitive to selected polyunsaturated fatty acids including eicosapentaenoic acid, docosahexaenoic acid, gamma linolenic acid and dihomogamma linolenic acid. The growth and invasiveness of prostate cancer cells can be inhibited by these cancer cells. In contrast, alpha linolenic acid and linoleic acid may play converse role. These experimental evidence is probably supported by the epidemiological data that dietary linoleic acid and probably alpha linolenic acid are associated with the incidence of prostate cancer and progression of prostate cancer. However, we are still facing huge challenges to determine the impact of fatty acids on prostate cancer, particularly at the clinical front. We yet have to determine if fatty acids, particularly highly unsaturated fatty acids, have therapeutic value in prostate cancer. With recent rapid progress in areas such as PPAR and identification of fatty acid desaturases, it may prompt further advance in this area.

REFERENCES

1. Sinclair HM. The diet of canadian indians and eskimos. Proc Nutr Soc 1953, 12:69–82.
2. Lancet. Eskimo diets and diseases. Lancet 1983, i:1139–41.
3. Carroll KK. Dietary factors in hormone dependent caners, In: *Nutrition and Cancer*. Winick M, ed., New York: John Weley & Sons, 1977.
4. Horrobin DF, ed. Essential fatty acids, lipid peroxidation, and cancer. In 'omega-6 essential fatty acids. New York: Wiley-Liss, 1990:351–78.
5. Burr GO, Burr MM. A new deficiency disease produced by the rigid exclusion of fat from the diet. J Biol Chem 1929, 82:345–67.
6. Burr GO, Burr MM. On the nature of the fatty acids essential in nutrition. J Biol Chem 1930, 86:587–621.
7. Hartop PJ, Prottey C. Changes in transepidermal water loss and the somposition of epidermal lecitin after applications of pure fatty acid triglycerides to the skin of essential fatty acid dificient rats. Br J Dermatol 1976, 95:255–64.
8. Basnayake V, Sinclair HM. Skin permeability in deficiency of essential fatty acids. J Physiol 1954, 126:55P–6P.
9. Hansen AE, Holmes SG, Wiese. HF. Fat in the diet in relation to nutrition of the dog. IV. Histologic features of the skin from animals fed diets with and without fat. Texas Rep Biol Med 1951, 9:491– 515.
10. Kingery FAJ, Kellum. RE. Essential fatty acid deficiency. Histochemical changes in the skin of rats. Arch Dermatol 1965, 91:272–9.
11. Nasr AN, Shostak S. Mitotic activity in the skin of mice deficient in EFA. Nature 1965, 207:1935.
12. Elías PM. The essential fatty acid deficient rodent: Evidence for a direct role for intercellular lipid in barrier function. In: *Models in Dermatology, Vol 1*. Maibach HI, Lowe NJ, eds, Karger: Basel, 1985:272–85.
13. Eynard AR, Monis B, Kalinec F, Leguizamón. RO. Increased proliferation of the epithelium of the proximal alimentary tract of EFA-deficient rats. A light and electron microscopy study. Exp Mol Pathol 1982, 36:135–43.
14. Kramar J, Levine. VE. Influence of fats and fatty acids on capillaries. J Nutr 1953, 50:149–60.
15. Jiang WG, Eynard AE, Mansel. RE. The pathology of essential fatty acid deficiency, a cell adhesion mediated phenomenon. Med Hypoth 2000, 55:257–62.
16. Jiang WG, Puntis MCA, Hallett MB. The molecular and cellular basis of cancer invasion and metastasis and its implications for treatment. Br J Surg 1994, 81:1576–90.
17. Jiang WG. Regulation of cell adhesion, a central mechanism in the anticancer action of essential fatty acids. Int J Mol Med 1998, 1:621–6.

18. Horrobin DF. Nutritional and medical importance of gamma-linolenic acid. Prog Lipid Res 1992, 31:163–94.
19. Karmali RA, Choi K, Otter G *et al*. Eicosanoids and metastasis. Experimental aspects in lewis lung carcinoma. Cancer Biochem Biophys 1986, 9:97–104.
20. Karmali RA, Marsh H, Fuchs C. Effect of omega-3 fatty acids on growth of a rat mammary tumor. J Natl Cancer Inst 1984, 73:457–61.
21. Begin ME, Ells G, Das UN, Horrobin DF. Differential killing of human carcinoma cells supplemented with n-3 and n-6 polyunsaturated fatty acids. J Natl Cancer Inst 1986, 77:1053–62.
22. Jiang WG, Bryce RP, Horrobin DF. Essential fatty acids, the molecular and cellular mechanisms of their anticancer action and clinical implications. Crit Rev Oncol Haematol 1998, 27:179–209.
23. Lai PBS, Ross JA, Fearon KCH *et al*. Cell-cycle arrest and induction of apoptosis in pancreatic- cancer cells exposed to eicosapentaenoic acid in-vitro. Br J Cancer 1996, 74:1375–83.
24. Cheeseman KH. Lipid peroxidation and cancer. In: *DNA, Free Radicals.*, Halliwell BH, Aruoma OI, eds, Sussex: Ellis Horwood Publishers, 1993:109–44.
25. Reddy N, Everhart A, Eling T, Glasgow W. Characterization of a 15-lipoxygenase in human breast carcinoma BT-20 cells: Stimulation of 13-HODE formation by TGF(alpha)/EGF. Biochem Biophys Res Commun 1997, 231:111–16.
26. Bougnoux P, Koscielny S, Chajes V *et al*. Alpha-linolenic acid content of adipose breast-tissue - a host determinant of the risk of early metastasis in breast-cancer. Br J Cancer 1994, 70:330–4.
27. Lanson M, Bougnoux P, Besson P *et al*. N-6 polyunsaturated fatty acids in human breast carcinoma phophatidylethanolamine and early relapse. Br J Cancer 1990, 61:776–8.
28. Narayan P, Dahiya R. Alterations in sphingomyelin and fatty-acids in human benign prostatic hyperplasia and prostatic-cancer. Biomed Biochim Acta 1991, 50:1099–108.
29. Fernandezbanares F, Esteve M, Navarro E *et al*. Changes of the mucosal n3 and n6 fatty-acid status occur early in the colorectal adenoma-carcinoma sequence. Gut 1996, 38:254–9.
30. Chaudry A, Mcclinton S, Moffat LEF, Wahle KWJ. Essential fatty-acid distribution in the plasma and tissue phospholipids of patients with benign and malignant prostatic disease. Br J Cancer 1991, 64:1157–60.
31. Chaudry AA, Wahle KWJ, McClinton S, Moffat LEF. Arachidonic-acid metabolism in benign and malignant prostatic tissue in-vitro - effects of fatty-acids and cyclooxygenase inhibitors. Int J Cancer 1994, 57:176–80.
32. Nakazawa I, Iwaizumi M, Ohuchi K. A difference in prostaglandin-producing ability between cancer- cells metastasized into liver and kidney. Tohoku J Exp Med 1991, 165:299–304.
33. Rigas B, Goldman IS, Levine L. Altered eicosanoid levels in human colon-cancer. J Lab Clin Med 1993, 122:518–23.
34. Shimizu S, Yamane M, Abe A *et al*. Omega-hydroxylation of docosahexaenoic acid or arachidonic-acid in human colonic well-differentiated adenocarcinoma homogenate. Biochim Biophys Acta 1995, 1256:293–6.
35. Cho HP, Nakamura MT, Clarke SD. Cloning, expression, and nutritional regulation of the mammalian delta-6 desaturase. J Biol Chem 1999, 274:471–7.

36. Cho HP, Nakamura M, Clarke SD. Cloning, expression, and fatty acid regulation of the human delta-5 desaturase. J Biol Chem 1999, 274:37333–9.
37. Hansen-Petrik MB, McEntee MF, Johnson BT, Obukowicz G, Masferrer J, Zweifel B et al. Selective inhibition of delta-6 desaturase impedes intestinal tumorigenesis. Cancer Lett 2002, 175:157–63.
38. Alvares K, Carrillo A, Yuan PM et al. Identification of cytosolic peroxisome proliferator binding-protein as a member of the heat-shock protein HSP70 family. Proc Natl Acad Sci USA 1990, 87:5293–7.
39. Issemann I, Green S. Activation of a member of the sterioid hormone receptor superfamily by peroxisome proliferators. Nature 1990, 347:645–9.
40. Beck F, Plummer S, Senior PV et al. The ontogeny of peroxisome-proliferator-activated receptor gene- expression in the mouse and rat. Proc R Soc Lond 1992, 247:83–7.
41. Zhang BW, Marcus SL, Sajjadi FG et al. Identification of a peroxisome proliferator-responsive element upstream of the gene encoding rat peroxisomal enoyl-coa hydratase 3-hydroxyacyl-coa dehydrogenase. Proc Natl Acad Sci USA 1992, 89:7541–5.
42. Nunez SB, Medin JA, Braissant O et al. Retinoid X receptor and peroxisome proliferator-activated receptor activate an estrogen responsive gene independent of the estrogen receptor. Mol Cell Endocrinol 1997, 127:27–40.
43. Pineau T, Hudgins WR, Liu L et al. Activation of a human peroxisome proliferator-activated receptor by the antitumor agent phenylacetate and its analogs. Biochem Pharmacol 1996, 52:659–67.
44. Lehmann JM, Lenhard JM, Oliver BB, Ringold GM, Kliewer SA. Peroxisome proliferator-activated receptors α and γ are activated by indomethacin and other non-steroidal anti-inflammatory drugs. J Biol Chem 1997, 272:3406–10.
45. Jump DB, Clarke SD. Regulation of gene expression by dietary fat. Annu Rev Nutr 1999, 19:63–90.
46. Forman BM, Chen J, Evans RM. Hydropipidemic drugs, polyunsaturated fatty acids, and eicosanoids are ligands for peroxisome proliferator activated receptors and. Proc Natl Acad Sci USA 1997, 94:4312–17.
47. Kliewer SA, Sundeth SS, Jones SA, Brown PJ, Wisely GB, Koble CS et al. Fatty acids and eicosanoids regulate gene expression through direct interactions with peroxisome proliferator activated receptor and. Proc Natl Acad Sci USA 1997, 94:4318–23.
48. Krey G, Braissant O, Lhorset F, Kalkhoven E, Perroud M, Parker MG, Wahli W. Fatty acids, eicosanoids, and hypolipidemic agents identified as ligands of peroxisome proliferator-activated receptors by coactivator-dependent receptor ligand assay. Mol Endocrinol 1997, 11:779–91.
49. Jiang CY, Ting AT, Seed B. PPAR-gamma agonists inhibit production of monocyte inflammatory cytokines. Nature 1998, 391:82–6.
50. Ricote M, Li AC, Willson TM, Kelly CJ, Glass CK. The peroxisome proliferator-activated receptor-gamma is a negative regulator of macrophage activation. Nature 1998, 391:79–82.
51. Devchand PR, Keller H, Peters JM, Vazquez M, Gonzalez FJ, Wahl W. The ppara leukotriene B4 pathway to inflammation control. Nature 1996, 384:39–43.
52. Yokomizo T, Izumi T, Chang K, Takuwa Y, Shimizu G-protein-coupled receptor for leukotriene that mediates chemotaxis. TAB-4. Nature 1997, 387:620–4.

53. Ren B, Thelen AP, Peters JM, Gonzalez FJ, Jump DB. Polyunsaturated fatty acid suppression of hepatic fatty acid synthase and S14 gene expression does not require peroxisome proliferator-activated receptor alpha. J Biol Chem 1997, 272:26827–32.
54. Kilgore MW, Tate PL, Rai S, Sengoku E, Price TM. MCF-7 and T47D human breast cancer cells contain a functional peroxisomal response. Mol Cell Endocrinol 1997, 129:229–35.
55. Jiang WG, Bryce RP, Horrobin DF, Mansel RE. Peroxisome proliferator activated receptor-γ mediates the effects of gamma linolenic acid in cancer cells. Prostaglandins Leukot Essent Fatty Acids 2000, 62:119–27.
56. Hart IR, Goode NT, Wilson RE. Molecular aspects of the metastatic cascade. Biochim Biophys Acta 1989, 989:65–84.
57. Johanning GL, Lin TY. Unsaturated fatty-acid effects on human breast-cancer cell-adhesion. Nutr Cancer 1995, 24:57–66.
58. Meterissian SH, Forse RA, Steele GD, Thomas P. Effect of membrane free fatty-acid alterations on the adhesion of human colorectal-carcinoma cells to liver macrophages and extracellular-matrix proteins. Cancer Lett 1995, 89:145–52.
59. Rose DP, Connolly JM, Liu XH. Effects of linoleic-acid on the growth and metastasis of 2 human breast-cancer cell-lines in nude-mice and the invasive capacity of these cell-lines in-vitro. Cancer Res 1994, 54:6557–62.
60. Varner JA, Cheresh DA. Integrins and cancer. Curr Opin Cell Biol 1996, 8:724–30.
61. Furukawa T, Watanabe M, Kumota T et al. Significance of in vitro attachment of human colon cancer to extracellular matrix proteins in experimental and clinical liver metastasis. J Surg Oncol 1993, 53:10–16.
62. Giancotti FG, Mainiero F. Integrin mediated adhesion and signlling in tumorigenesis. Biochim Biophys Acta 1994, 1198:47–64.
63. Johanning GL. Modulation of breast cancer cell adhesion by unsaturated fatty acids. Nutrition 1996, 12:810–16.
64. Rose DP, Connolly JM, Liu XH. Effects of linoleic-acid and gamma-linolenic acid on the growth and metastasis of a human breast-cancer cell-line in nude-mice and on its growth and invasive capacity in-vitro. Nutr Cancer 1995, 24:33–45.
65. Rose DP, Connolly JM, Rayburn J, Coleman M. Influence of diets containing eicosapentaenoic or docosahexaenoic acid on growth and metastasis of breast-cancer cells in nude-mice. J Natl Cancer Inst 1995, 87:587–92.
66. Hubbard NE, Erickson KL. Effect of dietary linoleic acid level on lodgement, proliferation and survival of mammary tumor metastases. Cancer Lett 1989, 44:117.
67. Jiang WG, Hiscox S, Puntis MCA et al. Gamma linolenic acid (GLA) inhibits tyrosine phosphorylation of focal adhesion kinase (FAK) and paxillin and tumour cell-matrix interaction. Int J Oncol 1996, 8:583–7.
68. duToit PJ, Vanaswegen CH, Duplessis DJ. The effect of essential fatty-acids on growth and urokinase-type plasminogen-activator production in human prostate DU-145 cells. Prostaglandins Leukot Essent Fatty Acids 1996, 55:173–7.
69. Reich R, Royce L, Martin GR. Eicosapentaenoic acid reduces the invasive and metastatic activities of malignant tumor cells. Biochem Biophys Res Commun 1989, 160:559–64.
70. Kariko D, Rosenbaum H, Kuo A et al. Stimulatory effect of unsaturated fatty acids on the level of plasminogen activator inhibitor I mRNA in cultured human endothelial cells. FEBS Lett 1995, 361:118–22.

71. Liu XH, Connolly JM, Rose DP. Eicosanoids as mediators of linoleic acid-stimulated invasion and type-IV collagenase production by a metastatic human breast-cancer cell-line. Clin Exp Metastasis 1996, 14:145–52.
72. Liu XH, Rose DP. Suppression of type-IV collagenase in MDA-MB-435 human breast-cancer cells by eicosapentaenoic acid in-vitro and in-vivo. Cancer Lett 1995, 92:21–6.
73. Zou Z, Anisowicz A, Hendrix MJC et al. Maspin, a serpin with tumor-suppressing activity in human mammary epithelial cells. Science 1994, 263:526–9.
74. Hopkins PCR, Whisstock J, Sager R. Function of maspin. Science 1994, 265:1893–4.
75. Sheng S, Carey J, Seftor EA et al. Maspin acts at the cell membrane to inhibit invasion and motility of mammary and prostatic cancer cells. Proc Natl Acad Sci USA 1996, 93:11669–74.
76. Jiang WG, Hiscox S, Horrobin DF et al. Expression of maspin in cancer cells and its regulation by gamma linolenic acid. Biochem Biophys Res Commun 1997, 237:639–44.
77. Jiang WG, Bryce RP, Horrobin DF, Mansel RE. Gamma linolenic acid regulates gap junction communications in endothelial cells and their interaction with tumour cells. Prostaglandins Leukot Essent Fatty Acids 1997, 56:307–16.
78. Weber C, Erl W, Pietsch A, Danesch U, Weber PC. Docosahexaenoic acid selectively attenuates induction of vascular cell adhesion molecule -1 and subsequent monocytic cell adhesion to human endothelial cells stimulated by tumor necrosis factor alpha. Arterioscler Thromb Vasc Biol 1995, 15:622.
79. De Caterina R, Cybulsky MI, Clinton SK et al. The omega-3 fatty acid docosahexaenoate reduces cytokine induced expression of proatherogenic and proinflammatory proteins in human endothelail cells. Atheroscler Thromb 1994, 14:1829.
80. De Caterina R, Cybulsky MA, Clinton SK et al. Omega -3 fatty acids and endothelial leukocyte adhesion molecules. Prostaglandins Leukot Essen Fatty Acids 1995, 52: 191–5.
81. Jiang WG, Hiscox S, Hallett MB et al. Inhibition of membrane ruffling and ezrin translocation by gamma linolenic acid. Int J Oncol 1996, 9:279–84.
82. Hennig B, Lipke DW, Boissonneault GA, Ramasamy S. Role of fatty-acids and eicosanoids in modulating proteoglycan metabolism in endothelial-cells. Prostaglandins Leukot Essent Fatty Acids 1995, 53:315–24.
83. McCarty MF. Fish-oil MAY impede tumor angiogenesis and invasiveness by down-regulating protein-kinase-c and modulating eicosanoid production. Med Hypoth 1996, 46:107–11.
84. Cai J, Jiang WG, Mansel RE. Inhibition of vascular endothelial cell motility and angiogenesis by gamma linolenic acid. Prostaglandins Leukot Essent Fatty Acids 1997, 57:247.
85. Ormerod LD, Garsd A, Abelson MD et al. Effects of altering the eicosanoid precursor pool on neovascularization and inflammation in the alkali-burned rabbit cornea. Am J Pathol 1990, 137:1243–52.
86. Kanayasu T, Morita I, Nakao-Hayashi J et al. Eicosapentaenoic acid inhibits tube formation of vascular endothelial cells in vitro. Lipid 1991, 26:271–6.
87. Cai J, Jiang WG, Mansel RE. Gamma linolenic acid inhibits expression of VE-cadherin and tube formation in human vascular endothelial cells. Biochem Biophys Res Commun 1999, 258:113–18.

88. Jiang WG, Bryce RP, Horrobin DF, Mansel RE. Gamma linolenic acid regulates gap junction communications in endothelial cells and their interaction with tumour cells. Prostaglandins Leukot Essent Fatty Acids 1997, 56:307–16.
89. Giovannucci E, Rimm EB, Colditz GA, Stampfer MJ, Ascherio A, Chute CC, Willett WC. A prospective-study of dietary-fat and risk of prostate-cancer. J Natl Cancer Inst 1993, 85:1571–9.
90. Gann PH, Hennekens CH, Sacks FM, Grodstein F, Giovannucci EL, Stampfer MJ. Prospective-study of plasma fatty-acids and risk of prostate-cancer. J Natl Cancer Inst 1994, 86:281–6.
91. Michaud DS, Augustsson K, Rimm EB, Stampfer MJ, Willett WC, Giovannucci E. A prospective study on intake of animal products and risk of prostate cancer. Cancer Causes Control 2001, 12:557–67.
92. Godley PA, Campbell MK, Miller C, Gallagher P, Martinson FE, Mohler JL, Sandler RS. Correlation between biomarkers of omega-3 fatty acid consumption and questionnaire data in african american and causcasian united states males with and without prostatic carcinoma. Cancer Epidemiol Biomarkers Prev 1996, 5:115–19.
93. Godley PA, Campbell MK, Gallagher P, Martinson FEA, Mohler JL, Sandler RS. Biomarkers of essential fatty acid consumption and risk of prostatic carcinoma. Cancer Epidemiol Biomarker Prev 1996, 5:889–95.
94. Bakker N, vantVeer P, Zock PL, Aro A, DelgadoRodriguez M, GomezAracena J et al. Adipose fatty acids and cancers of the breast, prostate and colon: An ecological study. Int J Cancer 1997, 72:587–91.
95. Harvei S, Bjerve KS, Tretli S, Jellum E, Robsahm TE, Vatten L. Prediagnostic level of fatty acids in serum phospholipids: Omega-3 and omega-6 fatty acids and the risk of prostate cancer. Int J Cancer 1997, 71:545–51.
96. Zock PL, Katan MB. Linoleic acid intake and cancer risk: A review and meta-analysis. Am J Clin Nutr 1998, 68:142–53.
97. Yang YJ, Lee SH, Hong SJ, Chung BC. Comparison of fatty acid profiles in the serum of patients with prostate cancer and benign prostatic hyperplasia. Clin Biochem 1999, 32:405–9.
98. Norrish AE, Skeaff CM, Arribas GLB, Sharpe SJ, Jackson RT. Prostate cancer risk and consumption of fish oils: A dietary biomarker-based case-control study. Br J Cancer 1999, 81:1238–42.
99. Rose DP, Connolly JM. Effects of fatty-acids and eicosanoid synthesis inhibitors on the growth of 2 human prostate-cancer cell-lines. Prostate 1991, 18:243–54.
100. Connolly JM, Rose DP. Interactions between epidermal growth factor-mediated autocrine regulation and linoleic acid-stimulated growth of a human prostate-cancer cell-line. Prostate 1992, 20:151–8.
101. Griffiths G, Jones HE, Eaton CL, Stobart AK. Effect of n-6 polyunsaturated fatty acids on growth and lipid composition of neoplastic and non-neoplastic canine prostate epithelial cell cultures. Prostate 1997, 31:29–36.
102. Motaung E, Prinsloo SE, van Aswegen CH, du Toit PJ, Becker PJ, du Plessis DJ. Cytotoxicity of combined essential fatty acids on a human prostate cancer cell line. Prostaglandins Leukot Essent Fatty Acids 1999, 99:331–7.
103. Hughes-Fulford M, Chen YF, Tjandrawinata RR. Fatty acid regulates gene expression and growth of human prostate cancer PC-3 cells. Carcinogenesis 2001, 22:701–7.

104. Pandian SS, Sneddon AA, Bestwick CS, McClinton S, Grant I, Wahle KWJ, Heys SD. Fatty acid regulation of protein kinase C isoforms in prostate cancer cells. Biochem Biophys Res Commun 2001, 283:806–12.
105. Chung BH, Mitchell SH, Zhang JS, Young CYF. Effects of docosahexaenoic acid and eicosapentaenoic acid on androgen-mediated cell growth and gene expression in LNCaP prostate cancer cells. Carcinogenesis 2001, 22:1201–6.
106. Ghosh J, Myers CE. Inhibition of arachidonate 5-lipoxygenase triggers massive apoptosis in human prostate cancer cells. Proc Natl Acad Sci USA 1998, 98: 13182–7.
107. Myers CE, Ghosh J. Lipoxygenase inhibition in prostate cancer. Eur Urol 1999, 35:395–8.
108. Cave WT. Dietary n-3 (omega-3) polyunsaturated fatty-acid effects on animal tumorigenesis. FASEB J 1991, 5:2160–6.
109. Tjandrawinata RR, HughesFulford M. Up-regulation of cyclooxygenase-2 by product-prostaglandin E-2. Adv Exp Med Biol 1997, 407:163–70.
110. Samid D, Wells M, Greene ME, Shen WY, Palmer CAN, Thibault A. Peroxisome proliferator-activated receptor gamma as a novel target in cancer therapy: Binding and activation by an aromatic fatty acid with clinical antitumor activity. Clin Cancer Res 2000, 6:933–41.
111. Shappell SB, Gupta RA, Manning S, Whitehead R, Boeglin WE, Schneider C et al. 15s-hydroxyeicosatetraenoic acid activates peroxisome proliferator-activated receptor gamma, inhibits proliferation in PC3 prostate carcinoma cells. Cancer Res 2001, 61: 497–503.
112. Collett GP, Betts AM, Johnson MI, Pulimood AB, Cook S, Neal DE, Robson CN. Peroxisome proliferator-activated receptor alpha is an androgen-responsive gene in human prostate and is highly expressed in prostatic adenocarcinoma. Clin Cancer Res 2000, 6:3241–8.
113. Nwankwo JO, Robbins MEC. Peroxisome proliferator-activated receptor-gamma expression in human malignant and normal brain, breast and prostate-derived cells. Prostaglandinns Leukot Essent Fatty Acids 2001, 64:241–51.
114. Freeman VL, Meydani M, Yong S, Pyle J, Flanigan RC, Waters WB, Wojcik EM. Prostatic levels of fatty acids and the histopathology of localized prostate cancer. J Urol 2000, 164:2168–72.
115. De Stefani E, Deneo-Pellegrini H, Boffetta P, Ronco A, Mendilaharsu M. Alpha-linolenic acid and risk of prostate cancer: A case-control study in uruguay. Cancer Epidemiol Biomarkers Prev 2000, 9:335–8.
116. Ramon JM, Bou R, Romea S, Alkiza ME, Jacas M, Ribes J, Oromi J. Dietary fat intake and prostate cancer risk: A case-control study in spain. Cancer Causes Control 2000, 11:679–85.
117. Newcomer LM, King IB, Wicklund KG, Stanford JL. The association of fatty acids with prostate cancer risk. Prostate 2001, 47:262–8.
118. Fearon KCH, Falconer JS, Ross JA, Carter DC, Hunter JO, Reynolds PD, Tuffnell Q. An open-label phase I/II dose escalation study of the treatment of pancreatic cancer using lithium gammalinolenate. Anticancer Res 1995, 16:867–74.
119. Barber MD, Fearon KCH, Tisdale MJ, McMillan DC, Ross JA. Effect of a fish oil-enriched nutritional supplement on metabolic mediators in patients with pancreatic cancer cachexia. Nutr Cancer 2001, 40:118–24.

120. Johnson CD, Puntis M, Davidson N, Todd S, Bryce R. Randomized, dose-finding phase III study of lithium gamolenate in patients with advanced pancreatic adenocarcinoma. Br J Surg 2001, 88:662–8.
121. Lockwood K, Moesgaard S, Hanioka T, Folkers K. Apparent partial remission of breast-cancer in high-risk patients supplemented with nutritional antioxidants, essential patty acids and coenzyme q(10). Mol Asp Med 1994, 15:231–40.
122. Das UN, Prasad VVSK, Reddy DR. Local application of gamma-linolenic acid in the treatment of human gliomas. Cancer Lett 1995, 94:147–55.
123. Reddy DR, Prassad VSSV, Das UN. Intratumoural injection of gamma leinolenic acid in malignant gliomas. J Clin Neurosci 1998, 5:36–9.
124. Anti M, Armelao F, Marra G *et al.* Effects of different doses of fish-oil on rectal cell-proliferation in patients with sporadic colonic adenomas. Gastroenterology 1994, 107:1709–18.
125. McIllmurray MB, Turkie W. Controlled trial of gamma linolenic acid in Duke's colorectal cancer. Br Med J 1987, 294:1260.
126. Vandermerwe CF, Booyens J, Katzeff IE. Oral gamma-linolenic acid in 21 patients with untreatable malignancy- an ongoing pilot open clinical-trial. Br J Clin Pract 1987, 41:907–15.
127. Vandermerwe CF, Booyens J. Essential fatty-acids and their metabolic intermediates as cytostatic agents - the use of evening primrose oil (linoleic and gamma-linolenic acid) in primary liver-cancer - a double-blind placebo controlled trial. S Afr Med J 1987, 72:79.
128. Vandermerwe CF, Booyens J, Joubert HF *et al.* The effect of gamma-linolenic acid, an in vitro cytostatic substance contained in evening primrose oil, on primary liver-cancer - a double-blind placebo controlled trial. Prostaglandins 1990, 40: 199–202.
129. Aronson WJ, Glaspy JA, Reddy ST, Reese D, Heber D, Bagga D. Modulation of omega-3/omega-6 polyunsaturated ratios with dietary fish oils in men with prostate cancer. Urology 2001, 58:283–8.

Chapter 5

ROLE OF PROSTAGLANDIN SYNTHESIS AND CYCLOOXYGENASE-2 IN PROSTATE CANCER AND METASTASIS

Alaa F. Badawi
Division of Population Science, Fox Chase Cancer Center, Philadelphia, PA, USA

Abstract: Metabolites of arachidonic acid, inclusive of prostatglandins (PGs), have been implicated in cancer for a number of years. In this overview, the evidence of the role of PGs and their interaction with endogenous hormones and exogenous (environmental) influences, predominately dietary factors, in the development and metastasis of prostate cancer, the mechanisms of action and approaches toward facilitating the design of effective strategies for the prevention and intervention of prostate cancer are considered. Included herein and apart from their traditionally thought of metabolic effects, PGs have been shown to function as biological response modifiers as evidenced from their effects on proliferation, apoptosis and immune responses.

Key words: arachidonic acid, cyclooxygenases (COX-1, COX-2), eicosanoids, prostaglandins

1. INTRODUCTION

The involvement of prostaglandins (PGs) and other eicosanoids in the development of human cancer has been known for more than two decades (1). Early knowledge focused on the role of PGs as mediators of thyroid carcinomas and on its participation in hypercalcemia (1). It was also demonstrated that the elevation in PG synthesis may influence tumor growth in humans and experimental animals (2). Numerous studies were further carried out to describe the effect of PG synthesis on carcinogen metabolism and tumor cell proliferation and metastatic potential (3–5). Additionally, the efficacy of inhibiting PG synthesis was examined as a means for preventing tumor development (4, 5). The role of PGs in the genesis of cancer was elucidated from observations demonstrating that: a) there is a direct relationship between the level of PGs synthesized and cancer incidence in both humans and animal models; b) the influence of various cancer-causing agents can be linked to their effect on PG synthesis; and c) the inhibition of PG synthesis hinders the development of tumor in animal models and in some human cancers (see below).

Prostate cancer is a leading cause of death in the world. In 2004, it was estimated that about 230,000 new cases (30% of all new cancers in men) were diagnosed and more than 30,000 patients died of prostate cancer in the USA (6). In UK, about 12,000 new cases of prostate cancer are diagnosed each year and the incidence has jumped 66% in the past 15 years (7). Among all European countries, only Switzerland has a higher fatality rate of 44.2 deaths per 100,000 compared with 34 in the UK (7). Over the past few decades, therefore, extensive research was directed towards understanding the mechanism(s) of prostate cancer development and providing practical measures for cure, prevention, and early detection. This effort enabled researchers to identify several candidate molecules, genes, and proteins that are linked to prostate cancer. Among these, PGs have emerged as possible promoters or growth enhancers, furnishing a promising tool that could be implemented or, at least, integrated into an effective strategy for prevention.

The present chapter reviews the evidence suggesting a possible role of PGs in the genesis of prostate cancer and discusses the mechanisms by which these lipid molecules may contribute to tumor development. Understanding this relationship may ultimately indicate new avenues of approach that might facilitate designing effective strategies for prostate cancer prevention and intervention.

2. PG SYNTHESIS

Arachidonic acid (AA) metabolites such as PGs, prostacyclins, thromboxanes and various lipoxygenase products, collectively known as eicosanoids, are produced in many tissues and modulate diverse physiological and pathophysiological responses. These bioactive lipids are potent mediators of a number of signal transduction pathways that modulate cellular adhesion, growth and differentiation (8). Cyclooxygenase (COX), also known as prostaglandin H-synthase, is the rate limiting enzyme in the metabolic conversion of AA to PGs and related eicosanoids (Figure 1). AA released from membrane phospholipids by phospholipase A_2 is converted to PGH_2 through the action of COX. COX enzymes contain two moieties: a) the cyclooxygenase moiety, which introduces two molecules of oxygen into AA to form the hydroperoxy endoperoxide PGG_2 and b) the endoper-

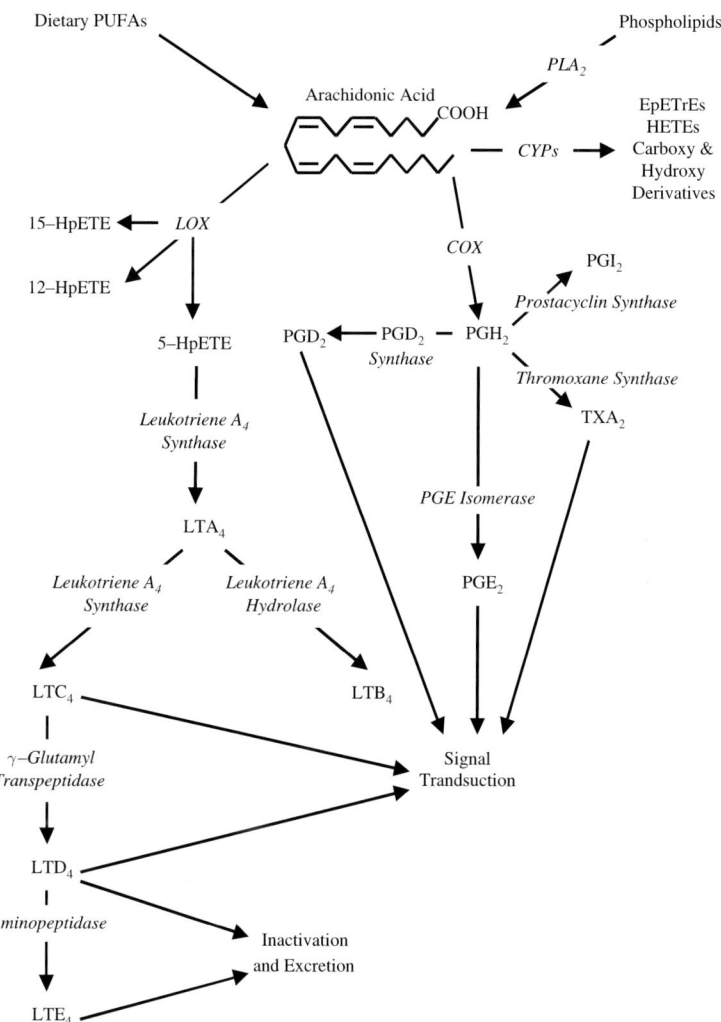

Figure 1. The metabolic conversion of arachidonic acid to prostaglandins and related eicosanoids. COX, cyclooxygenases (1 and 2); CYPs, cytochrome P450 enzymes; EpETrEs, epoxyeicosa-tetraenoic acids; HETEs, hydroxyeicosatetraenoic acids; HpETEs, hydroperoxyeicosa-tetraenoic acids; LOX, lipoxygenases; LT, leukotrienes; PG, prostaglnadins; PLA2, phospholipase A2; PUFAs, polyunsat-urated fatty acids; and TX, thromboxanes.

oxidase moiety, which reduces PGG_2 to the hydroxy endoperoxide PGH_2. Subsequently, PGH_2 is converted by cell-specific synthases to products such as PGE_2, $PGF_{2\alpha}$, PGI_2 or thromboxanes (9).

Table 1. Characteristics of cyclooxygenase-1 and cyclooxygenase-2

Characteristic	COX-1	COX-2
Expression	Constitutive	Inducible
Range of induction	2- to 4-fold	10- to 80-fold
Site of PG synthesis	ER[a]	ER & NE[a]
C terminus (18 aa cassette)[b]	(−)	(+)
Aspirin acetylation site	Ser^{530}	Ser^{516}
Chromosome (Human)	9	1
Protein size	72 kDa	72 & 74 kDa
Gene size	(single band)	(doublet)
mRNA size	22 kb (11 exons)	8.3 kb (10 exons)
	2.7 kb	4.5 kb

[a]ER: Endoplasmic Reticulum, NE: nuclear envelope
[b]Absent (−) or present (+). aa denotes amino acid.

Two COX isoforms, COX-1 and COX-2, have been identified (Table 1). COX-1 is constitutively expressed in many tissues (9, 10), although its expression can vary with the state of differentiation or following stimulation with cytokines or tumor promoters (10–13). PGs produced by COX-1 are thought to mediate "housekeeping" functions such as cytoprotection of the gastric mucosa, regulation of renal blood flow and platelet aggregation (14–16).

The recently discovered COX-2 message and protein (17), in contrast to COX-1, are normally undetectable in most tissues (for review see Ref. (18)). COX-2, however, is an inducible enzyme and it is expressed in response to proinflammatory agents, including cytokines, endotoxins, growth factors, tumor promoters and mitogens (19–22). COX-2 is expressed in a few specialized tissues such as brain, testes and macula densa of the kidney in the apparent absence of any activation. Because of its rapid induction by mitogens, the gene encoding COX-2 (*COX-2*) has been termed an immediate-early, or primary, response gene like c-*myc,* c-*fos* and c-*jun* ((20), 23–25).

The discovery of *COX-2* has stimulated a great deal of research in the field, much of which was to rationalize the redundancy between *COX-1* and *-2* and to understand the role of the *COX-2* gene in cancer development. COX-1 and COX-2 are encoded by separate genes, but the enzymes are structurally similar (Figure 2). The amino acid sequence of COX-2 is 61% identical to the COX-1 protein in humans (17). As indicated in Figure 2, the N-terminal signal peptide region is shorter in COX-2 than in COX-1. However, the two N-linked glycosylation sites at residues 53 and 130, the two heme ligands His-295 and His-374, the putative transmembrane

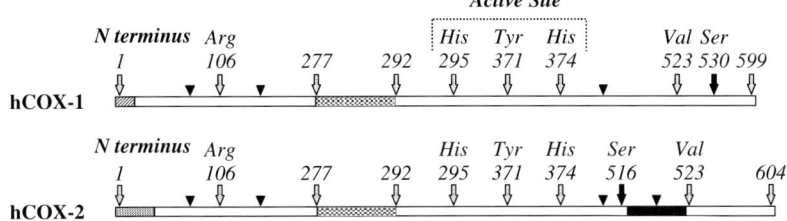

Figure 2. A diagram for COX-1 and COX-2 enzymes. The diagram highlights the putative N-terminal signal peptide region (//); the transmembrane domain residue 277–292 (✥); the 18-amino acid cassette insertion at the C-terminus (■); the putative N-linked glycosyl-ation sites (▼); the serine amino acid residue, the aspirin acetylation site (⇓); the axial (His-295) and the distal (His-374) heme ligands and the active site residue, Tyr-371, (17, 26, 27).

domain residues 277–292, the active-site residue Tyr-371, and the sequence surrounding the serine residue, the aspirin-acetylation site, at the C-terminus are conserved between COX-1 and COX-2 (17). There is an 18-amino acid insertion containing a putative N-glycosylation site at the C-terminal region of hCOX-2 (Figure 2 and Table 1). Apparently the important difference between the two isoenzymes is the substitution of Ile-523 in COX-1 by Val-523 in COX-2 (26). The presence of this smaller Val residue in COX-2 creates a larger active site (27) and allows for the appearance of a new pocket in the channel that accommodates the sulfur-containing side chains of selective COX-2 inhibitors (26).

Although COX-1 and -2 catalyze the conversion of AA to PGH_2 with similar kinetics (25), they utilize different phospholipase systems or lipid stores of AA (29). Moreover, COX-1 produces PGs only on the endoplasmic reticulum, while COX-2 forms products within or on the nuclear envelope as well as on the endoplasmic reticulum ((30), Table 1). It has been suggested that the COX-1 pathway is part of an acute signaling system because of its generalized constitutive expression (31). On the other hand, the COX-2 pathway, because of its inducible nature and the time lag required for expression, produces PGs that are likely to be employed in the secondary elaboration of various physiological events such as inflammation and mitogenesis (31).

During the metabolism of AA by COX-1 and -2, many chemicals, including carcinogenic agents, are oxidized. The oxidation of these xenobiotics occurs via either the peroxidase activity of the COX enzymes, the peroxyl radicals generated during AA oxygenation, or a combination of these two mechanisms (32). In many cases these reactions result in the formation of reactive intermediates that have mutagenic and carcinogenic activity (see 33). There is no adequate evidence to support a definitive role of xenobiotic metabolism in the genesis of prostate cancer. Nevertheless, carcinogen activation that occurs during AA oxygenation can participate in the initiation of carcinogenesis in various extra-hepatic tissues (including prostate) where the mixed function monooxygenase enzymatic system exists in a relatively low capacity (see below).

The COX isoforms are the primary targets of the non-steroidal anti-inflammatory drugs (NSAIDs) which act by inhibiting the activity of the two isoenzymes. The best known of these are aspirin, indomethacin, ibuprofen, piroxicam and sulindac. Aspirin inhibits the cyclooxygenase (but not the endoperoxidase) activity of COX-1 or -2 by acetylating a particular serine residue (Ser-530 in COX-1 and Ser-516 in COX-2) and thus blocking the channel that leads to the active site. This acetylation results in an irreversible inhibition of PG synthesis (34). Indomethacin forms a tight, slowly dissociable complex with COX that induces an inhibitory conformational change (35). Ibuprofen and piroxicam, on the other hand, compete with AA for the active site (36, 37). In general, most of these "classical" NSAIDs are better inhibitors of COX-1 than COX-2, although some, like flurbiprofen and ibuprofen, have nearly equal IC_{50} values (38). Since PGs produced by COX-2 are formed particularly at the sites of inflammation while PGs synthesized by COX-1 are required for the protection of mucosal membranes, inhibiting both COX-1 and COX-2 by the classical NSAIDs may lead to gastrointestinal and genitourinary toxicity. Therefore, reducing the inflammatory effects of COX-2 while retaining the cytoprotective actions of COX-1 is a desirable outcome that is achieved by specific COX-2 inhibitors (39). A variety of these inhibitors have become available recently such as NS-398, which blocks COX-2 expression and completely inhibit PG synthesis in inflammatory cells with no influence on PGs synthesized from COX-1 (39, 40). Generally, COX-2 inhibitors cause conformational changes in the protein and irreversible loss of activity (41).

3. PGS, COX-2 AND PROSTATE CANCER DEVELOPMENT AND METASTASIS

The role of PGs in the development of prostate cancer has been substantiated from several experimental evidence in both human and animal models (Section 3.1) as well as from epidemiological associations between a lower risk of prostate cancer with the intake of inhibitors of PG synthesis (Section 3.2). Moreover, various evidence concerning a role of PGs in the development of prostate cancer was derived from the possible involvement of these lipid molecules in the carcinogenic effects of fats and hormones on the gland (Section 3.3).

3.1 Experimental Evidence

Prostate exhibits the highest levels of COX-2 mRNA among other human tissues (10). Additionally, in the adult rat male reproductive system, COX-2 is the predominant isoform. It is heavily localized in the epithelium of the distal *vas deferens*, whereas COX-1 expression was many-fold greater than COX-2 in the other body organs (42). Intracellular PGE_2 has been shown to be involved in the mitogenic effects of estradiol (43) and testosterone (44) in the rat seminal vesicles but not in the ventral prostate (43, 44). It was suggested recently that PGE_2 plays a major role in the growth of prostate cancer cells through the activation of *COX-2* gene expression (45, 46). Elevated levels of PGs have been widely reported in malignant human prostate tumors (47–51) as well as in carcinogen-induced rat and mouse prostate cancers (52–54). *In vitro* studies with tissue explants or primary cultures of prostate tumor cells have also demonstrated higher PG production in malignant tissue compared to benign or normal (46, 50). Increased synthesis of PGs was associated with advancing prostate cancer and the concentrations raised as the degree of tumor differentiation progressed, *i.e.*, worse prognosis (50). We have found that PG synthesis and COX-2 mRNA and protein expression are significantly higher in prostate cancer tissues compared to controls (Figure 3, Badawi Personal Communication) Although the pathophysiologic significance of this correlation in the context of a role for PGs and COX-2 in prostate cancer is unclear, several studies with murine prostate cancer models indicate that PGs may indeed play a multifunctional role in controlling growth, metastasis, aggressiveness and host immune responses (47–53, 55).

Various studies of the inhibitory effects of NSAIDs on prostate carcinogenesis further implicate a function of PG synthesis in the development of prostate cancer. Rose and Connolly (56) reported inhibition in the growth of androgen-responsive and -unresponsive human prostate cancer cells by indomethacin. They concluded that NSAIDs have a significant protective activity when administered either during the early stage (initiation) or late stage (promotion) of prostate carcinogenesis. Similar results were obtained in Nb rats bearing subcutaneous implants of an androgen-insensitive prostate adenocarcinomas (57) and in estradiol-induced rat prostate tumor (43).

In *COX-2* stably transfected rat intestinal epithelial cells, over-expression of the gene has been accompanied by several phenotypic changes such as

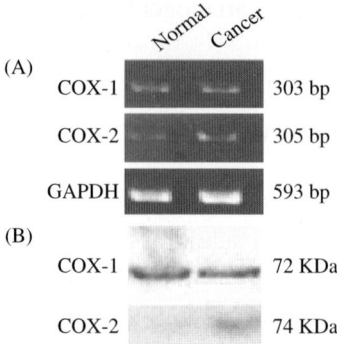

Figure 3. Expression of COX-2 mRNA and protein in human prostate cancer. Levels of COX-2 mRNA (A) in the prostate tissue were measured by RT-PCR. Single stranded cDNA was reverse transcribed from total RNA and used for PCR amplification with COX-1 (upper panel), COX-2 (middle panel) and GAPDH (lower panel) primers. Expression of COX-1 and COX-2 protein (B) was carried out by Western blot analysis. The blots represent n = 20 specimens in each group.

elevated levels of E-cadherin leading to increased adhesion to the extracellular matrix proteins and elevated bcl-2 protein expression with resistance to apoptosis (58). Furthermore, cells transformed with the Ha-*ras* oncogene showed an enhanced expression of *COX-2* accompanied by an increased production of PGE$_2$ (59). Similar changes may occur in prostate epithelial cells and would enhance the growth or reduce the loss of initiated or preneoplastic cells. Indeed, LNCaP, the human prostate cancer cell line that overexpresses *COX-2*, exhibited induction in apoptosis and down-regulation in *bcl-2* gene expression when treated with NS-398 (60).

3.2 Epidemiologic Evidence

In contrast to the experimental findings, the epidemiologic evidence for a protective effect of NSAIDs (*e.g.,* aspirin) in prostate cancer development is, at the moment, equivocal (61). The association between prostate cancer risk and the use of NSAIDs was investigated in a population-based case-control study in Auckland, New Zealand (62). A total of 317 newly diagnosed prostate cancer cases and 480 age-matched controls were recruited. The study reported a trend toward reduced risks of advanced prostate cancer associated with regular use of total NSAIDs (relative risk, RR = 0.73; 95% confidence intervals, CI = 0.50 – 1.07) and total aspirin (RR = 0.71; 95% CI = 0.47 – 1.08). Although these associations were statistically non-significant, the authors concluded that the findings support an etiological role for COX enzymes in prostate cancer progression (62).

A more recent study examined the effect of NSAIDs on tumor prevalence in abusers of analgesics, including aspirin (63). A group of 618 patients were compared to matched controls without evidence of aspirin abuse. The study concluded that the use of aspirin and other analgesics was associated with an overall risk of 0.4-fold of having developed malignancy relative to the control individuals. However, no statistically significant effect was found for patients with prostate cancer. Another prospective study that was carried out on 73 patients with chronic prostatitis showed that therapy with ibuprofen proved effective in alleviating the symptoms in about 70% of the patients (64).

Generally, the epidemiologic evidence for a protective effect of NSAIDs in prostate cancer development is inconsistent and still inconclusive. These inconsistencies are perhaps attributed to the nature and the limitations of epidemiologic studies. Conflicting observations may be due to a number of factors, such as the characteristics of the evaluated population, the choice of the control groups, the sample size, or various other biases that may result in random or systematic inaccuracies. Changes in the profile of NSAIDs use over time particularly with recent use, exclusion of the socioeconomic status that influences cancer risk, and the lack of information concerning NSAIDs other than aspirin all may combine and consequently contribute to misinterpretation of the protective role of NSAIDs in prostate cancer. Indeed, the promising experimental evidence and the inconclusive epidemiologic findings reflect the gaps in our understanding of the protective effects of NSAIDs.

One explanation for the inconsistent epidemiologic findings may relate to individual differences in NSAID metabolism due to genetic polymorphisms in enzymes (*e.g.*, cytochrome P450 2C9; CYP2C9) known to be involved in NSAID metabolism. Recently, we indicated that the failure to examine these molecular biomarkers of individual susceptibility and response may have contributed to the contradictory epidemiologic findings on the effects of NSAIDs in prostate cancer (69).

3.3 Evidence Derived from the Carcinogenic Action of Hormones and Dietary Fats

It is known that prostate cancer results from an interplay between endogenous hormones (65–69) and exogenous (environmental) influences that include, most prominently, dietary factors ((56), 69–71). The influence of hormones and diet, particularly fat consumption, on prostate cancer can be mediated, at least in part, by their effects on PG synthesis in the gland. Recent studies in the rat mammary gland suggest that the influence of hormones (72, 73) and dietary fat (73–75) on cancer development may be mediated, at least partly, by their effects on *COX-2* and PG synthesis (72–75). These effects can also be operative in the case of prostate cancer.

3.3.1 Hormones and PGs

Hormones such as androgens are crucial for the normal development of the prostate gland and the maintenance of its functional state in the adult. However, prolonged presence of androgens may be a risk factor in the development of prostate cancer (66, 76). For example, it is evident that both androgens and estrogens play an integral role in the growth of benign prostatic hypertrophy (77). Moreover, testosterone was found to be positively associated with human prostate cancer (78) and various epidemiologic studies suggest that the racial differences in the susceptibility and incidence of prostate carcinomas are partially related to hormonal influences (79). In animal studies, chronic exposure of adult mice and hamsters and prenatal exposure of mice to estrogenic compounds increased the incidence of prostate cancer (for review see Ref. (65)). Stimulation of prostate cancer growth was also evident in a variety of animal models following treatment with pituitary hormones such as prolactin (65). Further support for the role of hormones in prostate cancer was derived from studies showing androgen withdrawal as an effective approach in prostate cancer therapy (80, 81).

There is some evidence linking hormonal effects on prostate carcinogenesis to PG synthesis (48–50, 55). Administration of testosterone to male dogs results in a significant increase in PGs synthesized in the prostate (82). Androgen induced elevation in PGE_2 levels in the mouse genitourinary tract *in vivo* (83). Furthermore, PGs were suggested to be acting as second messengers for prolactin effects on prostate cancer development (84) and to mediate the mitogenic potential of testosterone in rat prostate (46). The acute effect of testosterone on the prostate was presumed to be related to its ability to increase the synthesis of $PGF2_\alpha$ in the gland (82). PGE_2 was also suggested to play a role in the mitogenicity of estradiol (43) and testosterone (44) in the rat seminal vesicles but not in the ventral prostate (43, 44). Finally, elevated levels of PGE_2 were associated with the aggressive, metastatic, androgen receptor-negative tumors (52, 53).

3.3.2 Dietary Fats and PGs

Dietary fatty acids are known to modulate prostate gland carcinogenesis in experimental animals (48, 85, 86) and may have similar effects in humans

(69, 70, 86). Numerous studies in rodents have shown that vegetable oils rich in n-6 polyunsaturated fatty acids (PUFAs) promote prostate cancer, whereas similar levels of marine oils rich in n-3 PUFAs inhibit (48, 85, 86, see below). n–6 PUFAs also stimulate, and n-3 inhibit, human prostate cancer cells in culture (56, 70). Feeding diets rich in marine oils suppresses the growth of human prostate cancer cells as solid tumors in athymic nude mice (70). Concerning the levels of fatty acids in human prostatic tissue, it has been shown that patients with malignant prostatic disease have significantly lower levels of AA concentration in the tissue phospholipids compared to the normal glands (87). The production of PGs by prostate cancer tissue was 10-fold higher than normal (87). Therefore, it can be suggested that the decreased levels of AA in prostate tumors are not due to its lower rate of formation but rather its elevated conversion to PGs. The relationship between prostate cancer incidence and dietary fat intake was estimated by international comparisons and epidemiological studies, which suggest that marine oil is an effective preventive factor (88).

Evidence linking the effects of dietary fat on prostate carcinogenesis to PG synthesis derives mainly from the observation that NSAIDs generally inhibit the promoting effects of diets rich in n-6 PUFAs (56). Furthermore, n-6 PUFAs are precursors of the PGs 2 series that are known to be mitogenic in both human and rodent prostate models (70). On the other hand, n-3 PUFAs are precursors of the PGs 3 series that lack a mitogenic effect (70). In support, PGs 3 series are 10-fold higher in the urine of volunteers after ingestion of n-3 PUFAs for 12 weeks compared to controls (89), suggesting their contribution to the observed favorable effects of marine oils on renal pathogenesis (88, 89).

4. FUNCTION OF PGS AND COX-2 IN PROSTATE CANCER DEVELOPMENT AND METASTASIS

Various theories were proposed to explain the exact mechanism(s) by which high rates of PG synthesis foster prostate cancer development and growth. These theories include the effects of PGs on cell proliferation, apoptosis, host immune response, and carcinogen metabolism.

4.1 Proliferation

PGs appear to be functioning as endogenous biological modifiers in different tissues and cells. PGs act, at least in part, through specific

G-protein-linked receptors to modulate the levels of the second messengers cAMP and Ca^{++} (8, 9) and, therefore, are involved in a variety of biological functions. The role of PG synthesis in controlling cell growth was substantiated from studies showing that these lipid molecules are not mitogens *per se* but act as permissive factors allowing the mitogenic action of various growth factors. For example, the epidermal growth factor-dependent proliferation of Balb/c 3T3 cells is inhibited by the COX inhibitor indomethacin (90). Moreover, $PGF_{2\alpha}$ stimulated the proliferation of the MC3T3-E1 osteoblast cells by increasing the number of insulin-like growth factor (IGF)-I binding sites (91). Additionally, human keratinocytes (92) and colon cancer cells (93) required PGE_2 for normal cell growth and proliferation. This proliferation was inhibited by NSAIDs in a manner that was overcome by the addition of PGE_2 (92).

12-*O*-tetradecanylphorbol-13-acetate (TPA) is a cancer-promoting agent that is usually used in mouse skin cancer models and induces a considerable PG synthesis at the site of administration (94). Topical application of TPA to mice caused epidermal hyperproliferation that was inhibited by indomethacin, an inhibition that was reversed by topical application of PGE_2 (94–96). In this model, PGE_2 was not a mitogen *per se* but rather acted as a co-mitogenic factor when applied with TPA (97). The marked increases in DNA, RNA and protein synthesis observed in rat skin treated topically with PGE_2 (98) suggest that PGs are regulatory factors in cell growth. These growth stimulating effects of PGs appear to be linked to biological modifiers such as polyamines. Elevated polyamines result from induced activity of ornithine decarboxylase (ODC) and are associated with increased DNA synthesis required for tumor growth. It is likely that tumor promoters enhance ODC activity in a PGE_2-dependent fashion (99), since inhibitors of AA metabolism inhibit both ODC activity and tumor development (58). This observation implies a possible link between PG synthesis, proliferation and tumorigenesis.

4.2   Apoptosis

COX-2 overexpression is associated with cell resistance to apoptosis, as observed in rat intestinal epithelial cells stably transfected with the gene (58) and in human prostate cancer cells (60). Several recent studies established a direct role of PGs in rendering cells resistant to apoptosis (100–104). For example, PGs effectively inhibited apoptosis in various animal (100, 101) and human (102) neuronal cell lines. This antiapoptotic effect of PGs was achieved by inhibitory signals following uptake through the PG transporter (101) or due to its role as a cAMP-elevating agent (102). Moreover, in rat hepatocytes, PGI_2, PGD_2 and PGE_1 decreased the frequency of apoptotic nuclei in a dose-dependent manner by up to 80% and suppressed internucleosomal DNA fragmentation (104). In human colon cancer cells, PGE_2 inhibited programmed cell death caused by the selective COX-2 inhibitor SC-58125 (104). Therefore, decreased apoptosis caused by PGs could lead to enhanced growth and/or decreased loss of initiated or preneoplastic cells and may explain how NSAIDs prevent cancer. The biochemical basis for the anti-proliferative characteristics of NSAIDs was generally attributed to their ability to reduce PG synthesis. More recently, however, these characteristics were partially linked to the ability of NSAIDs to induce apoptotic cell death (105–107). Although it can be argued that NSAIDs, by inhibiting COX expression, can mediate the induction of apoptosis, recent evidence refutes this presumption and suggests that the two mechanisms are not related (108). In fact, the anti-proliferative effect of NSAIDs can be ascribed to their influence on a variety of membrane processes that influence apoptosis and may not be linked to PG synthesis, such as the inhibition of superoxide anion generation and the coupling of mitochondrial oxidative phosphorylation (for review see 108).

The relationship between PG synthesis and apoptosis was examined by adopting three main approaches. *a*) Using human colon cancer cells that express *COX-2* and synthesize PGs (*e.g.*, HT-29) and cells that do not exhibit these characteristics (*e.g.*, HT-15). In these studies NSAIDs inhibited the proliferation of both cell lines regardless of their ability to synthesize PGs (93); *b*) Using sulindac and its metabolites: the reduced form that inhibits COX (*i.e.*, sulindac sulfide) (109, 110) and the oxidized form that is not known to inhibit COX (110), lipoxygenase or phospholipase A2 (111) (*i.e.*, sulindac sulfone). This approach showed that in spite of their ability to inhibit PG synthesis, both sulindac metabolites induced apoptosis (112) and inhibited tumor growth (115, 112, 113). *c*) Using chiral NSAIDs which exist in *S* and *R* enantiomeric forms (*e.g.*, flurbiprofen and carprofen) that inhibit or do not affect COX activity, respectively. These studies demonstrated that regardless of the ability of the enantiomeric forms to inhibit COX, they had equal anti-proliferative activity (4). Taken together, it can be concluded that the anti-proliferative potency of NSAIDs (*via* apoptosis) is likely to be a PG-independent mechanism although *COX-2* over-expression is associated with resistance to apoptosis (58, 60, 114).

4.3 Immune Suppression

The growth of various tumors is frequently associated with reduced immune response (115, 116). Suppression of immune surveillance (117) as well as inhibition of natural killer cell activity (118) were found to be mediated by high levels of PGE_2. It was suggested that PGs regulate immune function by acting as a negative feedback inhibitor for various processes including T cell proliferation, lymphokine production and macrophage and natural killer cell cytotoxicity (116–120). Moreover, colony stimulating factor, released by tumor cells, can cause monocytes and macrophages to synthesize PGE_2 as a contributory factor to the tumor-associated immune suppression (116, 121). This elevation in PGE_2 synthesis inhibited both the blastogenesis of the T cells and the activity of the natural killer cells (116, 121). Therefore, inhibition of COX activity may be associated with an enhanced immune response (118, 119) and reduced tumorigenesis. In support, indomethacin reduced the size of bone tumors in Moloney sarcoma virus infected mice (122). Moreover, administering PGE_2 to syngeneic mice bearing transplanted squamous cell carcinomas enhanced tumor transplantability (123). This inhibitory effect of NSAIDs on transplanted tumors is usually lost as growth progresses. In this case, immunosuppression results from the production of bone marrow-derived monocyte-like suppressor cells rather than from PG production (124).

4.4   Xenobiotic Metabolism

The effect of PGs and its precursor AA on xenobiotic oxidation catalyzed by human recombinant CYP enzymes and by human liver microsomes has been investigated recently (125). AA significantly inhibited CYP1A1- and 1A2-dependent O-deethylation and CYP1A2-, 2C8- and 2C19-dependent hydroxylation. AA also inhibited xenobiotic oxidation catalyzed by CYP1B1, 2B6, 2C9, 2D6, 2E1 and 3A4 in recombinant systems. Additionally, AA inhibited the activity of alkaline phosphatase in rat chondrocytes due to PG, but not to leukotriene, production (126).

Although the intracellular AA and the resultant PGs may inhibit xenobiotic metabolism, the peroxidase component of COX itself can oxidize a wide range of chemical carcinogens (*e.g.*, heterocyclic and aromatic amines and polycyclic aromatic hydrocarbons) besides metabolizing AA *via* a co-oxidation reaction (5, 127, 128). This reaction is inhibited by NSAIDs by preventing the COX-catalyzed generation of hydroperoxide substrate. Inhibiting carcinogen activation by NSAIDs hindered the growth of bladder cancer induced by *N*-[4,5-nitro-2-furyl]-2-thiazole] formamide (129) and colon cancer initiated by heterocyclic aromatic amines (130). This observation further supports the notion that inhibiting COX by NSAIDs may have a direct preventive effect on tumorigenesis independent of its effect on PG synthesis.

Peroxy radicals are generated during AA metabolism. These stable oxy radicals cause epoxidation for a variety of chemical carcinogens to their ultimate reactive forms. Carcinogen active metabolites produced by COX activity can bind to the cellular macromolecules, including DNA, to form a wide range of DNA adducts leading to mutagenesis and carcinogenesis (127, 128). There is a stereospecific difference between DNA adducts formed as a result of COX activation and those formed *via* CYP-catalyzed pathway. Analysis of these two types of DNA adducts may allow a precise characterization for the contribution of each metabolic pathway to the process of chemical carcinogenesis in extra-hepatic tissues (32). COX-mediated carcinogen activation offered a valid explanation for the influence of cigarette smoking in susceptibility to human bladder cancer (33) and may be relevant to carcinogen-induced prostate cancer both in human and animal models.

5. CONCLUDING COMMENTARY

Endogenous hormones and dietary fatty acids that are known to promote the development of prostate adenocarcinogenesis in rats following carcinogen treatment may induce the expression of the *COX-2* gene in the prostate gland (58, 59). However, the possibility that the induction of *COX-2* gene expression and the resulting increase in PG synthesis can enhance susceptibility of the prostate gland to cancer remains to be clarified. Further studies should be carried out to examine this hypothesis in rodent models and to determine whether a similar mechanism could be operative in the development of human prostate cancer. Studies utilizing transgenic animal models can be employed to examine prostate transformation under the influence of *COX-2* over-expression. The transgenic animal model has been used for a number of years and has yielded valuable information regarding the process of cancer development (131, 132). Moreover, mice with a targeted disruption of the *COX-2* gene have been constructed from the C57B116 background (133, 134) that is susceptible to prostate carcinogenesis (132, 135). Using this model will determine whether prostate tumorigenesis in animals lacking the *COX-2* is promoted by factors that are known to influence the formation of prostate cancer to an extent different from that in normal animals. The role of *COX-2* gene expression in prostate cancer can also be examined in human prostate epithelial cells that are stably transfected with and constitutively express the gene. Generating these cells will further clarify whether constitutive expression of *COX-2* is associated with increased susceptibility to neoplastic transformation and whether there are accompanied cellular and molecular changes that might be linked to the enhanced tumorigenic potential.

Elucidating the relationship between PG synthesis, *COX-2* expression, and prostate cancer development is critical for understanding the molecular basis of the disease and may suggest new views concerning scheduling chemotherapy. Comprehending the extent to which *COX-2* is involved in prostate cancer development may shed some light on the possibility of including NSAIDs that specifically inhibit COX-2 as an integral part of a reliable and effective strategy for cancer prevention.

ACKNOWLEDGMENTS

This publication was supported by grants CA06927 and CA57708 from the National Cancer Institute and by an appropriation from the Commonwealth of Pennsylvania. Its contents are solely the responsibility of the author and do not necessarily represent the official view of the National Cancer Institute. The author would like to thank Ms. Maureen Climaldi for her assistance during the preparation of this manuscript.

REFERENCES

1. Jaffe BM. Prostaglandins and cancer: An update. Prostaglandins 1974, 6:453–61.
2. Karmali RA. Prostaglandins and cancer. Review. Prostaglandins 1980, 5:11–28.
3. Marnett LJ. Aspirin and the potential role of prostaglandins in colon cancer. Cancer Res 1992, 52:5575–89.
4. Levy. GN. Prostaglandin H synthases, nonsteroidal anti-inflammatory drugs, colon cancer. FASEB J 1997, 11:234–47.
5. Marnett LJ. Prostaglandin synthase-mediated metabolism of carcinogens and a potential role for peroxyradicals as positive intermediates. Environ Health Perspect 1990, 88:5–12.
6. Landis SH, Murray T, Bolden S, Wingo PA. Cancer statistics, 1998. CA Cancer J Clin 1998, 48:6–29.
7. Anonymous. Prostate cancer in the UK. J R Soc Health 1997, 117:156.
8. Xie WL, Robertson DL, Simmons DL. Mitogen-inducible prostaglandin G/H synthase: A target for non-steroidal anti-inflammatory drugs. Drug Dev Res 1992, 25:245–65.
9. Simmons D, Xie W, Chipman JG, Evett GE. Multiple cyclooxygenases: Cloning of a mitogen-inducible form, In: *Prostaglandin, Leukotreines, Lipoxins and Paf.* Bailey JM, ed., New York: Plenum Press, 1991:67–78.
10. O'Neill GP, Ford-Hutchinson AW. Expression of mRNA for cyclooxygenase-1 and cyclooxy-genase-2 in human tissue. FEBS Lett 1993, 330:156–60.
11. Smith CJ, Morrow JD, Roberts LJ, Marnett LJ. Differentiation of monocytoid THP-1 cells with phorbol ester induces expression of prostaglandin endoperoxide synthase-1 (COX-1). Biochem Biophys Res Commun 1993, 192:787–93.

12. Samet JM, Fasano MB, Fonteh AN, Chilton FH. Selective induction of prostaglandin G/H synthase I by stem cell factor and dexamethasone in mast cells. J Biol Chem 1995, 270:8044–9.
13. Murakami M, Matsumoto R, Urade Y, Austen KF, Arm JP. C-kit ligand mediates increased expression of cytosolic phospholipase A2, prostaglandin endoperoxide synthase-1, and hematopoietic prostaglandin D2 synthase and increased ige-dependent prostaglandin D2 generation in immature mouse mast cells. J Biol Chem 1995, 270:3239–46.
14. DeWitt DL, Smith WL. Primary structure of prostaglandin G/H synthase from sheep vesicular gland determined from the complementary DNA sequence. Proc Natl Acad Sci USA 1988, 85:1412–6.
15. Merlie JP, Fagan D, Mudd J, Needleman P. Isolation and characterization of the complementary DNA for sheep seminal vesicle prostaglandin endoperoxide synthase (cyclooxygenase). J Biol Chem 1988, 283:3550–5.
16. Funk CD, Funk LB, Kennedy ME, Pong AS, Fitzgerald CA. Human platelet/erythroleukemia cell prostaglandin G/H synthase: CDNA cloning, expression, and gene chromosomal assignment. FASEB J 1991, 5:2304–12.
17. Hla T, Neilson K. Human cyclooxygenase-2 cDNA. Proc Natl Acad Sci USA 1992, 89:7384–8.
18. Jouzeau J-Y, Terlain B, Abid A, Nédélec E, Netter P. Cyclo-oxygenase isoenzymes: How recent findings affect thinking about nonsteroidal anti-inflammatory drugs. Drugs 1997, 53:563–82.
19. O'Banion MK, Winn VD, Young DA. CDNA cloning and functional activity of a glucocorticoid-regulated inflammatory cyclooxygenase. Proc Natl Acad Sci USA 1992, 89:4888–92.
20. Fletcher BS, Kujubu DA, Perrin DM, Herschman HR. Structure of the mitogen-inducible TIS 10 gene and demonstration that the TIS 10-encoded protein is a functional prostaglandin G/H synthase. J Biol Chem 1992, 267:4338–4.
21. DuBois RN, Awad J, Morrow J, 2nd, Roberts U, Bishop PR. Regulation of eicosanoid production and mitogenesis in rat intestinal epithelial cells by transforming growth factor-alpha and phorbol ester. J Clin Invest 1994, 93:493–8.
22. Smith WL, Meade EA, DeWitt DL. Interactions of PGH synthase isoenzymes 1 and 2 with NSAIDs. Ann NY Acad Sci 1994, 744:50–7.
23. Simmons DL, Levy DB, Yannoni Y, Erikson RL. Identification of a phorbol ester-repressible v-*src*-inducible gene. Proc Natl Acad Sci USA 1989, 86:1178–82.
24. Maier JA, Hla T, Maciag T. Cyclooxygenase is an immediate-early gene induced by interleukin-l in human endothelial cells. J Biol Chem 1990, 265:10805–8.
25. Ryseck RP, Raynoschek C, Macdonald-Bravo H, Dorfman K, Mattei MG, Bravo R. Identification of an immediate early gene, pghs-B, whose protein product has prostaglandin synthase/cyclooxygenase activity. Cell Growth Differ 1992, 3:443–50.
26. Needleman P, Isakson PC. Selective inhibition of cyclooxygenase 2. Sci Med 1998:26–35.
27. Wong E, Bayly C, Waterman HL, Riendeau D, Mancini JA. Conversion of prostaglandin G/H synthase-1 into an enzyme sensitive to PGHS-2-selective inhibitors by a double HIS513>arg and ILE523>val mutation. J Biol Chem 1997, 272:9280–6.
28. Smith WL, DeWitt DL. Biochemistry of prostaglandin endoperoxide H synthase-1 and synthase-2 and their differential susceptibility to nonsteroidal anti-inflammatory drugs. Semin Nephrol 1995, 15:179–84.

29. Murakami M, Matsumoto R, Austen KF, Arm JP. Prostaglandin endoperoxide synthase-1 and -2 couple to different transmembrane stimuli to generate prostaglandin D2 in mouse bone marrow-derived mast cells. J Biol Chem 1994, 269:22269–75.
30. Morita I, Schindler M, Regier MK, Otto JC, Hon T, DeWitt DL, Smith WL. Different intracellular locations for prostaglandin endoperoxide H synthase-1 and -2. J Biol Chem 1995, 270:10902–8.
31. DeWitt D, Smith WL. Yes, but do they still get headaches. Cell 1995, 83:345–8.
32. Eling TE, Curtis JF. Xenobiotic metabolism by prostaglandin H synthase. Pharmacol Ther 1992, 53:261–73.
33. Badawi AF, Abadi AA, Habib SL, Mohammed MA, Michael MS. Influence of cigarette smoking on prostaglandin synthesis and cyclooxygenase-2 expression in human urinary bladder cancer. Cancer Invest 2002, 20:651–656.
34. Meade EA, Smith WL, DeWitt DL. Differential inhibition of prostaglandin endoperoxide synthase (cyclooxygenase) isozymes by aspirin and other non-steroidal anti-inflammatory drugs. J Biol Chem 1993, 268:6610–4.
35. Kulmacz RJ, Lands WEM. Stoichiometry and kinetics of the interaction of prostaglandin H synthase with anti-inflammatory agents. J Biol Chem 1985, 260:12572–8.
36. Mitchell JA, Akarasereenont P, Thiemermann C, Flower RJ, Vane JR. Selectivity of nonsteroidal antiinflammatory drugs as inhibitors of constitutive and inducible cyclooxygenase. Proc Natl Acad Sci USA 1994, 90:11693–7.
37. Rome LH, Lands WEM. Structural requirements for time-dependent inhibition of prostaglandin biosynthesis by anti-inflammatory drugs. Proc Natl Acad Sci USA 1975, 72:4863–5.
38. Vane JR, Botting RM. New insights into the mode of action of anti-inflammatory drugs. Inflamm Res 1995, 44:1–10.
39. Masferrer JL, Zweifel BS, Manning PT, Hauser SD, Leahy KM, Smith WG et al. Selective inhibition of inducible cyclooxygenase 2 in vivo is anti-inflammatory and nonulcerogenic. Proc Natl Acad Sci USA 1994, 91:3228–32.
40. Futaki N, Takahashi S, Yokoyama M, Arai I, Higuchi S, Otoma S. NS-392, a new anti-inflammatory agent, selectively inhibits prostaglandin G/H synthase/cyclooxygenase (COX-2) activity in vitro. Prostaglandins 1994, 47:55–9.
41. Copeland RA, Williams JM, Giannaras J, Nurnberg S, Covington M, Pinto D et al. Mechanisms of selective inhibition of the inducible form of prostaglandin G/H synthase. Proc Natl Acad Sci USA 1994, 94:11202–6.
42. McKanna JA, Zhang MZ, Wang JL, Cheng H, Harris RC. Constitutive expression of cyclooxygenase-2 in rat vas deferens. Am J Physiol 1998, 275:R227–33.
43. Lyson K. Indomethacin suppression of the estradiol-induced proliferative response of the seminal vesicals. Exp Clin Endocrinol 1984, 84:223–7.
44. Lyson K, Pawlikowski M. Suppression of proliferative response of the seminal vesicles to testosterone by inhibitors of prostaglandin synthesis. Testosterone, indomethacin, and proliferation in seminal vesicles. J Androl 1983, 4:167–70.
45. Tjandrawinata RR, Hughes-Fulford M. Up-regulation of cyclooxygenase-2 by products-prostaglandin E2. Adv Exp Med Biol 1997, 407:163–70.
46. Tjandrawinata RR, Dahiya R, Hughes-Fulford M. Induction of cyclo-oxygenase-2 mRNA by prostaglandin E2 in human prostate carcinoma cells. Br J Cancer 1997, 75:1111–8.

47. Faas FH, Dang AQ, Pollard M, Hong XM, Fan K, Luckert PH, Schutz M. Increased phospholipid fatty acid remodeling in human and rat prostatic adenocarcinoma tissues. J Urol 1996, 156:243–8.
48. Karmali RA. Eicosanoids in neoplasia. Prev Med 1987, 16:493–502.
49. Ablin RJ, Shaw MW. Prostaglandin modulation of prostate tumor growth and metastases. Anticancer Res 1986, 6:327–8.
50. Khan O, Hensby CN, Williams G. Prostacyclin in prostatic cancer: A better marker than bone scan or serum acid phosphatase. Br J Urol 1982, 54:26–31.
51. Dunzendorfer U, Zahradnik HP, Grster K. 13, 14-Dihydro-15-keto-prostaglandin $F_{2\alpha}$ in patients with urogenital tumors. Urol Int 1980, 35:171–5.
52. Rubenstein M, Shaw MW, McKiel CF, Ray, PS, Guinan. PD. Immunoregulatory markers in rats carrying dunning R3327 H G, or MAT-LYLU prostatic adenocarcinoma variants. Cancer Res 1987, 47:178–82.
53. Shaw MW, Ablin RJ, Ray P, Rubenstein M, Guinan PD, McKiel CF Immunology of the Dunning R-. 3327 Rat prostate adenocarcinoma sublines: Plasma and tumor effusion prostaglandins. Am J Reprod Immunol Microbiol 1985, 8:77–9.
54. Smith BI, Wills MR, Savory J. Prostaglandins and cancer. Ann Clin Lab Sci 1983, 13:359–65.
55. Ablin RJ. Prostaglandins affect the tumor immune response in prostatic carcinoma. J Urol 1982, 127:997–8.
56. Rose DP, Connolly JM. Effects of fatty acids and eicosanoid synthesis inhibitors on the growth of two human prostate cancer cell lines. Prostate 1991, 18:243–54.
57. Drago JR, AI-Mondhiry HA. The effect of prostaglandin modulators on prostate tumor growth and metastasis. Anticancer Res 1984, 4:391–4.
58. Tsujii M, DuBois RN. Alteration in cellular adhesion and apoptosis in epithelial cells overexpressing prostaglandin endoperoxide synthase 2. Cell 1995, 83:493–501.
59. Subbaramaiah K, Telang N, Ramonetti JT, Araki R, DeVito B, Weksler BB, Dannenberg AJ. Transcription of cyclooxygenase-2 is enhanced in transformed mammary epithelial cells. Cancer Res 1996, 56:4424–9.
60. Liu XH, Yao S, Kirschenbaum A, Levine AC. NS398, a selective cyclooxygenase-2 inhibitor, induces apoptosis and down-regulates *bcl*-2 expression in LNCaP cells. Cancer Res 1998, 58:4245–9.
61. Swan DK, Ford B. Chemoprevention of cancer: Review of literature. Oncol Nutr Forum 1997, 24:719–27.
62. Norrish AE, Jackson RT, McRae CU. Non-steroidal anti-inflammatory drugs and prostate cancer progression. Int J Cancer 1998, 77:511–5.
63. Bucher C, Jordan P, Nickeleit V, Torhorst J, Mihatsch MJ. Relative risk of malignant tumors in analgesic abusers: Effect of intake of aspirin. Clin Nephrol 1999, 51:67–72.
64. Magoha GA. Ten years experience with chronic prostatitis in africans. East Afr Med J 1996, 73:176–8.
65. Bosland MC. Hormonal factors in carcinogenesis of the prostate and testis in human and in animal models. Prog Clin Biol Res 1996, 394:309–52.
66. Armstrong B. Endocrine factors in human carcinogenesis. IARC Sci Publ 1982, 39:193–221.
67. Henderson BE, Ross RK, Pike MC, Casagrande JT. Endogenous hormones as a major factor in human cancer. Cancer Res 1982, 42:3232–9.

68. Rioja LA, Sanz J. Carcinomas of the prostate: General concepts. Semin Oncol 1991, 18:2–8.
69. Badawi AF, El-Sohemy A. Non-steroidal anti-inflammatory drugs in chemoprevention of breast and prostate cancer. Med Hypoth 2001, 57:167–8.
70. Rose DP, Connolly JM. Dietary fat, fatty acids and prostate cancer. Lipids 1992, 27:798–803.
71. Pienta KJ, Esper PS. Is dietary fat a risk factor for prostate cancer. J Natl Cancer Inst 1993, 85:1538–40.
72. Badawi AF, Archer MC. Effect of hormonal status on the expression of the cyclooxygenase 1 and 2 genes and prostaglandin synthesis in rat mammary gland. Prostaglandins Other Lipid Mediat 1998, 56:167–81.
73. Badawi AF, El-Sohemy A, Stephen LL, Archer MC. Modulation of the expression of cyclooxygenase 1 and 2 genes in the mammary gland: Role of dietary fat and hormonal status. Adv Exp Med Biol 1999, 469:119–24.
74. Archer MC, el-Sohemy A, Stephen LL, Badawi AF. Molecular studies on the role of dietary fat and cholesterol in breast cancer induction. Adv Exp Med Biol 1997, 422:39–46.
75. Badawi AF, El-Sohemy A, Stephen LL, Ghoshal AK, Archer MC. Effects of dietary n-3 and n-6 polyunsaturated fatty acids on the expression of cyclooxygenase-1 and -2 and P21RAS in rat mammary glands. Carcinogenesis 1998, 19:905–10.
76. Wilding G. Endocrine control of prostate cancer. Cancer Surv 1995, 23:43–62.
77. Castagnetta LA, Carruba G. Human prostate cancer: A direct role for estrogens. Ciba Found Symp 1995, 191:269–89.
78. Signorello LB, Tzonou A, Mantzoros CS, Lipworth L, Lagiou P, Hsieh C *et al.* Serum steroids in relation to prostate cancer risk in case-control study (greece). Cancer Causes Control 1997, 8:632–6.
79. Montie JE. A glimpse at the future of some endocrine aspects of prostate cancer. Prostate Suppl 1996, 6:57–61.
80. Dearnaley DP. Cancer of the prostate. Br Med J 1994, 308:780–4.
81. Srinivasan G, Campbell E, Bashirelahi N. Androgen, estrogen, and progesterone receptors in normal and aging prostates. Microsc Res Techn 1995, 30:293–304.
82. Klein LA, Stoff JS, Ellis J. Acute effects of testosterone on serum PG levels in male dogs. Prostaglandins 1982, 24:467–73.
83. Gupta C. The role of prostaglandins in masculine differentiation: Modulation of prostaglandin levels in the differentiating genital tract of the fetal mouse. Endocrinology 1989, 124:129–33.
84. Rui II, Gordeladze JO, Gutvik KM, Purvis K. Prolactin desensitizes the prostaglandin el-dependent adenylyl cyclase in the rat prostate gland. Mol Cell Endocrinol 1984, 38:53–60.
85. Takai K. Promotional effects of high fat diet on chemical carcinogenesis of the prostate. Japan J Urol 1991, 82:871–0.
86. Bosland MC, Oakley-Girvan I, Whittemore AS. Dietary fat, calories, and prostate cancer risk. J Natl Cancer Inst 1999, 91:489–91.
87. Chaudry AA, Wahle KW, McClinton S, Moffat LE. Arachidonic acid metabolism in benign and malignant prostatic tissue in vitro: Effects of fatty acids and cyclooxygenase inhibitors. Int J Cancer 1994, 57:176–80.
88. Kuller LH. Dietary fat and chronic diseases: Epidemiologic overview. J Am Diet Assoc 1997, 97:9–15.

89. Fischer S, von Schacky C, Schweer H. Prostaglandins E3 and $F_{3\alpha}$ are excreted in human urine after ingestion of n-3 polyunsaturated fatty acids. Biochem Biophys Acta 1988, 963:501–8.
90. Nolan RD, Danilowicz RM, Eling TE. Role of arachidonic acid metabolism in the mitogenic response of balb/c 3T3 fibroblasts to epidermal growth factor. Mol Pharmacol 1988, 33:650–6.
91. Hakeda Y, Harada S, Matsumoto T, Tezuka K, Higashino K, Kodama H et al. Prostaglandin $F_{2\alpha}$ stimulates proliferation of clonal osteoplastic MC3T3-E1 cells by up-regulation of insulin-like growth factor 1 receptors. J Biol Chem 1991, 266:21044–50.
92. Pentland AP, Needleman P. Modulation of keratinocyte proliferation *in vitro* by endogenous prostaglandin synthesis. J Clin Invest 1986, 77:246–51.
93. Hanif R, Pittas A, Feng Y, Koutsos MI, Qiao L, Staiano-Coico L et al. Effects of non-steroidal anti-inflammatory drugs on proliferation and induction of apoptosis in colon cancer cells by a prostaglandin-independent pathway. Biochem Pharmacol 1996, 52:237–45.
94. Fürstenberger G, Marks F. Indomethacin inhibition of cell proliferation induced by the phorbol ester TPA is reversed by prostaglandin E2 in mouse epidermis *in vivo*. Biochem Biophys Res Commun 1987, 84:1103–8.
95. Fürstenberger WC, Marks F. Prostaglandins, epidermal hyperplasia and skin tumor promotion. Arachidonic Acid Metabolism and Tumor Promotion 1985, 49–72.
96. Verma AK, Ashendel CL, Boutwell RK. Inhibition by prostaglandin synthesis inhibitors of the induction of epidermal ornithine decarboxylase activity, the accumulation of prostaglandins and tumor promotion caused by 12-*O*-tetradecanoylphorbol-13-acetate. Cancer Res 1980, 40:708–15.
97. Fürstenberger G, Gross M, Marks F. Involvement of prostaglandins in the process of skin tumor promotion. In: *Ecosanoids and Cancer*. Thaler-Dao H, Crastes de Paulet A, Paoletti R, eds, New York: Raven Press, 1984:91–100.
98. Lupulescu A. Cytologic and metabolic effects of prostaglandins on rat skin. J Invest Dermatol 1977, 68:138–45.
99. Craven PA, Saito R, DeRubertis FR. Role of local prostaglandin synthesis in the modulation of proliferative activity of rat colonic epithelium. J Clin Invest 1983, 72:1365–75.
100. Kawamura T, Akira T, Watanaba M, Kagitani Y. Prostaglandin E1 prevents apoptotic cell death in superficial dorsal horn of rat spinal cord. Neuropharmacology 1997, 36:1023–30.
101. Kawamura T, Horie S, Maruyama T, Akira T, Imagawa T, Nakamura N. Prostaglandin E1 transported into cells blocks the apoptotic signals induced by nerve growth factor deprivation. J Neurochem 1999, 72:1907–4.
102. Ottonello L, Gonella R, Dapino P, Sacchetti C, Dallegri F. Prostaglandin E2 inhibits apoptosis in human neutrophilic polymorphonuclear leukocytes: Role of intracellular cyclic AMP levels. Exp Hematol 1998, 26:895–902.
103. Kroll B, Kunz S, Tu N, Schwarz LR. Inhibition of transforming growth factor-β1 and UV light-induced apoptosis by prostanoids in primary cultures of rat hepatocytes. Toxicol Appl Pharmacol 1998, 152:240–50.
104. Sheng H, Shao J, Morrow JD, Beauchamp RD, DuBois RN. Modulation of apoptosis and bcl-2 expression by prostaglandin E2 in human colon cancer cells. Cancer Res 1998, 58:362–6.

105. Hixson L, Alberts D, Krutzsch M, Einspahr J, Brendel K, Gross PH et al. Antiproliferative effect of nonsteroidal anti-inflammatory drugs (NSAIDs) against human colon cancer cells. Cancer Epidemiol Biomarker Prev 1994, 3:433–8.
106. Lu S, Xie W, Reed T, Bradshaw WS, Simmons DL. Nonsteroidal anti-inflammatory drugs cause apoptosis and induce cyclooxygenases in chicken embryo fibroblasts. Proc Natl Acad Sci USA 1995, 92:7961–5.
107. Elder DJE, Hague A, Hicks DJ, Paraskeva C. Different growth inhibition by the aspirin metabolite salicylate in human colorectal tumor cell lines: Enhanced apoptosis in carcinoma and *in vitro*-transformed adenoma relative to adenoma cell lines. Cancer Res 1996, 56:2273–6.
108. Abramson SB, Weissmann G. The mechanisms of action of antiinflammatory drugs. Arthritis Rheum 1989, 32:1–9.
109. Duggan DE, Hooke HF, Riskley AE, Shen TY, van Arman CG. Identification of the biologically active form of sulindac. J Pharmacol Exp Ther 1977, 201:8–13.
110. Shiff SJ, Qiao L, Rigas B. Sulindac sulfide, an aspirin-like compound, inhibits cell proliferation, causes cell cycle quiescence, and induces apoptosis in HT-29 colon adenocarcinoma cells. J Clin Invest 1995, 96:491–503.
111. Piazza GA, Alberts DS, Hixson LJ, Paranka NS, Li H, Finn T et al. Sulindac sulfone inhibits azoxymethane-induced colon carcinogenesis in rats without reducing prostaglandin levels. Cancer Res 1997, 57:2909–15.
112. Piazza GA, Kulchak-Rahm AL, Krutzsch M, Sperl G, Shipp-Puranka N, Gross PH et al. Antineoplastic drugs sulindac sulfide and sulfone inhibit cell growth by inducing apoptosis. Cancer Res 1995, 55:3110–6.
113. Thompson HJ, Briggs S, Paranka NS, Piazza GA, Brendel K, Gross PH et al. Inhibition of mammary carcinogenesis in rats by sulfone metabolite of sulindac. J Natl Cancer Inst 1995, 87:1259–60.
114. Battu S, Rigaud M, Beneytout JL. Resistance to apoptosis and cyclooxygenase-2 expression in a human adenocarcinoma cell line HT29CL.19a. Anticancer Res 1998, 18:3579–83.
115. Plescia O, Racis S. Prostaglandins as physiological immunoregulators. Prog Allergy 1988, 44:153–71.
116. Goodwin JS, Bankhurst AD, Messner RP. Suppression of human T-cell mitogenesis by prostaglandin; existence of a prostaglandin-producing suppressor cell. J Exp Med 1977, 146:1719–34.
117. Baich CM, Doghert PA, Cloud GA, Tilden AB. Prostaglandin E2-mediated suppression of cellular immunity in colon cancer cancer patients. Surgery 1984, 95:71–7.
118. Brunda MJ, Heberman RB, Holden HT. Inhibition of murine natural killer cell activity by prostaglandins. J Immunol 1980, 124:2682–7.
119. Goodwin JS. Immunological effects of nonsteroidal anti-inflammatory drugs. Am J Med 1984, 77:7–15.
120. Cantrow WD, Cheuing HT, Sundharadas G. Effects of prostaglandins on the spreading, adhesion and migration of mouse peritoneal macrophages. Prostaglandins 1978, 63:39–46.
121. Bockman RS. PGE inhibition of T-lymphocyte colony formation. J Clin Invest 1972, 64:812–21.
122. Strausser HR, Humes JL. Prostaglandin synthesis inhibition: Effect on bone changes and sarcoma tumor induction in BALB/c mice. Int J Cancer 1975, 15:724–30.

123. Lynch NR, Salomon JC. Tumor growth inhibition and potentiation of immunotherapy by indomethacin in mice. J Natl Cancer Inst 1979, 62:117–21.
124. Young MR, Duffie GP, Lozano Y, Young ME, Wright MA. Association of a functional prostaglandin E2-protein kinase A coupling with responsiveness of metastatic lewis lung carcinoma variants to prostaglandin E2 and to prostaglandin E2-producing nonmetastatic lewis lung carcinoma variants. Cancer Res 1990, 50:2973–8.
125. Yamazaki H, Shimada T. Effects of arachidonic acid, prostaglandins, retinol, retinoic acid and cholecalciferol on xenobiotic oxidations catalyzed by human cytochrome P450 enzymes. Xenobiotica 1999, 29:231–41.
126. Schwartz Z, Sylvia VL, Curry D, Luna MH, Dean DD, Boyan BD. Arachidonic acid directly mediates the rapid effects of 24,25-dihydroxyvitamin D3 via protein kinase C and indirectly through prostaglandin production in resting zone chondrocytes. Endocrinol 1999, 140:2991–3002.
127. Eling TE, Thompson DC, Foureman GL, Curtis JF, Hughes MF. Prostaglandin H synthase and xenobiotic oxidation. Ann Rev Pharmacol Toxicol 1990, 30:1–45.
128. Smith BJ, Curtis JF, Eling TE. Bioactivation of xenobiotics by prostaglandin *H* synthetase. Chem Biol Interact 1991, 79:245–64.
129. Murasaki G, Zenser TV, Davia BB, Cohen SM. Inhibition by aspirin of *N*-[4-(5-nitro-2-furyl-2-thiazoyl]formamide-induced bladder carcinogenesis. Carcinogenesis 1984, 5:53–5.
130. Wild, D, Degan GH. Prostaglandin H synthetase-dependent mutagenic activity of heterocyclic aromatic amines of the IQ type. Carcinogenesis 1987, 8:541–5.
131. Bosland MC. Animal models for the study of prostate carcinogenesis. J Cell Biochem 1992, 16H:89–98.
132. Thomson TC, Truong LD, Timme TL, Kadmon D, McCune BK, Flanders KC *et al*. Transgenic models for the study of prostate cancer. Cancer 1993, 71:1165–71.
133. Dinchuk JE, Car BD, Focht RJ, Johnston JJ, Jaffee BD, Covington MB *et al*. Renal abnormalities and an altered inflammatory response in mice lacking cyclooxygenase II. Nature 1995, 378:406–9.
134. Morham SG, Langenbach R, Loftin CD, Tiano HF, Vouloumanos N, Jennette JC *et al*. Prostaglandin synthase 2 gene disruption causes severe renal pathology in the mouse. Cell 1995, 83:473–82.
135. Waymouth C, Coman DR, Ward-Baily PF. Spontaneous tumors of the prostate gland in inbred strains of mice. J Natl Cancer Inst 1983, 70:199–20.

Chapter 6

CELL CYCLE REGULATION

Ruchi M. Newman[1] and Bruce R. Zetter[1,2]
[1]*Department of Surgery, Children's Hospital, Boston, MA, USA*
[2]*Department of Cell Biology, Harvard Medical School, Boston, MA, USA*

Abstract: Progression of the cell cycle is a tightly controlled process that is governed by several overlapping regulatory mechanisms. However, during the onset of prostate cancer and progression to malignancy, these stringent controls are cast aside and cell proliferation continues unchecked. Among the factors shown to contribute to aberrant cell proliferation and progression to malignancy in prostatic carcinoma are those that directly influence the cell cycle, such as androgen receptor and CDK inhibitors, as well as others that indirectly influence cell cycle control such as PTEN and polyamines. Here we discuss the mechanisms by which these factors manipulate the cell cycle and their contributions to the progression of prostate carcinoma.

Key words: cell cycle control, metastasis, androgen receptor, CDK inhibitors, PTEN, polyamines, antizyme

1. INTRODUCTION

1.1 Prostate Cancer

Prostate cancer is the most prevalent form of cancer in males. Although it is the second leading cause of death among older males, the incidence of latent prostate carcinoma is high, with only a small percentage of patients developing metastases to secondary sites (1). Development of prostate cancer at the primary site is a slow process, with the formation of a palpable mass capable of dissemination to secondary sites often taking decades (2, 3). Once prostate cancer does metastasize, usually to bone, tumor growth tends to become rapid, and is generally fatal within a few years. A question of crucial importance is why prostatic carcinomas have such a low apparent growth rate at the primary site, yet are capable of rapid growth at secondary sites. This switch from slow growth in normal cells or in localized prostate tumors to rapid growth is triggered, in part, by a many complex cellular changes that lead to unchecked growth. Deregulated growth is just one factor in the multistep processes which ultimately lead to tumor formation and malignancy (reviewed in 4–7). In the following review we will consider those factors which have been shown to have a direct role in dysregulation of the cell cycle leading to metastatic prostatic carcinoma.

1.2   Cell Cycle

As with most other processes, induction of aberrant growth during the induction of prostate carcinoma results in a shift in the precarious balance between those cellular factors which influence cell growth and those that influence cell death. To ensure faithful progression through the four defined phases of the cell cycle, cells utilize a series of checkpoints that prevent them from advancing to the next phase until they have successfully completed the previous phase. The cyclins, cyclin dependent kinases (CDKs), and CDK inhibitors are all guardians of these checkpoints and monitor mitogenic signals from the cellular environment to ensure that cell cycle progression occurs only during favorable circumstances. One key milestone in the progression from the G1 phase of the cell cycle is phosphorylation of the retinoblastoma protein (Rb) by the cyclin/CDK complexes. During the M and G0 phases of the cell cycle the Rb protein prevents transcription of genes involved in cell cycle progression by binding to a variety of substrates involved in cell cycle progression including the E2F family of transcription factors, rendering them inactive. Upon sequential phosphorylation by CDK4/6-cyclin D and CDK2-cyclin E complexes, Rb releases its substrates and cell cycle progression can ensue.

Cell cycle regulators are frequently mutated in many human tumors resulting in overexpression of cyclins and CDKs to promote cellular proliferation. Additionally, mutation or loss of CDK inhibitors is frequently seen in cancer and serves to prevent inhibiton of aberrant growth. In the majority of tumors, these mutations result in chromosomal alterations such as amplifications, translocations and deletions or from epigenetic inactivation such as methylation of promoters (reviewed in 6–8). In addition to these types of mutations, there is emerging evidence that seemingly unrelated factors can influence cell cycle progression in a variety of ways during the initiation and progression of metastatic prostate disease.

2. FACTORS INFLUENCING CELL CYCLE DYSREGULATION IN PROSTATE CANCER

2.1 Androgen Receptor

Androgens are required for growth of the prostatic epithelium as well as for maintenance of the prostate gland. Androgens are required for the onset of prostate cancer and this dependence persists in many stages of the disease as well. As a result, newly diagnosed cases of metastatic prostate cancer are often treated with androgen ablation therapy. With time, however, many patients develop androgen-independent tumors, which can grow unabated by anti-androgen therapy.

Androgens exert their effect on prostate cell proliferation by signalling through the androgen receptor (AR), a key nuclear transcription factor in the prostate. The AR regulates proliferation of prostate cancer cells by stimulation of cyclin-dependent kinases. However, in some prostate tumors AR stimulates expression of cell cycle inhibitors, thus leading to down-regulation of cellular proliferation (reviewed in 9, 10). The AR is a member of the nuclear receptor superfamily of transcription factors and is composed of a C-terminal ligand-binding domain (LBD), a DNA binding domain, and a variable N-terminal region. Normally, the AR is kept in an inactive state by heat-shock proteins which bind to the LBD region of the protein (11). In the presence of androgen, which in the case of the prostate is dihydrotestosterone (DHT), the heat shock proteins bound to the LBD of the AR are displaced by the androgen resulting in a conformational change. This new conformation allows the androgen-bound receptors to dimerize and form a functionally active complex (12). The active AR/androgen homodimer then moves to the nucleus, binds DNA and stimulates transcription of target genes. The best known target of the AR is prostate-specific antigen (PSA), whose expression levels are monitored clinically to diagnose aberrant prostate growth (13, 14).

There is emerging evidence which indicates that specific AR-mediated activation of transcription also requires the recruitment of transcriptional co-activators such as SRC1, TIF-1 and GRIP2 as well as co-repressors which include proteins with histone deacetylase (HDAC) activity or proteins which recruit HDACs to the receptor complex (15–17). In addition to these co-repressors, Knudsen et al., have identified cyclin D1 as an additional repressor of androgen receptor activation (18). They have shown that cyclin D1 interacts with the AR *in vivo* and inhibits its transactivation potential, without affecting AR expression. This inhibition is independent of CDK4 and thus also independent of the role of cyclin D1 in RB phosphorylation (19). They had previously shown that androgen induces cyclin D1 expression in prostatic adenocarcinoma cells as part of its mitogenic signal (20). These potentially opposing roles of cyclin D1 in response to androgen pose a paradox wherein cyclin D1 accomodates a mitogenic, androgen-responsive function (induction of CDK4 activity) (20) as well as an anti-mitogenic function (repression of AR activity) that occurs independent of CDK4 (18). The authors propose a model whereby androgen-mediated induction of cyclin D1 expression activates CDK4, and cell cycle progression ensues. However, this cell cycle progression selects against any anti-mitogenic function of cyclin D1. It has long been known that the retinoblastoma tumor suppressor protein, Rb, is the main cell cycle target of cyclin D-CDK4 complexes (21). Even after CDK4 mediated RB phosphorylation in early G1, cyclin D1 expression persists (22) even though D1 is no longer associated with CDK4. The authors show that ectopic expression of cyclin D1 or CDK4-refractory cyclin D1 actually inhibits cell cycle progression. These findings support the model that after Rb inactivation, androgen-induced cyclin D1 expression serves, presumably, to negatively regulate AR activity and thereby limit the rate of future mitogenic activation and cell cycle progression (19). These findings demonstrate that cyclin D1 contains two opposing functions in androgen-dependent cells and encourage further study of these roles in the progression of prostate carcinoma.

Studies on prostate cancer patients treated with androgen ablation therapy, as well as in castrated patients, have revealed that while the majority of androgen dependent cells undergo apoptosis after such treatments, a subset of androgen-responsive cells survives and that these cells can proliferate in the absence of androgen. Both androgen dependent and independent tumors continue to express AR, even in the absence of androgen. It is these cells that give rise to aggressive, treatment refractory metastatic tumors.

2.2 CDK Inhibitors

2.2.1 p27/Kip

The p27/Kip protein is best known as an inhibitor of cell cycle progression due to its ability to the block the cyclin/CDK complex formation required for normal cell progression. However, there is an emerging role for p27 as a tumor suppressor (reviewed in 23). Loss of heterozygosity in the region of chromosome 12p13, where p27 is located, commonly occurs in several human cancers, including prostate cancer (24–26). However, several investigators have shown that somatic mutations in p27 are rarely seen.

Despite these findings, there is a clear inverse correlation between p27 levels and survival rates in several human malignancies (reviewed in 27). Low levels of p27 presumably allow unchecked cell growth (28) leading to a malignant transformation.

Loss of p27 expression has been linked to development and progression of prostate cancer thus making it an attractive candidate as an independent prognostic marker for prostate cancer. Immunohistochemical analysis of primary prostate tumors and lymph node metastases found decreased p27 staining to coincide with a high tumor grade and proliferative index (29, 30). Additionally, several studies have shown that decreased levels of p27 correlate with poor prognosis for patients with prostate cancer (31–35).

In addition to regulating growth, p27 has recently been shown to have a role in cell adhesion and contact inhibition of cell growth (36–38). Most adherent, non-transformed cell lines are able to arrest growth in response to cell-cell contact. Loss of this contact-dependent growth inhibition is often seen in tumor cell lines grown in two-dimensional cultures. Upon transfer to three- dimensional culture (such as is found in solid tumors), cell lines derived from a variety of cancers again showed contact inhibition of growth which coincided with an upregulation of p27 (23, 37). Ablation of p27 expression by anti-sense oligonucleotides in these three-dimensional cultures resulted in loss of contact inhibited growth. Loss of p27 may thus allow unchecked cell proliferation (23).

The mechanism by which p27 is downregulated in prostate carcinoma is believed to involve its increased proteolysis by the SCF^{SKP2} ubiquitin ligase complex. Recent studies in androgen-sensitive LNCap cells have shown that androgen-induced G1-cell cycle arrest seen in these cells coincides with inhibition of cdk2 activity and an accumulation of p27 protein due to reduced ubiquitinylation. This androgen-dependent decrease in ubiquitinylated p27 is accompanied by a specific loss of the SKP2 F-box protein suggesting that SKP2 is responsible for regulating p27 levels in these cells. Furthermore, SKP2 overexpression is sufficient to overcome p27 accumulation in androgen arrested cells by stimulating cellular p27 ubiquitylation (39). Taken together, these results suggest that overexpression of SKP2 may be one of the mechanisms that allow prostate cancer cells to escape growth control mediated by p27.

2.2.2   p16/INK4A

The cyclin dependent kinase inhibitor p16 (INK4A/MTS1/CDKN2) functions to prevent activation of the CDK4/cyclin D kinase complex by sequestering the CDK4 component. This inhibition results in the accumulation of hypophosphorylated retinoblastoma protein (Rb) which arrests cell cycle progression. Like other CDK inhibitors, inactivation or loss of p16 is a common event in many types of cancer including prostate cancer (40–44). Restoration of p16 protein expression in prostate cancer cells inhibits growth both *in vivo* and *in vitro* (45).

The mechanism by which p16 exerts its inhibitory effect on tumor growth has not been elucidated although some studies indicate that overexpression of p16 in prostate cancer may induce cell senescence in an Rb-dependent manner (46). Additionally, in the absence of Rb, p16 can still induce growth inhibition, through an as yet unidentified mechanism (46).

2.3 Genetic Determinants

2.3.1 PTEN/MMAC1

The PTEN tumor suppressor (also known as MMAC1) is often mutated or lost in prostate cancer as well as in several other types of sporadic cancers. The PTEN protein is a phosphatase that can dephosphorylate the important second messenger phosphatidylinositol (3, 4, 5)-triphosphate, thereby antagonizing the cell survival signaling mediated by the PI-3-kinase/AKT pathway. The Akt/PKB proto-oncogene, which acts as a serine-threonine kinase, has been shown to be a critical regulator of many cellular processes including cell cycle progression, apoptosis, angiogenesis and metabolism. Loss of PTEN results in constitutive activation of Akt/PKB (47–49) leading to activation of mitogenic and pro-survival signaling molecules.

Numerous studies have implicated the loss of MMAC/PTEN in prostate cancer progression. Although multiple cytogenetic studies of prostate tumors detected low rates of mutation and deletion of MMAC/PTEN in organ-confined prostate cancers (50–52), 60% of metastatic prostate cancers demonstrated loss of heterozygosity for MMAC/PTEN. This loss is accompanied by a significant rate of alterations of the second allele (48, 53). Overexpression of PTEN in certain cell types has been shown to suppress colony formation, growth in soft agar and tumor formation in nude mice (54, 55). Most recently, Davies et al., have shown that MMAC/PTEN expression in PC3 cells decreased the level of phospho-Akt but not that of phospho-Mapk or FAK. Expression of MMAC/PTEN inhibited the *in vitro* growth of PC3 cells primarily by blocking cell cycle progression (56). In a nude mouse model, the *ex-vivo* expression of MMAC/PTEN in orthotopically implanted PC3 cells did not inhibit tumorigenicity. However, *ex-vivo* expression of MMAC/PTEN did significantly reduce local tumor size by inhibiting cellular proliferation, a result that is consistent with the *in vitro* experiments. Additionally, *ex-vivo* expression of MMAC/PTEN completely inhibited the development of lymph node metastases by PC3 cells. Thus, these experiments suggest that MMAC/PTEN is not a critical regulator of prostate tumor formation but rather a critical regulator of aggressive local prostate tumor growth and metastasis (56)

2.3.2 KLF6

The Kruppel-like factor 6 (KLF6/Zf9/CPBP) is a ubiquitously expressed transcription factor of unknown function (57–59). The KLF6 gene is located on chromosome 10 in a region that is frequently deleted in sporadic prostate adenocarcinoma and several mutations in KLF6 have recently been isolated from primary prostate tumors (60). Potential *in vivo* targets for KLF6-mediated transcriptional activation include collagen $\alpha 1(1)$ (58), types I and II TGFβ receptors (61), urokinase type plasminogen activator (uPA) (62), and the cyclin dependent kinase inhibitor p21 (WAF/CIP) (60). Overexpression of KLF6 in NIH3T3 cells has been shown to inhibit cell growth in a p53-independent manner (60). This growth inhibition is due to the upregulation of p21 expression by KLF6 (60). Furthermore, a variety of tumor-derived mutations in KLF6 fail to suppress growth of PC3 cells and do not transactivate p21 promoter constructs. Taken together, these data implicate KLF6 as a potential tumor suppressor gene in prostate cancer.

2.4 Polyamines

A question of crucial importance is why prostatic carcinomas have such a low apparent growth rate at the primary site, yet are capable of rapid growth upon metastasis to secondary sites such as bone. One possible explanation is that there are growth factors at the secondary sites that promote tumor formation. In fact, previous results from our laboratory show that high concentrations of transferrin in the bone marrow may facilitate the growth of prostate cancer and metastases at that site (63).

If locally high concentration of growth factors contribute to the growth of prostate carcinoma metastases in bone, what causes the relatively slow growth and progression of prostate carcinoma in the prostate? The most obvious possibilities include a) that stimulatory growth factors are absent in the prostate or b) that the normal prostate contains growth inhibitory molecules that suppress or retard the growth of primary prostate carcinomas. While there is little direct evidence for the first assumption, we have previously purified a growth inhibitor from normal human prostate and identified it as the polyamine spermine (64), a molecule made in abundance in the normal human prostate and then secreted into the prostatic fluid (65)

Polyamines are produced by virtually all cells in the body and are required for cell proliferation and differentiation although many of their specific biologic functions are still unknown. They were initially identified in prostatic secretions and the concentration of polyamines in prostatic tissue is 50–100 fold greater than in any other tissue (65). Modulation of polyamine levels is critical for many processes including protein synthesis and growth control. Accordingly, there is a tightly regulated mechanism for maintenance of polyamine levels (reviewed in 66). The enzyme ornithine decarboxylase (ODC) is the rate-limiting enzyme in polyamine biosynthesis and production of the enzyme is under negative feedback inhibition by polyamines such that it is rapidly suppressed by increased cellular polyamine levels (67).

Cell cycle regulation is intimately related to polyamine biosynthesis. Polyamine levels rise during the cell cycle and are required for passage through the cell cycle (68). It might be expected that high levels of polyamines would be growth stimulatory. Indeed, development of polyamine analogs, which interfere with tumor growth by depleting cellular polyamine levels is currently being widely investigated as a treatment for a variety of cancers including androgen-independent prostate carcinoma.

While it might then be expected that high levels of polyamines would be growth stimulatory, the reverse has been seen, especially for spermine and spermidine. Spermine has been previously shown to inhibit the growth of several cell types (69–72). The reduction in cell proliferation in spermine or spermidine treated cells is often associated with the feedback inhibition of polyamine synthetic enzymes, especially ODC production is rapidly induced by various growth stimuli and there is evidence that overexpression of ODC plays an important role in prostate tumor growth and development (73, 74). Furthermore, ODC has been shown to have proto-oncogenic function in many other cancers (75–77)

In addition to being regulated by growth stimuli, levels of ODC are controlled by a unique enzyme called ornithine decarboxylase antizyme (reviewed in 66). Studies on degradation of ODC have shown that antizyme replaces ubiquitin in targeting ODC for degradation by the 26S proteasome (78). Protein synthesis of antizyme is itself tightly regulated by a distinctive polyamine-mediated ribosomal frameshifting mechanism (67, 79).

In the presence of high quantities of spermine, synthesis of antizyme (AZ) is induced by an unusual translational frameshift mechanism (Figure 1). In a variety of cell types this induces G1 cell cycle arrest. Antizyme is able to bind to ODC, an enzyme which catalyzes the rate-limiting step in polyamine synthesis. Upon binding to AZ, ODC is targeted for degradation

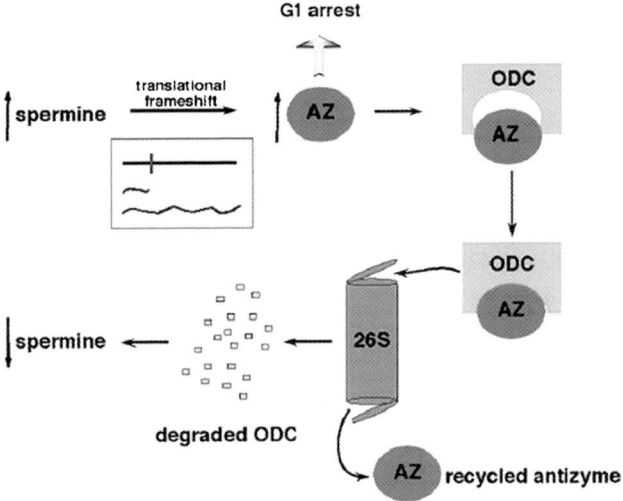

Figure 1. Feedback regulation of antizyme by spermine.

by the 26S proteasome in an ubiquitin-independent manner, while AZ is recycled. Degradation of ODC prevents synthesis of polyamines

Work from our laboratory has shown that the concentration of spermine equal to or lower than those present in the prostate can inhibit the growth of prostate carcinoma cells (64, 80). These concentrations of spermine also cause induction of AZ in the prostate carcinoma cells (80). Strikingly, spermine-independent overexpression of AZ is associated with growth inhibition and tumor regression in a number of cell types and animal models (81–84). Specifically spermine-mediated as well as ectopic induction of antizyme production arrests cells in the G1 phase of the cell cycle (80, 82). In one malignant oral keratinocyte model, ectopic overexpression of AZ results in reversion of the malignant phenotype and induces epithelial differentiation (82).

There are suggestions in the literature that levels of inducible AZ can vary with progression toward the metastatic phenotype. Because antizyme is a negative regulator of cell growth, one might predict that AZ levels would decrease as tumors progressed. In our own work with Dunning prostate carcinoma cell lines, we find that the more highly metastatic derivatives of these cell lines fail to produce AZ in response to exogenous polyamines. This would suggest increased capacity for cell growth in a polyamine-rich environment such as the prostate. Moreover, since synthesis of polyamines is so tightly regulated, a decrease in AZ levels would lead to an accumulation of ODC in the cell, a condition known to cause malignant transformation (75).

Intriguingly, AZ levels drop precipitously in carcinogen induced tumors in the hamster cheek pouch as the tumors become more malignant (85).

Polyamine analogues have been developed that interfere with different components of the polyamine pathway. Recently, Mitchell and colleagues (81) have shown that these compounds differ greatly in their ability to upregulate AZ treated cells. The authors have suggested that selecting agents for their ability to stimulate AZ production may optimize the possibility of choosing analogs with maximal growth arresting properties. These analogues chosen in this way may have the best chance of succeeding as anti-cancer drugs in animals and in humans (81).

The exact mechanism of AZ-mediated growth arrest remains unclear, however, it is tempting to speculate that since AZ overproduction induces a G1 cell cycle arrest it may be acting to dysregulate key cell cycle regulatory proteins. Given that AZ can target ODC for destruction by the 26S proteasome in the absence of ubiquitin, it may be that AZ could target cell cycle regulatory factors for degradation in the same manner. If true, this would be a completely novel mechanism of cell cycle regulation that relies on antizyme-targeted proteolyis of cell cycle proteins.

3. CONCLUSION

In the progression of cancer, the cell cycle is dysregulated such that cells no longer look to normal mitogenic signals for cues as to when to proliferate. Cancer cells tend to accumulate a variety of mutations that alter the regulatory mechanisms that tightly control the cell cycle. Although very little is known about how this concerted sabotage of a variety of diverse cellular processes is accomplished, factors specifically regulating cell cycle regulatory proteins are thought to be key players. An additional effect of a subset of these proteins is their effect on metastasis. Mutations in serine/threonine kinase PTEN/MMAC1 or the CDK inhibitory p27 have been shown to be involved not only subversion of the cell cycle machinery, but also in the progression of metastatic disease. Further *in vivo* study using animal models is required to elucidate how cells coordinate aberrant cell growth and proliferation with increased metastatic ability.

A question of crucial importance that remains to be answered is if the progression to metastatic disease is a necessary outcome of dysregulation of the cell cycle. In the case of many cancers including prostate cancer, early detection of localized disease presents a much better prognosis for the patient than that of metastatic disease. If we can determine how to prevent the cancer cells from progressing to metastatic disease simply by restoring the proper checkpoint to the cell cycle, then the number of deaths resulting from many types of cancer could be significantly reduced.

REFERENCES

1. Landis SH *et al.* Cancer statistics. CA Cancer J Clin 1999, 49:8–31, 1.
2. Schmid HP, McNeal JE, Stamey, TA. Observations on the doubling time of prostate cancer. The use of serial prostate-specific antigen in patients with untreated disease as a measure of increasing cancer volume. Cancer 1993, 71:2031–40.
3. Schmid HP, McNeal JE, Stamey, TA. Clinical observations on the doubling time of prostate cancer. Eur Urol 1993, 23(Suppl 2):60–3.
4. Green DR, Evan, GI. A matter of life and death. Cancer Cell 2002, 1:19–30.
5. Malumbres M, Barbacid, M. To cycle or not to cycle: A critical decision in cancer. Nat Rev Cancer 2001, 1:222–231.
6. Evan GI, Vousden, KH. Proliferation, cell cycle and apoptosis in cancer. Nature 2001, 411:342–8.
7. Hanahan D, Weinberg, RA. The hallmarks of cancer. Cell 2000, 100:57–70.
8. Malumbres M, Barbacid, M. To cycle or not to cycle: A critical decision in cancer. Nat Rev Cancer 2001, 1:222–31.
9. Culig Z *et al.* Androgen receptor–an update of mechanisms of action in prostate cancer. Urol Res 2000, 28:211–9.
10. Culig Z *et al.* Expression and function of androgen receptor in carcinoma of the prostate. Microsc Res Tech 2000, 51:447–55.
11. Pratt WB, Toft, DO. Steroid receptor interactions with heat shock protein and immunophilin chaperones. Endocr Rev 1997, 18:306–60.
12. Ohara-Nemoto Y *et al.* Characterization of the nontransformed and transformed androgen receptor and heat shock protein 90 with high-performance hydrophobic- interaction chromatography. J Steroid Biochem 1988, 31:295–304.
13. Pettaway CA. Prognostic markers in clinically localized prostate cancer. Tech Urol 1998, 4:35–42.
14. Cleutjens KB *et al.* Two androgen response regions cooperate in steroid hormone regulated activity of the prostate-specific antigen promoter. J Biol Chem 1996, 271:6379–88.
15. Jenster G, Coactivators, corepressors as mediators of nuclear receptor function: An update. Mol Cell Endocrinol 1998, 143:1–7.
16. Collingwood TN, Urnov FD, Wolffe, AP. Nuclear receptors: Coactivators, corepressors and chromatin remodeling in the control of transcription. J Mol Endocrinol 1999, 23:255–75.
17. Bevan C, Parker, M. The role of coactivators in steroid hormone action. Exp Cell Res 1999, 253:349–56.
18. Knudsen KE, Cavenee WK, Arden, KC. D-type cyclins complex with the androgen receptor and inhibit its transcriptional transactivation ability. Cancer Res 1999, 59:2297–301.
19. Petre CE *et al.* Cyclin D1: Mechanism and consequence of androgen receptor co-repressor activity. J Biol Chem 2002, 277:2207–15.

20. Knudsen KE, Arden KC, Cavenee, WK. Multiple G1 regulatory elements control the androgen-dependent proliferation of prostatic carcinoma cells. J Biol Chem 1998, 273:20213–22.
21. Lukas J et al. Cyclin D1 protein oscillates and is essential for cell cycle progression in human tumour cell lines. Oncogene 1994, 9:707–18.
22. Sherr CJ. Cancer cell cycles. Science 1996, 274:1672–7.
23. Philipp-Staheli J, Payne SR, Kemp, CJ. P27(KIP1): Regulation and function of a haploinsufficient tumor suppressor and its misregulation in cancer. Exp Cell Res 2001, 264:148–68.
24. Takeuchi S et al. Allelotype analysis of childhood acute lymphoblastic leukemia. Cancer Res 1995, 55:5377–82.
25. Hatta Y et al. Ovarian cancer has frequent loss of heterozygosity at chromosome 12P12.3-13.1 (Region of TEL and KIP1 loci) and chromosome 12Q23-ter: Evidence for two new tumour-suppressor genes. Br J Cancer 1997, 75:1256–62.
26. Kibel AS et al. Deletion mapping at 12P12-13 in metastatic prostate cancer. Genes Chromosomes Cancer 1999, 25:270–6.
27. Slingerland J, Pagano, M. Regulation of the cdk inhibitor P27 and its deregulation in cancer. J Cell Physiol 2000, 183:10–7.
28. Coats S et al. Requirement of P27KIP1 for restriction point control of the fibroblast cell cycle. Science 1996, 272:877–80.
29. Guo Y et al. Loss of the cyclin-dependent kinase inhibitor P27(KIP1) protein in human prostate cancer correlates with tumor grade. Clin Cancer Res 1997, 3(Pt1):2269–74.
30. Cheville JC et al. Expression of P27KIP1 in prostatic adenocarcinoma. Mod Pathol 1998, 11:324–8.
31. Yang RM et al. Low P27 expression predicts poor disease-free survival in patients with prostate cancer. J Urol 1998, 159:941–5.
32. Tsihlias J, Kapusta L, Slingerland, J. The prognostic significance of altered cyclin-dependent kinase inhibitors in human cancer. Annu Rev Med 1999, 50:401–23.
33. Cordon-Cardo C et al. Distinct altered patterns of P27KIP1 gene expression in benign prostatic hyperplasia and prostatic carcinoma. J Natl Cancer Inst 1998, 90:1284–91.
34. Cote RJ et al. Association of P27KIP1 levels with recurrence and survival in patients with stage C prostate carcinoma. J Natl Cancer Inst 1998, 90:916–20.
35. De Marzo AM et al. Prostate stem cell compartments: Expression of the cell cycle inhibitor P27KIP1 in normal, hyperplastic, and neoplastic cells. Am J Pathol 1998, 153:911–9.
36. Huang S, Chen CS, Ingber, DE. Control of cyclin D1, P27(KIP1), and cell cycle progression in human capillary endothelial cells by cell shape and cytoskeletal tension. Mol Biol Cell 1998, 9:3179–93.
37. St Croix B et al. E-cadherin-dependent growth suppression is mediated by the cyclin-dependent kinase inhibitor P27(KIP1). J Cell Biol 1998, 142:557–71.
38. Levenberg S et al. P27 is involved in N-cadherin-mediated contact inhibition of cell growth and S-phase entry. Oncogene 1999, 18:869–76.
39. Lifuang L, Schulz H, Wolf, DA. The F-box protein SKP2 mediated androgen control of P27 stability in LNCaP human prostate cancer cells. BCM Cell Biol 2002, 3:22.
40. Liggett WH Jr, Sidransky, D. Role of the P16 tumor suppressor gene in cancer. J Clin Oncol 1998, 16:1197–206.
41. Jen J et al. Deletion of P16 and P15 genes in brain tumors. Cancer Res 1994, 54:6353–8.

42. Kamb A et al. Analysis of the P16 gene (CDKN2) as a candidate for the chromosome 9p melanoma susceptibility locus. Nat Genet 1994, 8:23–6.
43. Nobori T et al. Deletions of the cyclin-dependent kinase-4 inhibitor gene in multiple human cancers. Nature 1994, 368:753–6.
44. Jarrard DF et al. Deletional, mutational, and methylation analyses of CDKN2 (P16/MTS1) in primary and metastatic prostate cancer. Genes Chromosomes Cancer 1997, 19:90–6.
45. Steiner MS et al. Adenoviral vector containing wild-type P16 suppresses prostate cancer growth and prolongs survival by inducing cell senescence. Cancer Gene Ther 2000, 7:360–72.
46. Steiner MS et al. P16/MTS1/INK4A suppresses prostate cancer by both pRb dependent and independent pathways. Oncogene 2000, 19:1297–306.
47. McMenamin ME et al. Loss of PTEN expression in paraffin-embedded primary prostate cancer correlates with high gleason score and advanced stage. Cancer Res 1999, 59:4291–6.
48. Suzuki H et al. Interfocal heterogeneity of PTEN/MMAC1 gene alterations in multiple metastatic prostate cancer tissues. Cancer Res 1998, 58:204–9.
49. Wu X et al. The PTEN/MMAC1 tumor suppressor phosphatase functions as a negative regulator of the phosphoinositide 3-kinase/akt pathway. Proc Natl Acad Sci USA 1998, 95:15587–91.
50. Dong JT et al. PTEN/MMAC1 is infrequently mutated in pT2 and pT3 carcinomas of the prostate. Oncogene 1998, 17:1979–82.
51. Pesche S et al. PTEN/MMAC1/TEP1 involvement in primary prostate cancers. Oncogene 1998, 16:2879–83.
52. Vlietstra RJ et al. Frequent inactivation of PTEN in prostate cancer cell lines and xenografts. Cancer Res 1998, 58:2720–3.
53. Cairns P et al. Frequent inactivation of PTEN/MMAC1 in primary prostate cancer. Cancer Res 1997, 57:4997–5000.
54. Cheney IW et al. Suppression of tumorigenicity of glioblastoma cells by adenovirus-mediated MMAC1/PTEN gene transfer. Cancer Res 1998, 58:2331–4.
55. Furnari FB et al. Growth suppression of glioma cells by PTEN requires a functional phosphatase catalytic domain. Proc Natl Acad Sci USA 1997, 94:12479–84.
56. Davies MA et al. Adenoviral-mediated expression of MMAC/PTEN inhibits proliferation and metastasis of human prostate cancer cells. Clin Cancer Res 2002, 8:1904–14.
57. Koritschoner NP et al. A novel human zinc finger protein that interacts with the core promoter element of a TATA box-less gene. J Biol Chem 1997, 272:9573–80.
58. Ratziu V et al. ZF9, a kruppel-like transcription factor up-regulated in vivo during early hepatic fibrosis. Proc Natl Acad Sci USA 1998, 95:9500–5.
59. Suzuki T et al. Isolation and initial characterization of GBF, a novel DNA-binding zinc finger protein that binds to the GC-rich binding sites of the HIV-1 promoter. J Biochem (Tokyo) 1998, 124:389–95.
60. Narla G et al. KLF6, a candidate tumor suppressor gene mutated in prostate cancer. Science 2001, 294:2563–6.
61. Kim Y et al. Transcriptional activation of transforming growth factor beta1 and its receptors by the kruppel-like factor ZF9/core promoter-binding protein and SP1. Potential mechanisms for autocrine fibrogenesis in response to injury. J Biol Chem 1998, 273:33750–8.

62. Kojima S et al. Transcriptional activation of urokinase by the kruppel-like factor ZF9/COPEB activates latent TGF-beta1 in vascular endothelial cells. Blood 2000, 95:1309–16.
63. Rossi MC, Zetter, BR. Selective stimulation of prostatic carcinoma cell proliferation by transferrin. Proc Natl Acad Sci USA 1992, 89:6197–6201.
64. Smith RC et al. Identification of an endogenous inhibitor of prostatic carcinoma cell growth. Nat Med 1995, 1:1040–1045.
65. Heston WDW. Prostatic polyamines, polyamine targeting as a new approach to therapy of prostatic cancer. Cancer. Surv 1991, 11:217–238.
66. Coffino P. Regulation of cellular polyamines by antizyme. Nat Rev Mol Cell Biol 2001, 2:188–94.
67. Matsufuji S et al. Autoregulatory frameshifting in decoding mammalian ornithine decarboxylase antizyme. Cell 1995, 80:51–60.
68. Laitinen J et al. Polyamines MAY regulate S-phase progression but not the dynamic changes of chromatin during the cell cycle. J Cell Biochem 1998, 68:200–12.
69. Facchiano F et al. Transglutaminase activity is involved in polyamine-induced programmed cell death. Exp Cell Res 2001, 271:118–29.
70. Seiler N et al. Spermine cytotoxicity to human colon carcinoma-derived cells (CACO-2). Cell Biol Toxicol 2000, 16:117–30.
71. Stefanelli C et al. Polyamines directly induce release of cytochrome c from heart mitochondria. Biochem J 2000, 347 Pt 3:875–80.
72. Segal JA, Skolnick, P. Spermine-induced toxicity in cerebellar granule neurons is independent of its actions at NMDA receptors. J Neurochem 2000, 74:60–9.
73. Mohan RR et al. Overexpression of ornithine decarboxylase in prostate cancer and prostatic fluid in humans. Clin Cancer Res 1999, 5:143–7.
74. Gupta S et al. Chemoprevention of prostate carcinogenesis by alpha- difluoromethylornithine in TRAMP mice. Cancer Res 2000, 60:5125–33.
75. Auvinen M et al. Ornithine decarboxylase activity is critical for cell transformation. Nature 1992, 360:355–58.
76. Hibshoosh H, Johnson M, Weinstein, IB. effects of overexpression of ornithine decarboxylase (ODC) on growth control and oncogene-induced cell transformation. Oncogene 1991, 6:739–43.
77. Tabib A, Bachrach, U. Role of polyamines in mediating malignant transformation and oncogene expression. Int J Biochem Cell Biol 1999, 31:1289–95.
78. Murakami Y et al. Ornithine decarboxylase is degraded by the 26s proteosome without ubiquitination. Nature 1992, 360:597–99.
79. Rom E, Kahana, C. Polyamines regulate the expression of ornithine decarboxylase antizyme in vitro by inducing ribosomal frame-shifting. Proc Natl Acad Sci USA 1994, 91:3959–63.
80. Koike C, Chao DT, Zetter, BR. Sensitivity to polyamine-induced growth arrest correlates with antizyme induction in prostate carcinoma cells. Cancer Res 1999, 59: 6109–12.
81. Mitchell JL et al. Antizyme induction by polyamine analogues as a factor in cell growth inhibition. Biochem J 2002, 366:663–71.
82. Tsuji T et al. Induction of epithelial differentiation and DNA demethylation in hamster malignant oral keratinocyte by ornithine decarboxylase antizyme. Oncogene 2001, 20:24–33.

83. Murakami Y *et al*. Forced expression of antizyme abolishes ornithine decarboxylase activity, suppresses, cellular levels of polyamines and inhibits cell growth. Biochem. J 1994, 304:183–87.
84. Feith DJ, Shantz LM, Pegg, AE. Targeted antizyme expression in the skin of transgenic mice reduces tumor promoter induction of ornithine decarboxylase and decreases sensitivity to chemical carcinogenesis. Cancer Res 2001, 61:6073–81.
85. Tsuji T *et al*. Reduction of ornithine decarboxylase antizyme (ODC-az) level in the 7,12-dimethylbenz(a)anthracene-induced hamster buccal pouch carcinogenesis model. Oncogene 1998, 16:3379–85.

Chapter 7

EPITHELIAL-MESENCHYMAL MOLECULAR INTERACTIONS IN PROSTATIC TUMOR CELL PLASTICITY

Mary J.C. Hendrix[1,4], Jun Luo[5], Elisabeth A. Seftor [1,4], Navesh Sharma[1,6], Paul M. Heidger Jr.[1,4], Michael B. Cohen[2,4], Robert Bhatty[1], Jirapat Chungthapong[1], Richard E.B. Seftor[1,4] and David Lubaroff[3,4]

[1]*Departments of Anatomy and Cell Biology, University of Iowa, Iowa City, IA, USA*
[2]*Pathology, University of Iowa, Iowa City, IA, USA*
[3]*Urology, College of Medicine, University of Iowa, Iowa City, IA, USA*
[4]*The Holden Comprehensive Cancer Center, University of Iowa, Iowa City, IA, USA*
[5]*Brady Urological Institute, Johns Hopkins Medical Institutions, Baltimore, MD, USA*
[6]*University Health Sciences, College of Osteopathic Medicine, Kansas City, MO, USA*

Abstract: Tumor cell plasticity poses a significant clinical challenge in that the fate and function of tumor cells can be elusive until a tumor mass is evident. An overview of key molecular events in prostate cancer, initiated by an epithelial-to-mesenchymal transition, highlights the cooperative interactions of diverse prostatic subpopulations within heterogeneous tumors. A remarkable example of plasticity is demonstrated by subpopulations of E-cadherin-positive and E-cadherin-negative tumor cells working in concert to form *de novo* vasculogenic-like networks while expressing vascular-associated genes, called vasculogenic mimicry, resulting in acquisition of the metastatic phenotype. A better understanding of the molecular mechanisms underlying prostate tumor cell plasticity may provide new prognostic markers for clinical diagnosis and novel therapeutic intervention strategies for disease management.

Key words: prostate cancer, plasticity, E-cadherin, epithelial-mesenchymal transition

1. INTRODUCTION

Prostate cancer is the most commonly diagnosed type of cancer and the second-leading cause of cancer-related deaths in American men. With the advent of the prostate-specific antigen (PSA) test, the number of newly diagnosed cases reached 200,000 in 2000, accounting for over 35% of all cancers affecting men (1). Statistics also indicate that after lung cancer, prostate cancer is the leading cause of cancer-related deaths among men in the U.S., with an estimated 30,000 deaths each year. Most remarkably, post-mortem examination has found that as many as 30% of men over age 50 harbor microscopic foci of prostate cancer, indicating the extremely high prevalence of latent prostate cancer which is not detected clinically during the life span of men (2, 3, 4). Although early-staged prostatic tumors are relatively benign, a subset of these tumors progresses to become invasive, metastatic, and life-threatening cancers. Thus, understanding the molecular mechanisms underlying prostate cancer progression is crucial to the development of therapeutic strategies to manage this disease.

Tumor metastasis involves a series of sequential steps, which include the acquisition of cellular motility and invasiveness (for review, see 5). A crucial event in prostate cancer progression is the transition from the noninvasive to the invasive phenotype, demonstrated by the epithelial-to-mesenchymal transition (6-8). This transition involves a series of molecular alterations, resulting in altered cell-substrate attachment, decreased cell-cell adhesion, and increased cellular motility and invasive ability.

Another significant clinical challenge in the detection and management of prostate cancer is tumor cell plasticity, in that the fate and function of tumor cells can be elusive until a tumor mass is evident. A remarkable example of tumor cell plasticity has recently been described as vasculogenic mimicry in aggressive uveal and cutaneous melanoma (9–13), ovarian (14) breast carcinoma (15, 16), and prostate cancer (17). This new concept suggests that aggressive tumor cells can mimic vascular cell phenotypes, such as endothelial cells, and possibly perform vascular functions (13). These observations may provide new prognostic markers for tumor detection, clinical diagnosis and novel therapeutic intervention strategies.

1.1 Importance of E-Cadherin in Prostate Biology

The majority of diagnosed prostate cancer remains localized and never produces dramatic clinical symptoms, while a subset of these cancers (roughly 1 in 5) progress to invasive and metastatic cancers that are life threatening. One of the key features of invasive and metastatic prostate cancer, as well as other carcinomas, is the downregulation of E-cadherin expression – a cell adhesion molecule responsible for normal epithelial maintenance. E-cadherin (originally called uvomorulin, L-CAM, cell-CAM 120/80, or Arc-1) is a 120 kDa glycoprotein mediating Ca^{2+}-dependent homophilic cell-cell adhesion between epithelial cells (18–20). As illustrated in Figure 1, the extracellular domain of the E-cadherin molecule

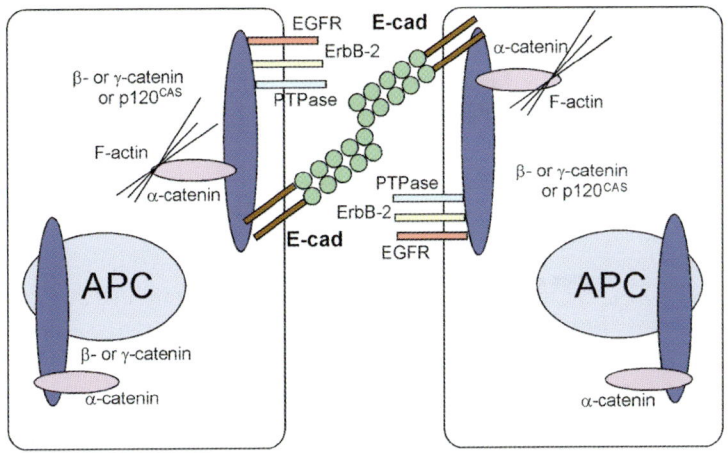

Figure 1. Molecules associated with the E-cadherin/catenin complex.

on the cell membrane binds to that of another molecule on the opposite membrane of another cell. Intracellularly, E-cadherin is linked to the cytoskeletal actin filaments through interactions with the catenins (α-, β-, γ-catenin/plakoglobin); (21). Interactions between E-cadherin and key cytoskeletal proteins through the catenins confer stability of the cell-cell adherens junctions. Disruption of these interactions results in the loss of cell adhesion and dissociation of epithelial sheets – the initiation of epithelial-mesenchymal molecular interactions. In fact, transgenic mice deficient in E-cadherin die *in utero* because of defective formation of the initial epithelium, the trophectoderm (22).

1.2 New Advances in the Dunning Rat Model for Prostate Cancer Biology

The field of prostate cancer research has been limited by the lack of reliable experimental models. Therefore, we devoted considerable effort to developing unique Dunning rat cancer cell lines that would allow the study of the heterogeneous components of prostate adenocarcinomas (23), using an integrated *in* vivo and *in* vitro experimental strategy (shown in Figure 2).

The heterogeneous tumor cell line R3327-5' arising from a subcutaneous injection of R3327-5, a cell line isolated from the original R3327 Copenhagen rat tumor, was generated and propagated in our laboratory. Cloning of individual populations from this heterogeneous cell line on a morphological basis yielded several homogeneous cell clones with different morphological,

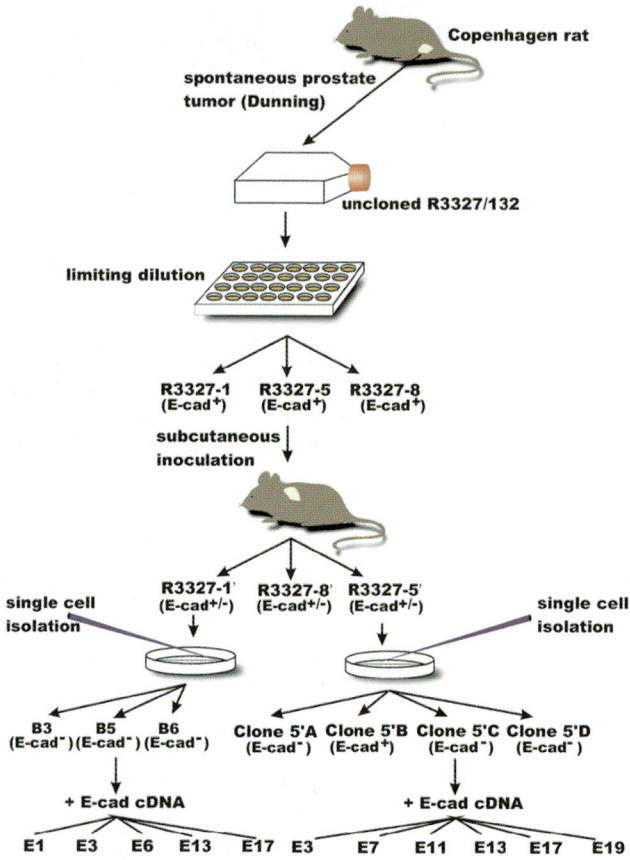

Figure 2. Experimental approach flow chart for the development of new Dunning rat cell lines. Cultured late passage cells from a spontaneous rat prostate tumor were cloned by a limiting dilution procedure. R3327-5, a poorly invasive E-cadherin-positive subline in vitro, was injected subcutaneously into the right flank of male Copenhagen rats. Single cells were cloned from the heterogeneous R3327-5' culture of the excised tumor to yield four morphologically distinct clones, which were subsequently assayed for differences in morphology, E-cadherin expression, and invasive and metastatic potential. In addition, select E-cadherin-negative clones were stably transfected with E-cadherin cDNA to yield several experimental cell clones.

tumorigenic, metastatic and invasive properties. The phenotypic characteristics distinguishing these subpopulations are demonstrated in Figure 3. R3327-5'B cells grow in clusters, are E-cadherin-positive, form large subcutaneous tumors but are poorly invasive and modestly metastatic compared with the R3327-5'A, R3327-5'C and R3327-5'D cells, which grow in individual fibroblast-like patterns, are E-cadherin-negative and are highly invasive and metastatic without being tumorigenic at subcutaneous injection sites.

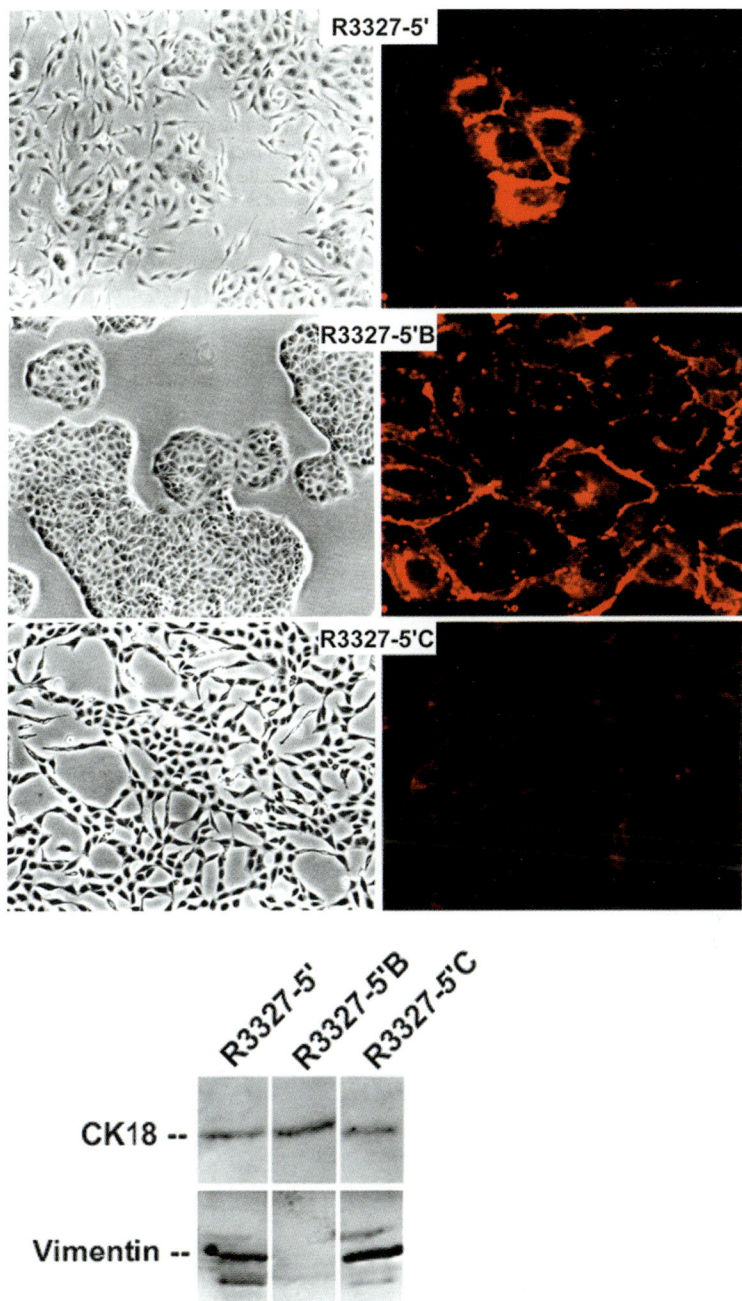

Figure 3. Left three panels show phase contrast, light micrographs of cell cultures: parental R3327-5'; and clones R3327-5'B and R3327-5'C. The cultures exhibited distinctive morphologies. Note the sparse, fibroblastic-like, spindle-shaped (continued on page 132)

Our previous studies utilizing these clones have shown differences in immunological response elicited by these tumor cells following inoculation into a syngeneic host (24). The parental cell lines and subpopulations were all cytokeratin positive; however, the fibroblastic-like subpopulation was vimentin-positive, while the E-cadherin-epithelial-like subpopulation was negative for the mesenchymal vimentin marker – indicating the phenotypic distinction between the two derivatives. Previous studies have shown the biological and clinical relevance of the coexpression of cytokeratin and vimentin intermediate filament proteins in several tumor types, including breast cancer and melanoma, which is indicative of an aggressive phenotype (25–28).

Although it is unlikely that E-cadherin is the sole determining factor for tumor invasion and metastasis, we have recently shown that E-cadherin plays a central role in reducing the cellular invasiveness of prostatic adenocarcinoma, due in part to the downregulation of matrix metalloproteinases-2 (MMP-2) activity (29), summarized in Table 1. These observations provide a direct connection between the re-expression of E-cadherin, a mesenchymal-to-epithelial phenotype transition, accompanied by changes in MMP activity – important biological targets for therapeutic intervention.

1.3   Prostatic Vasculogenic Mimicry

The recent observation of the cooperative interactions of the E-cadherin-positive (epithelial-like phenotype) and E-cadherin-negative (fibroblastic-like phenotype) subpopulations resulting in vasculogenic mimicry serve as an excellent example of prostatic plasticity – an epithelial-to-vascular phenotype transition (17), illustrated in Figure 4. In this study, Dunning rat R3327-5', R3327-5'A, R3327-5'B cells were assessed for their ability to form vasculogenic structures on 3-dimensional cultures of basement

Figure 3 (continued) cells mingled with epithelial-like, polygonal cells in the parental culture; the islands of closely adherent polygonal cells are the epithelial-like clone R3327-5'B; and the interlacing pattern of fibroblastic-like cells are characteristic of clone R3327-5'C cultures. (Magnification=220X). Right three panels show E-cadherin expression in cell cultures by immunofluorescence microscopy. Positive staining was only observed in R3327-5'B and in the epithelial clusters in the heterogeneous R3227-5' parental line. (Magnification=1400X). Western blot analysis, shown in the lowest right panel beneath the photomicrographs, demonstrated the presence of cytokeratin 18 (CK18) in all 3 cell lines tested, indicative of an epithelial marker. Vimentin, a mesenchymal marker, was found in the parental R3327-5' cells and in the fibroblastic-like R3327-5'C cells.

Table 1. Reduced invasive ability and MMP-2 activity in E-cadherin-transfected tumor cells

Cell Line	Invasive ability	MMP-2 activity
Clone5'C (sham)	20.1 ± 1.0^a	1.00^b
E7	6.8 ± 1.4	0.33
E11	6.7 ± 0.7	0.38
E13	6.6 ± 0.8	0.26
E19	6.0 ± 0.4	0.44

[a]Invasion is measured as the percentage of prostatic tumor cells capable of invading a basement membrane-coated polycarbonate membrane over 24 hours within a membrane invasion culture system (MICS) chamber compared with the total number of cells seeded (SE$\pm$; n = 6 wells per parameter and run in duplicate experiments). Clone 5'C (R3327-5'C) is an E-cadherin-negative Dunning cell clone that was stably transfected with E-cadherin cDNA and compared with the sham transfected control, as previously described [29]. Data from 4 of the experimental clones (E7, E11, E13 and E19) are presented.

[b]The zymograms were digitized and the area associated with the MMP-2 activity determined for each cell line and compared to the value for Clone 5'C (normalized to a value of 1.00).

membrane matrix (matrigel) or collagen I gels. Heterogeneous populations of rat parental R3327-5' cells formed vasculogenic-like tubular structures, which proceeded to anastomose, forming networks similar to embryonic vascular networks. Microscopic observations of the network evolution over three weeks revealed steady outgrowths which developed into tubular patterns interconnecting spheroidal nests of cells. Co-cultures of GFP-labeled R3327-5'B plus unlabeled R3327-5'A cells resulted in vasculogenic-like tubular networks identical in structure to those formed by the heterogeneous parental cell line, with the GFP-labeled R3327-5'B cells forming the tubular structures and the R3327-5'A cells forming the support background. Furthermore, microinjection of fluorescent dye into the tubular networks demonstrated that the dye followed the course of the vasculogenic-like networks, thus demonstrating the perfusability of the tubular networks. Most noteworthy was the finding that 3-D cultures of R3327-5'A and R3327-5'B, grown independently, did not yield vasculogenic-like networks until they were co-cultured to reflect the heterogeneous composition found in the parental R3327-5' cell line (17).

Scanning electron micrographs of the 3-D cultures demonstrated the presence of cell-lined tubular networks with widely varying lumenal diameters interconnecting nests of dense tumor cell clusters. Transmission electron microscopic analysis of these extending structures revealed that the tubular structures consisted of a lumen bound by tumor cells exhibiting a polarity

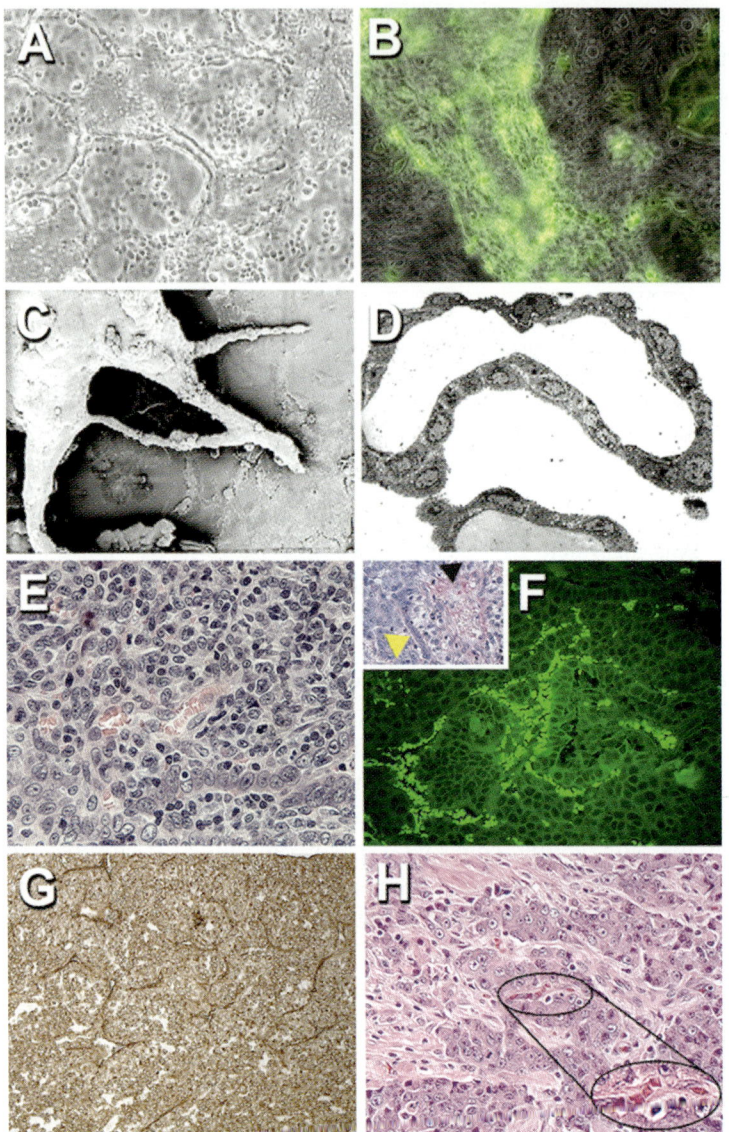

Figure 4. Microscopic demonstration of vasculogenic mimicry by rat prostatic tumor cells on 3-D matrices in culture and *in situ*. Phase and fluorescence microscopy of in vitro tubular network formation by the rat heterogeneous cancer cell line R3327-5' (A) and a co-culture of R3327-5'A with GFP-labeled R3327-5'B cells (B). Scanning electron microscopy (SEM; C) and transmission electron microscopy (TEM; D) micrographs of R3327-5' cells grown on a 3-D matrix. SEM shows the presence of tubular, cell-lined extensions or protrusions from a cluster of tumor cells (C), while TEM shows the presence of lumen within the tubular, cell-lined extensions (D). Evidence for putative *in vivo* vasculogenic mimicry following injection of Dunning tumor cells into Copenhagen rats is shown in E, F and G.

reversed from that expected in glandular epithelium. Polarized tumor cells were arranged with their basal aspects toward the tubular lumen and their microvillous apical surfaces toward the exterior. The lining cells were connected by desmosomal junctions on the outer aspect of the tubular wall, forming tubular, blood vessel-like structures.

In the *in vivo* studies, circumstantial evidence was presented in support of *in situ* vasculogenic mimicry by the presence of tumor cell-lined, erythrocyte-containing channels within rat tumors and various grades of human prostatic adenocarcinoma. Rat tumors arising from s.c. injection of the Dunning R3327-5' cell line into shoulder flanks averaged 15–20 mm in diameter and exhibited little-to-no necrosis. Several of the tumor-lined channels could be seen in the vicinity of conventional endothelial-cell lined vasculature. Presence of plasma and erythrocytes in rouleaux formation within many of these channels was clearly revealed using short wavelength fluorescence. Localization of laminin within the tumors arising from the injection of Dunning R3327-5' cells into nude mice demonstrated laminin-stained channels in regions of high vascularity (*i.e.*, erythrocytes) between clusters of laminin-positive prostatic tumor cells. In addition, eighteen histological sections of low and high grade human prostatic adenocarcinoma were examined for the presence of erythrocyte-containing channels or spaces. There was little-to-no evidence of tumor-lined channels in Gleason grades 2, 3 and 4 tumors. However, Gleason grade 5 tumors revealed some tumor-lined channels containing erythrocytes in rouleaux formation. Endothelial-lined blood vessels were identified in all cases, regardless of disease severity.

A multi-probe ribonuclease protection assay was used to characterize the expression of a series of vascular-associated markers by the Dunning rat prostate cancer cells. All of the cell lines assessed expressed at least some of

◄─────────────────

Figure 4. (continued) Subcutaneously (s.c.)injected R3327-5' tumor cells generated large tumors with little-to-no necrosis. Microscopic study of the tumors using brightfield (E and F, inset) and short wavelength fluorescence (F) to highlight erythrocyte containing spaces, revealed the presence of tumor cell-lined channels containing erythrocytes in rouleaux formation and plasma. These tumor cell-lined channels (yellow arrowhead) often occurred in close proximity to traditional endothelial-lined vessels (black arrowhead; F, inset). Localization of laminin expression in s.c. tumors arising from injection of R3327-5' cells into nude mice revealed the presence of laminin stained networks between clusters of laminin-positive tumor cells (G). While the presence of conventional endothelial-lined vasculature was predominantly seen in histopathological sections of human prostatic adenocarcinoma tumors from Gleason grades 2 to 4, erythrocyte containing tumor cell-lined channels were observed in Gleason grade 5 tumors (H). Original magnifications, X 100 (A), X 200 (B, F and F inset), X 300 (C), X 2250 (D), X 630 (E), X 400 (G and H).

the markers to varying degrees. Specifically, the results demonstrated that TIE-1, thrombin-receptor, TIE-2, CD-31, endoglin, angiopoietin, and VEGF were expressed by R3327-5'B cells, whereas endoglin, angiopoietin and VEGF were expressed at the message level by R3327-5'A and R3327-5'C cells at varying levels, as summarized in Table 2.

The recent prostatic vasculogenic mimicry findings lend further credence to previous reports on melanoma, breast and ovarian cancers showing vasculogenic-like networks formed by tumor cells *in vitro* and tumor cell-lined channels *in vivo* (9–17), which may account for a subcategory of highly aggressive, non-angiogenic tumors. *In situ*, the presence of tumor cell-lined channels containing erythrocytes in rouleaux formation (not random leakage from vasculature) or just plasma was confirmed in advanced rat and human prostatic adenocarcinoma, and may represent a potential alternative mode of dissemination and possibly tumor perfusion. Recent studies by Shirakawa and colleagues (16) have demonstrated unique hemodynamic imaging associated with vasculogenic mimicry in aggressive inflammatory breast cancer. This is the first study to provide experimental evidence characterizing the microcirculatory differences between angiogenesis and vasculogenesis in a cancer model. The molecular underpinnings of the vascular phenotype observed in various tumor models is slowly becoming elucidated through various molecular analyses. Studies with melanoma, ovarian and breast carcinoma, and most recently prostate cancer, are collectively revealing the expression of multiple molecular phenotypes by the aggressive tumor cells indicative of a genetically deregulated genotype, similar to an embryonic phenotype (9–15, 17, 30, 31). Interestingly, the formation of a microcirculation in the absence of endothelial cells has been observed in normal embryonic tissue. Adoption of an endothelial phenotype by cytotrophoblasts, including the expression of vascular markers, as they participate in the establishment of the human placenta and primordial circulation has been reported

Table 2. Expression of vascular/angiogenic markers by rat prostatic tumor cells

Cells	TIE-1	Thrombin Receptor	TIE-2	CD31	Endoglin	Angio-poietin	VEGF
R3327-5'A	$-^a$	−	−	−	++	+	+++
R3327-5'B	++	++	+	+	++	++	++
R3327-5'C	−	±	−	−	++	+	+++

[a] The amount of RNAse-protected mRNA was determined by digitizing the exposed film and determining the area of the markers that were then ranked from + → +++ relative to the most abundantly expressed mRNA (VEGF).

(32–34), which indicates the ability of more differentiated cells to perform embryonic vasculogenic-like functions (called pseudovasculogenesis).

Indeed, the intriguing differences in the expression of vascular genes, such that the R3327-5'B cells expressed more of an endothelial phenotype while the R3327-5'A cells produced higher levels of VEGF, may suggest important changes in the heterogeneous tumor phenotype as it evolves from a less aggressive state to a more aggressive state. These results strongly support the contention that cooperativity of multiple cell phenotypes is necessary for successful prostatic tumor development.

2. CONCLUSIONS

A hypothetical model depicting prostate tumor cell plasticity is illustrated in Figure 5, based on the interpretation of data derived from *in vitro* and *in vivo* models of prostatic adenocarcinoma. The importance of E-cadherin in maintaining the integrity of the epithelial phenotype is well known, and its transient downregulation coincides with observations of epithelial-to-mesenchymal transition. What is not well understood is the molecular trigger that catalyzes this event leading to sequential steps in the metastatic cascade, including acquisition of the invasive/aggressive phenotype involving the coordinate regulation of MMP activity and the initiation of remodeling the tumor microenvironment. The molecular signals involved in the dynamic reciprocity between the tumor cells and their microenvironment are the focus of intense investigation, and these studies are key to the development of new therapeutic strategies. The heterogeneity of prostatic adenocarcinomas poses an experimental challenge as well as an opportunity for experimental manipulation. Our investigative team has attempted to address this challenge by isolating distinct subpopulations of tumor cells with fibroblastic and epithelial phenotypes. The data indicate that these subpopulations cooperate to engage in vasculogenic mimicry, in which the epithelial-like subpopulation expressesendothelial/vascular-associated molecules, and the fibroblastic-like subpopulation expresses vascular-stimulating growth factors. It is tempting to speculate that these tumor cells have the potential to revert to an embryonic-like phenotype, based on their *de novo* formation of primitive vasculogenic-like networks reminiscent of embryologic events. However, the biological significance of this observation remains to be elucidated. In this regard, further ambiguity may result from studies attempting to document the increase in microvascularity with a corresponding increase in tumor burden and severity, in which the results have been somewhat perplexing and inconclusive. A contributing factor to

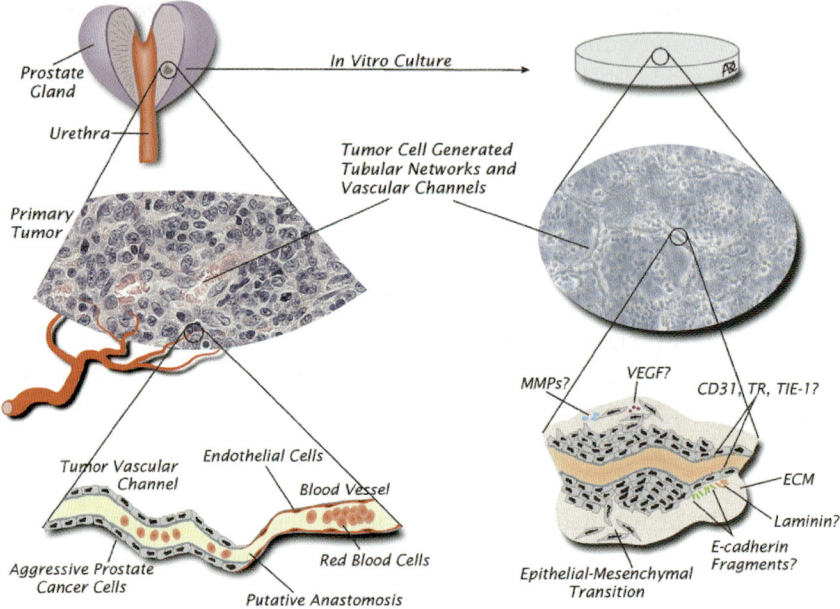

Figure 5. Hypothetical model for prostate tumor cell plasticity, including epithelial-mesenchymal molecular transition and embryonic-like vasculogenic mimicry by aggressive heterogeneous prostatic tumor cells. Synergistic biomechanical and molecular interactions of individual components in a primary, heterogeneous tumor result in the formation of tumor-lined, channel-like structures. These occur within the tumor (shown containing erythrocytes in rouleaux formation) in the vicinity of endothelial-lined vasculature. This phenomenon is observed in 3-D cultures *in vitro* where perfusable tumor cell-lined tubular networks connecting spheroids of tumor cells express laminin in addition to vascular-associated genes.

these mixed results has been the reliance on conventional endothelial and other vascular markers to identify tumor neovasculature (35) and tendency to ignore the staining of tumor-lined structures whose presence was hitherto unexplained. Our results suggest that a growing tumor mass may contain tumor-cell lined channels which express vascular markers that would stain for typical endothelial markers, in addition to conventional endothelial-lined vasculature. Whether this observation reflects vessel co-option, mosaic vasculature (tumor and endothelial cells; (36)), or putative anastomosis between tumor- and endothelial-lined vasculature remains enigmatic, and will require more precise tools of investigation. Also, investigations addressing the potential clinical relevance of tumor cell-lined vasculature are critical to our understanding of their significance. The field of tumor vascularization is rapidly evolving, and offers ample opportunity for new insights

(37). For example, recent observations showing aggressive melanoma cells forming new vasculature in ischemic tissues uniquely demonstrated the importance of the microenvironment in cell fate determination (13). Similar experimental approaches are encouraged in prostate cancer research to explore the extent of tumor cell plasticity and its profound ramifications, particularly with respect to detection, diagnosis and management.

ACKNOWLEDGEMENTS

This research has been supported by grants from the National Cancer Institute CA88043 and the Wallace Research Foundation. The authors gratefully acknowledge Dr. Dawn Kirschmann for her artistic contributions, and Katherine Walters of the University of Iowa Central Microscopy Research Facility for her electron microscopic expertise.

REFERENCES

1. Greenlee RT, Murray T, Bolden S, Wingo PA. Cancer statistics, 2000. CA Cancer J Clin 2000, 50:7–33.
2. Guileyardo JM, Johnson WD, Welsh RA, Akazaki K, Correa P. Prevalence of latent prostate carcinoma in two U.S. populations. J Natl Cancer Inst 1980, 65:311–16.
3. Sakr WA, Haas GP, Cassin BF, Pontes JE, Crissman JD. The frequency of carcinoma and intraepithelial neoplasia of the prostate in young male patients. J Urol 1993, 150:379–85.
4. Sakr WA, Haas GP, Grignon DJ, Crissman JD, Heilbrun LK, Cassin BJ et al. High grade prostatic intraepithelial neoplasia and prostatic adenocarcinoma between the ages of 20-69. An autopsy study of 249 cases. In Vivo 1994, 8:439–44.
5. Tímár J, Csuka O, Orosz Z, Jeney A, Kopper L. Molecular pathology of tumor metastasis. I. Predictive pathology. Pathol Oncol Res 2001, 7:217–30.
6. Bracke ME, Van Roy FM, Mareel MM. The E-cadherin/catenin complex in invasion, metastasis. Curr Top Microbiol Immunol 1996, 231:123–61.
7. Smith MEF, Pignatelli M. The molecular histology of neoplasia: The role of the cadherin/catenin complex. Histopathology 1997, 31:107–11.
8. Paul R, Ewing CM, Jarrard DF, Isaacs WB. The cadherin cell-cell adhesion pathway in prostate cancer progression. Br J Urol 1997, 79(s):37–43.
9. Maniotis AJ, Folberg R, Hess A, Seftor EA, Gardner LMG, Pe'er J et al. Vascular channel formation by human melanoma cells in vivo and in vitro: Vasculogenic mimicry. Am J Pathol 1999, 155:739–52.
10. Hess AR, Seftor EA, Gardner LMG, Carles-Kinch K, Schneider GB, Seftor REB et al. Molecular regulation of tumor cell vasculogenic mimicry by tyrosine phosphorylation: Role of epithelial cell kinase (ech/EPHA2). Cancer Res 2001, 61:3250–5.
11. Seftor REB, Seftor EA, Koshikawa N, Meltzer PS, Gardner LMG, Bilban M et al. Cooperative interactions of laminin 5 (2 chain, matrix metalloproteinase-2, and

membrane type-1/metalloproteinase are required for mimicry of embryonic vasculogenesis by aggressive melanoma. Cancer Res 2001, 61:6322–7.
12. Hendrix MJC, Seftor EA, Meltzer PS, Gardner LMG, Hess AR, Kirschmann DA et al. Expression and functional significance of VE-cadherin in aggressive human melanoma cells: Role in vasculogenic mimicry. Proc Natl Acad Sci USA 2001, 98:8018–23.
13. Hendrix MJC, Seftor REB, Seftor EA, Gruman LM, Lee LML, Nickoloff BJ et al. Transendothelial function of human metastatic melanoma cells: Role of the microenvironment in cell-fate determination. Cancer Res 2002, 22:3333-333.
14. Sood AK, Seftor EA, Fletcher MS, Gardner LMG, Heidger PM Jr, Buller RE et al. Molecular determinants of ovarian cancer plasticity. Am J Pathol 2001, 158:1279–88.
15. Hendrix MJC, Seftor EA, Kirschmann DA, Seftor REB. Molecular biology of breast cancer metastasis: Molecular expression of vascular markers by aggressive breast cancer cells. Breast Cancer Res 2000, 2:417–22.
16. Shirakawa K, Kobayashi H, Heike Y, Kawamoto S, Brechbiel MW, Kasumi F et al. Hemodynamics in vasculogenic mimicry and angiogenesis of inflammatory breast cancer xenografts. Cancer Res 2002, 62:560–6.
17. Sharma N, Seftor REB, Seftor EA, Gruman LM, Heidger PM Jr, Cohen MB et al. Prostatic tumor cell plasticity involves cooperative interactions of distinct phenotypic subpopulations: Role in vasculogenic mimicry. Prostate 2002, 50:189–201.
18. Edelman GM, Crossin KL. Cell adhesion molecules: Implications for a molecular histology. Annu Rev Biochem 1991, 60:155–90.
19. Holtfreter J, Townes PL. Directed movements and selective adhesion of embryonic amphibian cells. J Exp Zool 1955, 128:53–120.
20. Suzuki ST. Structural and functional diversity of cadherin superfamily: Are new members of cadherin superfamily involved in signal transduction pathway. J Cell Biochem 1996, 61:531–42.
21. Kelmer R. From cadherins to catenins: Cytoplasmic protein interactions and regulation of cell adhesion. Trends Genet 1993, 9:317–21.
22. Larue L, Ohsugi M, Hirchenhain J, Kemler R. E-cadherin null mutant embryos fail to form a trophectoderm epithelium. Proc Natl Acad Sci USA 1994, 91:8262–7.
23. Luo J, Sharma N, Seftor EA, De Larco J, Heidger PM, Hendrix MJC, Lubaroff DM. Heterogeneous expression of invasive and metastatic properties in a prostate tumor model. Pathol Oncol Res 1997, 3:264–71.
24. Sharma N, Luo J, Kirschmann DA, O'Malley Y, Robbins MEC, Akporiaye ET et al. A novel immunological model for the study of prostate cancer. Cancer Res 1999, 59:2271–6.
25. Hendrix MJC, Seftor EA, Seftor REB, Trevor KT. Experimental co-expression of vimentin and keratin intermediate filaments in human breast cancer cells results in phenotypic interconversion and increased invasive behavior. Am J Pathol 1997, 150:483–95.
26. Hendrix MJC, Seftor EA, Chu YW, Trevor KT, Seftor REB. Role of intermediate filaments in migration, invasion and metastasis. Cancer Metastas Rev 1997, 15:507–25.
27. Thomas PA, Kirschmann DA, Cerhan JR, Folberg R, Seftor EA, Sellers TA, Hendrix MJC. Association between keratin and vimentin expression, malignant phenotype, and survival in postmenopausal breast cancer patients. Clin Cancer Res 1999, 5:2698–703.

28. Hendrix MJC, Seftor EA, Seftor REB, Gardner LM, Boldt HC, Meyer M *et al.* Biologic determinants of uveal melanoma metastatic phenotype: Role of intermediate filaments as predictive markers. Lab Invest 1998, 78:153–63.
29. Luo J, Lubaroff DM, Hendrix MJC. Suppression of prostate cancer invasive potential and matrix metalloproteinase activity by E-cadherin transfection. Cancer Res 1999, 59:3552–6.
30. Bittner M, Meltzer P, Chen Y, Jiang Y, Seftor E, Hendrix M *et al.* Molecular classification of cutaneous malignant melanoma by gene expression profiling. Nature 2000, 406:536–40.
31. Sood AK, Fletcher MS, Hendrix MJC. The embryonic-like properties of aggressive human tumor cells. J Soc Gynecol Invest 2002, 9:2–9.
32. Damsky CH, Fisher SJ. Trophoblast pseudo-vasculogenesis: Faking it with endothelial adhesion receptors. Curr Opin Cell Biol 1998, 10:660–6.
33. Zhou Y, Damsky CH, Fisher SJ. Preeclampsia is associated with failure of human cytotrophoblasts to mimic a vascular adhesion phenotype. One cause of defective endovascular invasion in this syndrome. J Clin Invest 1997, 99:2152–64.
34. Zhou Y, Fisher SJ, Janatpour M, Benbacev O, Dejana E, Wheelock M, Damsky CH. Human cytotrophoblasts adopt a vascular phenotype as they differentiate. A strategy for successful endovascular invasion. J Clin Invest 1997, 99:2139–51.
35. Fregene TA, Khanuja PS, Noto AC, Gehani SK, Van Egmont EM, Luz DA, Pienta KJ. Tumor-associated angiogenesis in prostate cancer. Anticancer Res 1993, 13:2377–81.
36. Chang YS, diTomaso E, McDonald DM, Jones R, Jain RK, Munn LL. Mosaic blood vessels in tumors: Frequency of cancer cells in contact with flowing blood. Proc Natl Acad Sci USA 2000, 97:14608–13.
37. Klausner RD. Commentary: The fabric of cancer cell biology - weaving together the strands. Cancer Cell 2002, 1:3–1.

Chapter 8

ORTHOTOPIC METASTATIC MOUSE MODELS OF PROSTATE CANCER

Robert M. Hoffman
Department of Surgery, UCSD Medical Center, San Diego, CA, USA and AntiCancer, Inc., San Diego, CA, USA

Abstract: Orthotopic metastatic models of prostate cancer are reviewed here. Emphasis is placed on surgical orthotopic implantation models in nude mice. The advantages of surgical orthotopic implantation of tissue fragments are discussed with regard to resulting metastasis which reflect the clinical pattern of prostate cancer. The use of green fluorescent protein and red fluorescent protein to image primary tumor growth and metastasis, including whole-body imaging of prostate cancer, is discussed. The application of the models for gene expression studies, drug discovery, and gene therapy is also reviewed.

Key words: prostate cancer cell lines, surgical orthotopic implantation, green fluorescent protein, red fluorescent protein, whole-body imaging, metastasis, drug discovery

1. BACKGROUND OF METASTATIC ANIMAL MODELS OF PROSTATE CANCER

Prostate cancer is the most frequently occurring tumor in men and is the second leading cause of male death in the United States, accounting for about 30,000 deaths per year in the U.S. (1). Huggins and Hodges (2) observed the androgen dependence of prostatic carcinoma growth, and since that time androgen ablation has been an important feature of therapy for prostate carcinoma. However, for prostate carcinomas that have become hormone-independent, there is no effective systemic treatment (3).

A clinical report of over 600 patients suffering from stage D2 prostate cancer indicated an overall mean survival of 36 months in patients treated with combined androgen blockade (4). At the time of initial presentation, approximately 30–50% of prostate cancer patients have evidence of metastatic disease (5). The mechanism controlling prostate cancer progression and effective therapeutic strategies for metastatic prostate cancer are poorly understood. This is in part due to the lack of a suitable animal model that can mimic the clinical patterns of human prostate cancer growth and metastasis (6).

Prostate cancer occurs in a high percentage of men over 50 but is aggressive in only a small percentage of patients. It is, therefore, also necessary to develop models and markers to distinguish aggressive from non-aggressive tumors, and responsive from non-responsive ones, in order to make proper treatment decisions (7) and to develop new treatment strategies (3).

Nonhuman mammals have very rare incidence of prostate cancer (8), which limit the possibilities of using nonhuman mammal models to study human prostate cancer. With the first introduction of immunodeficient rodents in cancer research in the late 1960s (9, 10), xenografted human cancer models are now widely used. The inability to reject many of the xenografts implanted in these animals due to defect(s) in their immune system make them the only known tool for studying *in vivo* human cancer growth and metastasis outside the human body (6, 9, 10).

A number of cell lines from human prostatic carcinoma that grow in athymic nude mice (SCID), including LNCaP which is androgen-dependent (11), and the androgen-independent cell lines DU-145 (12) and PC-3 (13, 14) have been isolated (3). The Dunning R-3327 hormone-dependent rat prostatic adenocarcinoma has also been developed (15).

Experimental *in vivo* growth of human prostate carcinoma lines has usually followed subcutaneous (sc) transplantation, with occasional metastatic activity, as first observed by Ware et al. (16). Ware et al. (17) were the first to demonstrate that differential injection sites affected the behavior of PC-3. Intrasplenic injection (18) resulted in metastatic activity. The PC-3 line originated from a bone metastasis (4). When PC-3 was injected into the tail vein of the nude mice while the inferior cava was occluded, tumor growth in the lumbar vertebrae, pelvis, and femurs occurred (19). When PC-3 cells were injected into the peritoneal cavity, intra-abdominal growth resulted; when injected into the spleen, liver metastases resulted and when injected into the seminal vesicles, large tumors developed from there (20), when injected intracardiacly, bone metastasis could also result (19, 20, 21).

LNCaP is a cell line derived from a supraclavicular lymph node metastasis of human prostate carcinoma. LNCaP exhibits increased proliferation in response to androgens. When LNCaP cells were mixed with the reconstituted basement membrane matrigel and injected sc in nude mice, tumors grew in the mice by 12 weeks without observed metastases (22).

More realistic models of human cancer can be constructed through orthotopic transplantation of the human tumor to the animal host (23). Subsequent studies in a number of laboratories have shown that orthotopic injection of human tumor cells in immunodeficient mice can produce relevant metastatic patterns in comparison to ectopic transplantation (24–30).

The tumorigenicity and the incidence of metastasis of LNCaP after orthotopic (intraprostate) or sc injection in male nude mice were compared by Stephenson et al. (31). LNCaP cells produced tumors only when orthotopically implanted in the prostate. Viewig et al. (32) showed that orthotopic implantation of the rat R3327-MatLyLu prostate adenocarcinoma in in Copenhagen rats resulted in tumor growth in the prostate and metastasis to pelvic and retroperitoneal lymph nodes and lung.

In a subsequent study by Pettaway et al. (33), 56% of nude mice. injected orthotopically with a suspension of LNCaP cells formed prostate tumors. Twelve of 43 mice had microscopic metastases in the regional lymph nodes.

In another study, orthotopic injection of LNCaP in nude mice resulted in local growth in 7 of 10, and lymph node metastasis in 4 of 10 nude mice (34).

Hormone-independent cell lines (PC-3, PC-3-125-IL, and TSU-Pr1) were highly tumorigenic and had a higher rate of lymph node metastasis after orthotopic injection than after sc implantation. PC-3 cell lines consistently metastasized to the lungs (34).

Nude and SCID mice were injected either sc or orthotopically with LNCaP cell suspensions in a comparative study by Sato et al. (35). LNCaP tumor incidence after sc injection was 100% in SCID mice and 80% in nude mice. No lymph node or distant metastases were observed with sc tumors. After orthotopic injection in SCID and nude mice retroperitoneal or mediastinal lymph node metastases were found in 100% of SCID mice, and microscopic pulmonary metastases were identified in 40%. The nude mice had retroperitoneal lymph node metastasis in 25% of the animals but no other metastasis was found.

Thalmann et al. (36) reported a spontaneous bone metastasis model of androgen-independent human prostate cancer LNCaP derived sublines. The animals developed bone metastasis in 10% and 21.5% of intact and castrated hosts, respectively, after orthotopic injection of cell suspensions. These results provided some useful information to recognize the biological behavior of prostate cancer.

Transrectal ultrasonography (TRUS) was used to monitor mouse orthotopic prostate tumors. Orthotopic tumors were initiated by inoculation of RM-9 murine prostate cancer cells into the dorsal prostate of C57BL/6 male mice. By ultrasound, tumors became detectable 7 days after tumor cell inoculation. The tumor volume calculated by TRUS correlated significantly with the actual tumor weight measured at autopsy. Similarly, tumor growth suppression induced by cis-diamminedichloroplatinum (CDDP) was detected by TRUS with reasonable accuracy (37).

Injection of tumor cells into the prostate gland of nude mice, however, requires delicate, hard-to-control technical conditions, and spillage outside the prostate may generate rather variable results. Furthermore, some studies showed that artificial dissemination rather than spontaneous metastasis might occur following tumor cell injection, even when cells were not directly injected into the vasculature (38–40). It has been shown that tumor cells can enter the draining lymph or blood circulation within 10 minutes to 3 hours of injection, which will eventually form distant artificial metastases (41, 42). Most importantly, a cell suspension lacks tissue architecture, which seems critical for the full expression of the spontaneous metastatic potential of the transplanted human tumors.

Previous studies showed that the proliferation of tumor cells implanted in nude mice was preceded by the penetration of host stromal cells into the tumor (43, 44). Based on this important role of stroma in tumor growth, some investigators coinjected cultured fibroblasts with tumor cells and observed significant, growth-stimulating effects (45–47). Also, many studies demonstrated enhanced growth of tumor cells following co-injection of Matrigel (48–51), an extract of basement membrane components, which primarily consists of laminin, collagen IV and heparan sulfate proteoglycan (52). Current concepts suggest that Matrigel serves as a supportive matrix for the tumor cells. It collects tumor cells, allows paracrine factors to take effect, activates the release of angiogenic factors and stimulates the production of proteases and motility of tumor cells, thus facilitating growth and progression (53, 54).

We have developed surgical orthotopic-implantation (SOI) techniques utilizing histologically intact tissue, including surgical specimens, to develop metastatic models in immunodeficient mice for most types of human cancer including colon cancer (55, 56), human bladder cancer (57, 58), human lung cancer (59–62), and human pancreatic cancer (63). Surgical orthotopic implantation of histologically intact tumor tissue maintains the overall tissue architecture during implantation.

The histologically intact tumor tissue used in SOI possesses a large amount of supportive stromal cells, which are essential for maintaining the three-dimensional tumor architecture. The tissue architecture is believed to contribute to the difference in metastatic expression resulting from SOI and orthotopic injection of tumor cell suspensions, which have no three-dimensional architecture.

For all cancer types tested, intact-tissue orthotopic transplantation resulted in greater metastatic expression than orthotopic transplantation of cell suspensions (3, 55, 57, 58, 63–67).

We demonstrated orthotopic growth of prostate cancer line PC-3 with subsequent lymph node metastases by using the SOI technique (3). In a subsequent study, a large series of animals was implanted with PC-3 by improved SOI techniques (6). The patterns of growth and metastasis represented clinical prostate cancer. The advantages of this model for the study of prostate cancer and the possible mechanisms that underlie them are discussed below.

The early stages of tumor progression and micrometastasis formation have been difficult to visualize in current models due to the inability to identify small number of tumor cells against a background of many host tissues. We have developed new models of human and animal cancer by transfer of the *Aequorea victoria* jellyfish green fluorescent protein (GFP) gene to tumor cells that enabled visualization of fluorescent tumors and metastases at the microscopic level in fresh viable tissue and *in vivo* after transplantation (68–73), including prostate cancer (74). These models are discussed below.

2. DESCRIPTION OF METASTATIC PROSTATE CANCER MODELS

2.1 Orthotopic Models Implanted with Tumor-Cell Suspensions

Stephenson et al. (31), as mentioned above, reported lymph node metastasis but no lung metastasis of PC-3 after orthotopic injection of cell suspension in nude mice.

The tumorigenicity of and the incidence of metastasis of human prostate cancer PC-3M and LNCaP-FGC (LNCaP) cell lines subsequent to prostatic (orthotopic) or sc (ectopic) implantations in male nude mice was also determined (31). LNCaP cells produced tumors only in the prostate. Enhanced tumorigenicity at the orthotopic site was found for PC-3M cells, but not partental PC-3. Lymph node metastases were observed in practically all mice given an injection of PC-3M cells in the prostate, but they were uncommon with sc injection of these cells. LNCaP tumors in the mouse prostate (but not PC-3M tumors) produced detectable levels of human prostate-specific antigen (PSA) in the serum, even when tumors were small (1.5 mm in diameter). Immunohistochemistry analysis demonstrated the presence of the PSA marker in tissue sections of LNCaP but not of PC-3M tumors (31).

Previous studies have shown, as mentioned above, that the injected tumor cells may enter the lymphatic stream very shortly after injection (38–42). Therefore, the metastasis observed may be due to artificial dissemination.

Shevrin et al. (20) demonstrated lung metastasis of PC-3 cells, but this was achieved by injecting tumor cells directly into the tail vein of the nude mice, in which several steps of the metastatic process that naturally occur in patients were bypassed (75–77). Waters et al. (78) reported rather high lung metastasis of PC-3 cells after urinary bladder wall injection of cell suspensions. However, they concluded, on the other hand, that lung metastasis of PC-3 from orthotopic tumor cell injection was infrequent (1 of 10 mice).

Pettaway et al. (33) demonstrated that cells derived from the metastatic lesions of the orthotopically injected parental line of LNCaP, became increasingly metastatic after multiple selection cycles of orthotopic injection, subsequent isolation of metastatic cells and orthotopic reinjection. Even so, after a number of cycles of selection LNCaP still did not metastasize to the lung from the orthotopic site. Lung metastasis was only achieved by iv injection of the selected metastatic cells. Variants with increasing metastatic potential of PC-3M and LNCaP cells were selected by injection into the prostates of athymic mice. Tumors from the prostate or lymph nodes were harvested, and cells were reinjected into the prostate. This cycle was repeated three to five times to yield cell lines PC-3M-Pro4, PC-3M-LN4, LNCaP-Pro3-5, and LNCaP-LN3-4. Parental and variant cells were injected into the prostates of nude mice. PC-3M-LN4 cells produced enhanced regional lymph node and distant organ metastasis as compared to PC-3M-Pro4 or PC-3M cells. Orthotopically implantated LNCaP-LN3 cells produced a higher incidence of regional lymph node metastases than LNCaP-Pro5 or LNCaP cells. The metastatic LNCaP-LN3 cells exhibited clonal karyotypic abnormalities, were less sensitive to androgen (*in vitro* and *in vivo*), and produced high levels of PSA (33).

Histopathologic evidence from a murine prostate gland into which SP 3031 human prostate cancer cells had been injected indicated dysplastic glandular epithelium and carcinomatous areas. The human prostate tumors transformed host organ cells, with specific chromosomal alterations that may be associated with transformation (79).

Murine prostate cell lines were evaluated for growth and metastasis in orthotopic (dorso-lateral prostate) locations. Orthotopic tumors produced by cell lines derived from metastatic lesions tended to grow less rapidly but demonstrated greater spontaneous metastatic potential than the cell lines derived from primary tumors (80).

2.2 Surgical Orthotopic Implantation (SOI) of PC-3 in the Nude Mouse Prostate

The hormone-independent human prostate cancer line PC-3 was SOI as intact tissue which was harvested from nude-mouse sc -growing tissue (3). The orthotopic transplantation resulted in local growth and metastasis to the bladder and kidney, as well as distant metastasis to the inguinal, iliac, and mediastinal lymph nodes. Hydronephrosis was observed due to urinary blockage by the locally-growing tumor. The human genomic probe demonstrated by in situ hybridization that the tumors were of human origin showing a positive hybridization stain for the tumor cells but not for the stroma or lymphocytes, in the nude mouse lymph-node metastasis of PC-3. The histology of DU-145 and PC-3 growing and metastasizing in the nude mice matched published histologies of these tumors (12, 19). This orthotopic transplant model of prostate carcinoma resembled the clinical picture of growth within the prostate capsule, showing urinary obstruction, hydronephrosis, local invasion, and distant metastasis (3).

Using improved SOI of PC-3 in the ventral portion of the prostate (6), the take rate was 95% with only 1 of 20 mice having no orthotopic growth upon autopsy. Within the 3-month period following implantation, all tumors in the prostate reached more than 2 cm in diameter and usually disfigured the shape of the lower abdomen. The survival time of the animals ranged from 9 to 12 weeks. At time of euthanization, severe signs of cachexia could be observed in all the mice. Autopsy demonstrated that the orthotopically growing tumor usually protruded into the abdominal avity and very frequently invaded the lower abdominal wall. Distended urinary bladder and hydronephrosis due to blocked urethras were also frequently seen. The seminal vesicles, the bladder, and the lower abdominal wall were often invaded by the orthotopic primary tumors. Microscopic examination of the tissue sections demonstrated that 5 of 19 animals had lung metastases and 13 of 19 had periaortic lymph node metastases (6). Histopathology of the primary tumor showed sheets of densely packed, anaplastic epithelial cells with abundant, foamy, eosinophilic cytoplasm. The nuclei were pleomorphic and had varying amounts of unevenly dispersed chromatin. Many abnormal mitoses could be seen. The prostate gland was almost replaced by tumor cells and very few glandular structures could be seen (6). Microscopically, lymph node metastases were characterized by widespread infiltration of tumor cells in the subcapsular, the cortical and medullary area. In many of the lymph nodes analyzed, tumor cells occupied the whole node and lymphatic cells could barely be seen.

Microscopic examination of lung specimens showed that the metastases were disseminated. Small nests of tumor cells were observed in almost every high power field. When large tumor nests were seen, they often resided around the airway structures (6).

Intact tissue of the human prostate carcinoma cell line PC-3M was prepared by growth of this cell line subcutaneously in a nude mouse. One piece of $1.5\,\text{mm}^3$ intact tumor tissue was implanted by SOI in the ventral lateral lobes of the prostate gland of 10 nude mice. All 10 mice had tumors in the prostate gland and metastasis to periaortic lymph nodes. The time when mice with implanted PC-3M become moribund was 28–32 days after SOI (81).

2.3 Surgical Orthotopic Implantation of LNCaP in the Nude Mouse Prostate

LNCaP grew extensively after SOI in the ventral portion of the prostate. Eighteen of 20 implanted mice had orthotopic growth. Autopsy demonstrated that the orthotopically-growing tumors usually protruded into the abdominal cavity and very frequently invaded the lower abdominal wall. Distended urinary bladder and hydronephrosis due to blocked urethra were also frequently seen. The seminal vesicles, the bladder, and the lower abdominal wall were often invaded by the orthotopic primary tumors. Microscopic examination of the tissue sections demonstrated that 8 of 18 animals had lung metastases and 11 of 18 had periaortic lymph node metastases. Histopathology of the primary tumor showed densely packed, poorly differentiated cells. The prostate gland was almost replaced by tumor cells and very few glandular structures could be seen. Microscopically, lymph node metastases involved almost the whole node. Microscopic examination of lung specimens showed that the metastases were disseminated in small nests of tumor cells. The mean survival time of the animals was 72 days (82).

SOI eliminated the need to select highly metastatic cells through complex procedures from a parental tumor for the purpose of establishing metastatic animal models of human cancer as was necessary for the orthotopic models using cell suspensions, described above. Moreover, the SOI metastatic models more closely mimic the clinical pattern, thus providing better tools to study the biology of cancer metastasis and for evaluating novel therapeutics for prostate cancer (6).

2.4 Bone Metastasis Models of Prostate Cancer

Thalmann et al. (36) injected a mixture of human fibroblasts and LNCaP human prostate carcinoma cells into the dorsolateral lobe of the prostate gland of athymic mice. Metastases were selected that were apparently hybrids of the human fibroblasts and cancer cells. These variants developed bone metastasis in 10% and 21.3% of intact and castrated hosts, respectively.

A number of experimental bone metastasis models have also been developed in the last several years (19–21, 73). To establish these models, a high metastatic cell line was first selected and inoculated via the tail vein. In one study, in order to detect bone marrow metastases, isolation of total RNA from the bone marrow and subsequent RT-PCR was necessary (73). These types of models provide a useful tool for prostate cancer, but they do not mimic the natural history of this disease.

Using GFP-expressing PC-3 transplanted by SOI to the dorsolateral lobes of the nude mouse prostate, we established an imageable spontaneous bone metastasis mouse model of non-selected human prostate cancer. In this model, the GFP expression of the SOI-implanted PC-3 cell line enabled metastases to be visualized throughout the skeletal system and to other important organs as well. Extensive and widespread skeletal metastases, visualized by GFP expression, were found. The skeletal metastasis included the skull, rib, pelvis, femur, and tibia.

Metastases in the transplanted animals were also found in the lung, pleural membrane, liver, kidney, adrenal gland, brain and spinal cord. Thus, the metastatic pattern of human prostate cancer PC-3-GFP accurately reproduces the clinical course of advanced metastatic androgen-independent prostate cancer (74). These data demonstrate the far-reaching malignancy of this tumor (74).

Such a high incidence of skeletal and other metastases could not have been previously visualized before the development of the GFP-SOI model which provided the necessary tools. The bone microenvironment in the mouse provides a highly fertile soil for human prostate cancer matching the clinical situation (83). The PC-3-GFP model also revealed for the first time the extensive spontaneous liver metastasis potential of this tumor. This new metastatic model will be useful for studying the mechanism and developing therapy of skeletal and other metastases in prostate cancer (74).

The green fluorescent protein (GFP) gene was introduced into LNCaP cells by lipofection (84). Biological characteristics of a subline (LNCaP-GFP) that expressed GFP at high level were compared to those of the parental cells. LNCaP-GFP cells were orthotopically inoculated to the SCID mouse, and metastases to distant organs were chronologically examined under fluorescence microscopy. There was no difference in growth rates and androgen-responsiveness *in vitro* between LNCaP-GFP and LNCaP cells. LNCaP-GFP cells inoculated to SCID mice produced prostate specific antigen. Colonies consisting of a few LNCaP-GFP cells were detected in the lung under fluorescence microscopy as early as 4 weeks after orthotopic inoculation (84).

3. GENE EXPRESSION AND PROSTATE CANCER METASTASIS MODELS

A prostate cancer line (PC-3M) was engineered to overexpress hyaluronidases (hyal-1). Although the *in vitro* properties of the hyal-1 overexpressing cell line was indistinguishable from the parental cells, the orthotopic growth of hyal-1 expressing PC-3M cells in *nu/nu* mice resulted in significantly increased numbers of metastases, suggesting a role for hyal-1 in extravasation and metastasis (85).

The nuclear factor (NF)-kappaB/relA transcription factor is constitutively activated in human prostate cancer cells. It was determined that blocking NF-kappaB/relA activity in human prostate cancer cells affected their angiogenesis, growth, and metastasis in an orthotopic nude mouse model of PC-3M. Transfection with a mutated IkappaBalpha (IkappaBalphaM) blocks NF-kappaB activity. PC-3M control cells produced rapidly growing tumors and regional lymph node metastasis, whereas PC-3M-IkappaBalphaM cells produced slow-growing tumors with low metastatic potential. Inhibition of NF-kappaB inhibited expression of three major proangiogenic molecules, vascular endothelial growth factor (VEGF), interleukin (IL)-8, and matrix metalloproteinase (MMP)-9, and decreased tumore angiogenesis (86).

Subclones of the PC-3M and LNCaP cell lines were selected for increased metastatic potential after successive orthotopic implantation in the prostate of nude mice. Comparative genomic hybridization (CGH) was used to compare the chromosomal abnormalities between the parental cell lines and variants to determine whether specific chromosomal abnormalities can be associated with different growth properties. PC-3M-Pro4, a derivative line that produced significantly larger tumors in the prostate, had a unique gain of 3q13. PC-3M-LN4, a derivative line that produced significantly larger metastatic tumors in the lymph nodes and had higher incidences of distant metastases, had a specific gain of 1q21–q22 and losses of 10q23–qter and 18q12–q21. A derivative line of LNCaP that produced significantly larger tumors in the prostate, LNCaP-Pro5, had a unique gain on 13q12–q13. In comparison, LNCaP-LN3, a derivative line that had a significantly higher incidence of lymph node metastases and produced significantly larger metastatic tumors in the lymph nodes, had specific losses of 16q23–qter and 21q (87).

To investigate the potential genetic changes underlying the progression of human hormone-resistant prostate cancer, chromosomal alterations of the DU-145 cell line and a subline isolated form a metastasis in an orthotopic model were analyzed. DU-145 cells were injcted into the dorsal prostate. From a resulting paraaortic lymph node metastasis, a subline (DU-145 MN1), was isolated. After orthotopic implantation of DU-145 cells tumorigenicity was 100% but only 2 mice had lymphnode metastases. In contrast, the take rate after implantation of DU-145 MN1 was 100%, with frequent lymphnode metastases. There was gain of a chromosome 8 and only two copies of chromosome 17 in the DU-145 MN1 cells as compared to the parental cell line. The emergence of an i(9)(q10) in addition to two normal chromosome 9 homologues in the DU-145 MN1 cell line was confirmed by fluorescent *in situ* hybridization (FISH) using a chromosome 9-specific painting probe. Chromosomal changes, following repeated orthotopic implantation, may enable location of the genes involved in the progression and chemoresistance of human hormone-resistant prostate cancer (88).

After orthotopic intraprostatic injection of tumor cells into SCID mice, the metastatic DU-145 prostate carcinoma cells expressed 12-lipoxygenase (12-LOX) at a significantly higher level compared with the non-metastatic counterparts. The functional involvement of 12-LOX in the metastatic process was demonstrated when DU-145 cells were pretreated *in vitro* with the 12-LOX inhibitors N-benzyl-N-hydroxy-5-phenylpentamide (BHPP) or baicalein with subsequent inhibition of lung colonization in the orthotopic model (89).

IL-8 expression by human prostate cancer growing within the prostate of athymic nude mice regulates tumor angiogenesis, growth, and metastasis. Poorly metastatic PC-3P cells were transfected with the full-length sense IL-8 cDNA, whereas highly metastatic PC-3M-LN4 cells were transfected with the full-sequence antisense IL-8 cDNA. After orthotopic implantation, the sense-transfected PC-3P cells were highly tumorigenic and metastatic, with significantly increased neovascularity and IL-8 expression compared with either PC-3P cells or controls. Antisense transfection significantly reduced the expression of IL-8 and MMP-9 and tumor-induced neovascularity, resulting in inhibition of tumorigenicity and metastasis. These results demonstrate that IL-8 expression regulates angiogenesis and metastasis in prostate cancer, in part by induction of MMP-9 expression (90).

Human prostate PC-3 ML tumor cells transfected with IL-10 were examined for tumor growth and metastasis following orthotopic implantation

7.3 Histological and GFP Evaluation of Tumor Growth and Metastasis

Mice were euthanized if found moribund during the observation period. All mice were humanely sacrificed using CO_2 inhalation three months after tumor implantation and then immersed in 10% formalin for subsequent autopsy and microscopic examination. Regional and distant lymph nodes, the lung, the liver as well as other organs suspected of metastasis were routinely embedded, sectioned, and stained with hematoxylin and eosin using standard techniques for microscopic examination. The skeletal system was carefully examined grossly under a dissecting microscope (7×) with the removal of the soft tissue for possible bone metastasis (6).

7.3.1 GFP DNA Expression Vector

The RetroXpress vector pLEIN was purchased from Clontech Laboratories, Inc. (Palo Alto, CA). The pLEIN vector expresses enhanced green fluorescent protein (EGFP) and the neomycin resistance gene on the same bicistronic message which contains an IRES site (72).

7.3.2 Production of GFP Retrovirus

PT67, an NIH3T3-derived packaging cell line, expressing the 10 Al viral envelope, was purchased from Clontech Laboratories, Inc. PT67 cells were cultured in DME medium (Irvine Scientific, Santa Ana, CA) supplemented with 10% heat-inactivated fetal bovine serum (FBS) (Gemini Bio-products, Calabasas, CA). For vector production, packaging cells (PT67), at 70% confluence, were incubated with a precipitated mixture of DOTAP™ reagent (Boehringer Mannheim), and saturating amounts of pLEIN plasmid for 18 hours. Fresh medium was replenished at this time. The cells were examined by fluorescence microscopy 48 hours post-transfection. For selection, the cells were cultured in the presence of 500 – 2000 µg/ml of G418 (Life Technologies, Grand Island, NY) for seven days (72).

7.3.3 GFP Gene Transfection of Prostate Carcinoma Cells

For GFP gene transfection, 20%-confluent PC-3 cells were incubated with a 1:1 precipitated mixture of retroviral supernatants of PT67 cells and Ham's F-12 K (GIBCO) containing 7% fetal bovine serum (FBS) (Gemini Bio-products, Calabasas, CA) for 72 hours. Fresh medium was replenished at this time. PC-3 cells were harvested by trypsin/EDTA 72 hours higher incidence of lymph node metastases and produced significantly larger metastatic tumors in the lymph nodes, had specific losses of 16q23–qter and 21q (87).

To investigate the potential genetic changes underlying the progression of human hormone-resistant prostate cancer, chromosomal alterations of the DU-145 cell line and a subline isolated form a metastasis in an orthotopic model were analyzed. DU-145 cells were injcted into the dorsal prostate. From a resulting paraaortic lymph node metastasis, a subline (DU-145 MN1), was isolated. After orthotopic implantation of DU-145 cells tumorigenicity was 100% but only 2 mice had lymphnode metastases. In contrast, the take rate after implantation of DU-145 MN1 was 100%, with frequent lymphnode metastases. There was gain of a chromosome 8 and only two copies of chromosome 17 in the DU-145 MN1 cells as compared to the parental cell line. The emergence of an i(9)(q10) in addition to two normal chromosome 9 homologues in the DU-145 MN1 cell line was confirmed by fluorescent *in situ* hybridization (FISH) using a chromosome 9-specific painting probe. Chromosomal changes, following repeated orthotopic implantation, may enable location of the genes involved in the progression and chemoresistance of human hormone-resistant prostate cancer (88).

After orthotopic intraprostatic injection of tumor cells into SCID mice, the metastatic DU-145 prostate carcinoma cells expressed 12-lipoxygenase (12-LOX) at a significantly higher level compared with the non-metastatic counterparts. The functional involvement of 12-LOX in the metastatic process was demonstrated when DU-145 cells were pretreated *in vitro* with the 12-LOX inhibitors N-benzyl-N-hydroxy-5-phenylpentamide (BHPP) or baicalein with subsequent inhibition of lung colonization in the orthotopic model (89).

IL-8 expression by human prostate cancer growing within the prostate of athymic nude mice regulates tumor angiogenesis, growth, and metastasis. Poorly metastatic PC-3P cells were transfected with the full-length sense IL-8 cDNA, whereas highly metastatic PC-3M-LN4 cells were transfected with the full-sequence antisense IL-8 cDNA. After orthotopic implantation, the sense-transfected PC-3P cells were highly tumorigenic and metastatic, with significantly increased neovascularity and IL-8 expression compared with either PC-3P cells or controls. Antisense transfection significantly reduced the expression of IL-8 and MMP-9 and tumor-induced neovascularity, resulting in inhibition of tumorigenicity and metastasis. These results demonstrate that IL-8 expression regulates angiogenesis and metastasis in prostate cancer, in part by induction of MMP-9 expression (90).

Human prostate PC-3 ML tumor cells transfected with IL-10 were examined for tumor growth and metastasis following orthotopic implantation in the prostate gland of SCID mice. Volume and extent of metastasis were negatively correlated with the amount of IL-10 production. Controls showed that parental PC-3 ML grew rapidly and metastasized when implanted orthotopically and died by 14–16 weeks. In contrast, the PC-3 ML-IL10a or PC-3 ML-IL10b clones induced only 10–20% death after 23–24 weeks (91).

Transfection of primary human prostate tumor cell lines (HPCA-10a, 10b, 10c, and 10d) with the transforming growth factor (TGF)-beta-1 gene promoted tumor growth, angiogenesis, and metastasis after orthotopic implantation in SCID mice. In contrast, IL-10 transfected cells or cells co-transfected with these two genes exhibited reduced growth rates and significantly reduced angiogenesis and metastasis. TGF-beta1 expression induced MMP-2 expression, whereas IL-10 down-regulated MMP-2 expression while up regulating tissue inhibitor of matrix metalloproteinase (TIMP)-1 in the transfected cells. Mouse survival was zero after 4–6 months in mice bearing transforming growth factor-beta1 (TGF-β1) and MMP-2-expressing tumors. Survival increased significantly in mice implanted with IL-10- and TIMP-1-expressing tumors (92).

Prostate adenocarcinoma PC-3 and DU-145 cell lines express alphaII(b)beta3 integrin markers. Implantation in SCID mice determined that alphaII(b)beta3 mediates metastatasis. In DU-145 cells the integrin localizes to focal contact sites, whereas it is predominantly intracellular in PC-3 cells. Both tumor cell lines were tumorigenic when implanted subcutaneously or intraprostatically in SCID mice, but only DU-145 cells injected intraprostatically metastasized. There was higher expression of alphaII(b)beta3 in DU-145 tumor cell suspensions isolated from the prostate when compared to DU-145 tumor cells from the subcutis (93).

A nontumorigenic cell line isolated from the rat prostatic epithelium (NbE) transfected with the activated oncogene p185neu-T was used to investigate the role of this oncogene in tumor progression. When clones overexpressing p185neu-T were injected orthotopically into the dorsal-lateral prostates of nude mice, prostatic tumors were detected in all mice injected and metastasis was detected to the skeletal muscle in the rib area in 60–80% of the mice injected. Control cell lines produced no prostatic tumors or metastases. Clones overexpressing p185neu-T demonstrated an increased expression of epidermal growth factor receptor and p180erbB4 (94).

The expression level of several metastasis-regulating genes correlated with the metastatic potential of human prostate cancer cells implanted into the prostate of nude mice. Human PC-3M cells and selected cell variants with different metastatic potentials were evaluated. Human prostate cancer cells implanted in nude mice at an ectopic site (sc) expressed lower levels of epidermal growth factor receptor (EGFR), multidrug resistance (mdr)-1, basic fibroblast growth factor (bFGF), IL-8, and collagenase type IV than those implanted in an orthotopic site, indicating that the expression of these genes was dependent on the organ environment. Highly metastatic cells growing in the prostate expressed higher levels of EGFR, bFGF, type IV collagenase, and mdr-1 mRNA than low metastatic parental cells in the same site (95).

4. GENE THERAPY AND PROSTATE CANCER METASTASIS MODELS

Angiogenin, a mediator of neovascularization was targeted by an antisense oligodeoxynucleotide, designated JF2S, in human prostate tumors in nude mice in an orthotopic model. Systemic prophylactic administration of JF2S prevented, in 47% of mice, formation of regional iliac lymph node micrometastases arising from primary PC-3 tumors growing orthotopically in the prostate. Total protection from regional metastasis occurred in those mice in which JF2S diminished human angiogenin expression. Tumor angiogenesis was also impaired by JF2S treatment. These findings demonstrate that human prostate cancer metastasis in athymic mice is susceptible to disruption of human angiogenin gene expression (96).

The effects of interferon-beta (IFN-beta) gene transfer on the growth of PC-3MM2 human prostate cancer in nude mice were investigated. Intratumoral delivery of an adenoviral vector encoding murine IFN-beta (AdIFN-beta) suppressed orthotopic PC-3MM2 tumors and development of metastasis by 80%, and eradicated the tumors in 20% of mice. Immunohistochemical staining showed that AdIFN-beta-treated tumors contained fewer microvessels, fewer proliferating cells, and more apoptotic cells than did the control tumors. Compared with controls, tumors injected with AdIFN-beta expressed higher levels of IFN-beta and inducible nitric oxide synthase (iNOS) and lower levels of basic bFGF and TGF-β1 (86).

Highly metastatic PC-3M human prostate cancer cells were engineered to constitutively produce murine IFN-beta with a retroviral vector containing murine IFN-beta cDNA. Parental (PC-3M-P), control vector-transduced (PC-3M-Neo), and IFN-beta-transduced (PC-3M-IFN-beta) cells were injected into the prostate or subcutis of nude mice. PC-3M-P and PC-3M-Neo cells produced rapidly growing tumors and regional lymph node metastases, whereas PC-3M-IFN-beta cells did not. PC-3M-IFN-beta cells also suppressed the tumorigenicity of bystander non-transduced prostate cancer cells. PC-3M-IFN-beta tumors were homogeneously infiltrated by macrophages, whereas control tumors contained fewer macrophages at their periphery. PC-3M-IFN-beta tumors contained fewer proliferative cells and more apoptotic cells than controls. Staining with antibody against CD31 showed that control tumors contained more blood vessels than PC-3M-IFN-beta tumors. The data suggested that the suppression of tumorigenicity and metastasis of PC-3M-IFN-beta cells was due to inhibition of angiogenesis and activation of host effector cells (97).

The efficacy of a single injection of a recombinant adenovirus expressing murine IL-12 (AdmIL-12) was determined by direct injection into orthotopic mouse prostate carcinomas generated from a poorly immunogenic cell line (RM-9) derived from the mouse prostate reconstitution system. Significant growth suppression and increased mean survival time were observed compared with controls. Suppression of pre-established lung metastases was also observed. Cytolytic natural killer cell activity was markedly enhanced 1–2 days after virus injection. Immunohistochemical analysis showed significantly elevated intratumoral infiltration of CD4+ and CD8+ T-cells. Splenocyte-derived cytotoxic T-lymphocytes were also detected. Increased numbers of nitric oxide synthase-positive macrophages were also seen in the AdmIL-12 treated group. The antitumor efficacy of adenovirus-mediated IL-12 depends on the activation of nitric oxide synthase in macrophages and T-cell activation (98).

The effectiveness of an adenovirus that expresses both IL-12 and the costimulatory molecule B7-1 (AdmIL12/B7) or one that expresses IL-12 alone (AdmIL-12) were compared using the poorly immunogenic RM-9 orthotopic murine model of prostate cancer. A significant reduction in orthotopic tumor size and increased survival was demonstrated in mice treated with a single orthotopic injection of AdmIL-12/B7 compared with AdmIL-12 or controls. Orthotopic treatment of tumors with both vectors led to an infiltration of both CD4+ and CD8+ immunoreactive cells, with AdmIL-12/B7 treatment having a more prolonged infiltration of CD8+ cells. AdmIL-12/B7 was also more effective than AdmIL-12 or controls at suppression of pre-established metastases. A vaccine model based on sc injection of infected, irradiated RM-9 cells demonstrated that both AdmIL-12 and AdmIL-12/B7 were effective at suppressing the development and growth of challenge orthotopic tumors (99).

Mutation of the p53 tumor suppressor gene has been associated with the progression of prostate cancer. An orthotopic metastatic model for human prostate cancer was used to determine efficacy of the wild-type p53 gene using an adenoviral vector (rAd-p53). The human prostate cancer cell line

PC-3 has a homozygous loss of p53 expression in nude mice following orthotopic injection. A single injection of rAd-p53 into an established orthotopic prostate tumor resulted in primary tumor growth suppression and reduced the frequency of metastasis (100).

An orthotopic mouse model of metastatic prostate cancer using a cell line (RM-1) derived from the mouse prostate was developed. Adenovirus (ADV)-mediated transduction of the herpes simplex virus thymidine kinase (HSV-tk) gene in conjunction with ganciclovir (GCV) in this model led to significant suppression of growth and of spontaneous metastasis with a significant survival advantage and a continued suppression of metastatic activity for treated animals despite regrowth of the primary tumor (101).

Induction of potent antitumor natural killer (NK) cell activity by herpes simplex virus-thymidine kinase and ganciclovir therapy was observed in the orthotopic RM-1 mouse model of prostate cancer. *In vivo* depletion of NK cells resulted in a 20% reduction in growth suppression within the primary tumor and complete abrogation of the inhibition of preestablished lung metastases. Depletion of T-cells had no effect on either response. NK cells within adenovirus/HSV-tk- and ganciclovir-treated tumors, thus mediated both local and systemic antitumor activities in this model (102).

5. OTHER TREATMENT OF PROSTATE CANCER METASTASIS

Arsenic trioxide (As2O3) was administered to SCID mice inoculated orthotopically with PC-3 cells. The orthotopic metastasis model showed tumor growth inhibition in the primary and metastatic lesions with no signs of toxicity (103).

Caveolin-1 plays important roles in signal transduction and lipid transport. Injections of caveolin-1 antibody suppressed the orthotopic growth and spontaneous metastasis of a highly metastatic, androgen-insensitive caveolin-1-secreting mouse prostate cancer (104).

Prostate stem-cell antigen (PSCA) is a cell-surface antigen expressed in normal prostate and overexpressed in prostate cancer tissues. Anti-PSCA mAbs efficacy was evaluated on the androgen-dependent LAPC-9 and the androgen-independent recombinant cell line PC-3-PSCA. Orthotopic tumors were inhibited in a dose-dependent manner. Inhibition of metastasis to distant sites also occurred resulting in a significant prolongation in the survival of tumor-bearing mice (105).

6. ORTHOTOPIC DOG MODEL

A new canine prostate cancer epithelial cell line designated DPC-1 has been isolated from a poorly differentiated canine prostatic adenocarcinoma (106). Tumorigenicity was assessed in nude mice and in one adult immunodeficient dog. DPC-1 displays immunoreactivity to human PSA and prostate-specific membrane antigen (PSMA). DPC-1 was found to be highly tumorigenic not only in nude mice but also for the first time after orthotopic seeding in an immunodeficient dog.

7. MATERIALS AND METHODS IN THE AUTHOR'S LABORATORY

7.1 Animals

Outbred nu/nu mice, 4–6 weeks old, were used for sc and orthotopic transplantation of DU-145, PC-3, and LNCaP. All the mice were maintained in a pathogen-free environment. Cages, bedding, food, and water were autoclaved and changed regularly. All the mice were maintained in a daily cycle of 12 hr light and 12 hr darkness (3). They were maintained in a specific pathogen-free environment in compliance with USPHS guidelines governing the care and maintenance of experimental animals under Assurance Number A3873-01. Mice were fed with autoclaved laboratory rodent diet (Teklad LM-485, Western Research Products, Orange, CA) (6).

7.2 Surgical Orthotopic Implantation

PC-3 DU-145 and LNCaP cells were obtained initially from the American Tissue Type Culture Collection (Rockville, MD). Tumor tissue used for surgical orthotopic implantation was derived from a tumor growing subcutaneously after injection of prostate cancer cells in a nude mouse. Tissue from the periphery of the tumor was harvested in log phase and necrotic tissue was carefully removed under a dissecting microscope to minimize the amount of viable tissue for implantation. The viable tissue was then cut into small cubes of 1 mm^3 in standard tissue culture medium under sterile conditions. To minimize variation in subsequent tumor growth and metastasis, these tumor pieces were randomly mixed and an equal amount of pieces was implanted in each mouse as described below.

7.2.1 SOI to Ventral Lateral Lobes of Prostate

Mice were anesthetized by isoflurane (Ohmeda Caribe Inc., Guayama, PR) and positioned supinely. An opening was made right above the pubis symphysis to expose the prostate gland. The fascia surrounding the ventral portion of the prostate was carefully isolated and the two ventral lateral lobes of the gland were separated by a small incision using a pair of fine surgical scissors. Five of the above tissue pieces were sutured into the incision using an 8–0 nylon suture. The two parts of the separated lobes were then sutured together with the tumor pieces wrapped within. The surrounding fascia was then used to wrap this portion of the gland to consolidate the incision. The abdomen was closed using a 6–0 suture (6).

7.2.2 SOI to Dorsal Lateral Lobe of Prostate

Two tumor fragments (1 mm^3) from a sc tumor from a single animal were implanted by SOI in the dorsolateral lobe of the prostate in nude mice. After proper exposure of the bladder and prostate following a lower midline abdominal incision, the capsule of the prostate was opened and the two tumor fragments were inserted into the capsule. The capsule was then closed with an 8–0 surgical suture. The incision in the abdominal wall was closed with a 6–0 surgical suture in one layer (7, 8). The animals were kept under isoflurane anesthesia during surgery. All procedures of the operation described above were performed with a 7 × magnification microscope (Olympus) (74).

To confirm the human origin of the tumors growing in the nude mice, the Oncor total-human-genome probe (Oncor, Gaithersburg, MD) was used. Briefly, paraffin-embedded blocks of the nude-mouse tumor, both local and metastatic, were cut into 4-μm-thick sections and applied to silanized slides. After deparaffinization, protein digestion and dehydration, the Oncor biotinylated "Total-human DNA painting probe" was used for in situ hybridization. Avidin, anti-avidin antibody and horse-radish peroxidase-avidin complex with 3–3'-diaminobenzidine tetrahydrochloride (DAB) as the substrate was subsequently applied for the detection system according to the specifications supplied by Oncor. Hematoxylin was used in counter-staining. The nuclei of positive cells stained brown, indicating their human origin. Negative controls utilized the total procedure but without the human-genome-specific DNA probe. The human genomic probe was used to determine the human origin of the prostate tumors in the nude mice since neither DU-145 nor PC-3 produce PSA (3).

7.3 Histological and GFP Evaluation of Tumor Growth and Metastasis

Mice were euthanized if found moribund during the observation period. All mice were humanely sacrificed using CO_2 inhalation three months after tumor implantation and then immersed in 10% formalin for subsequent autopsy and microscopic examination. Regional and distant lymph nodes, the lung, the liver as well as other organs suspected of metastasis were routinely embedded, sectioned, and stained with hematoxylin and eosin using standard techniques for microscopic examination. The skeletal system was carefully examined grossly under a dissecting microscope ($7\times$) with the removal of the soft tissue for possible bone metastasis (6).

7.3.1 GFP DNA Expression Vector

The RetroXpress vector pLEIN was purchased from Clontech Laboratories, Inc. (Palo Alto, CA). The pLEIN vector expresses enhanced green fluorescent protein (EGFP) and the neomycin resistance gene on the same bicistronic message which contains an IRES site (72).

7.3.2 Production of GFP Retrovirus

PT67, an NIH3T3-derived packaging cell line, expressing the 10 Al viral envelope, was purchased from Clontech Laboratories, Inc. PT67 cells were cultured in DME medium (Irvine Scientific, Santa Ana, CA) supplemented with 10% heat-inactivated fetal bovine serum (FBS) (Gemini Bio-products, Calabasas, CA). For vector production, packaging cells (PT67), at 70% confluence, were incubated with a precipitated mixture of DOTAP™ reagent (Boehringer Mannheim), and saturating amounts of pLEIN plasmid for 18 hours. Fresh medium was replenished at this time. The cells were examined by fluorescence microscopy 48 hours post-transfection. For selection, the cells were cultured in the presence of $500 - 2000\,\mu g/ml$ of G418 (Life Technologies, Grand Island, NY) for seven days (72).

7.3.3 GFP Gene Transfection of Prostate Carcinoma Cells

For GFP gene transfection, 20%-confluent PC-3 cells were incubated with a 1:1 precipitated mixture of retroviral supernatants of PT67 cells and Ham's F-12 K (GIBCO) containing 7% fetal bovine serum (FBS) (Gemini Bio-products, Calabasas, CA) for 72 hours. Fresh medium was replenished at this time. PC-3 cells were harvested by trypsin/EDTA 72 hours post-transfection, and subcultured at a ratio of 1:15 into selective medium which contained 200 μg/ml of G418. The level of G418 was increased to 1000 μg/ml stepwise. PC-3 clones expressing GFP (PC-3-GFP) were isolated with cloning cylinders (Bel-Art Products, Pequannock, NJ) with trypsin/EDTA and were then amplified and transferred by conventional culture methods (74).

7.3.4 Doubling Time of Stable GFP Clones

PC-3-GFP or non-transfected cells were seeded at 1.5×10^4 in 35 mm culture dishes. The cells were harvested and counted every 24 hours using a hemocytometer (Reichert Scientific Instruments, Buffalo, NY). The doubling time was calculated from the cell-growth curve over a period of ten days (74).

7.4 Fluorescence Imaging

A Leica fluorescence stereo microscope model LZ12 equipped with a mercury 50W lamp power supply was used (107–109). To visualize both GFP and RFP fluorescence at the same time, excitation was produced through a D425/60 band pass filter and 470 DCXR dichroic mirror (110). Emitted fluorescence was collected through a long pass filter GG475 (Chroma Technology, Brattleboro, VT). Macroimaging was carried out in a light box (Lightools Research, Encinitas, CA). Fluorescence excitation of both GFP and RFP tumors was produced through an interference filter 440+/−20 nm using slit fiber optics for animal illumination. Fluorescence was observed through a 520 nm long pass filter (110). Images from the microscope and light box were captured on a Hamamatsu C5810 3-chip cool color CCR camera (Hamamatsu Photonics Systems, Bridgewater, NJ).

Images were processed for contrast and brightness and analyzed with the use of Image Pro Plus 4.0 software (Media Cybernetics, Silver Springs, MD). High resolution images of 1024×724 pixels were captured directly on an IBM PC or continuously through video output on a high resolution Sony VCR model SLV-R1000 (Sony Corp., Tokyo Japan) (107–109).

8. CONCLUSIONS AND PERSPECTIVES

Intraprostatic implantation of PC-3 cell suspensions in nude mice resulted in paraaortic lymph node metastases in 10 of 10 mice with prostatic tumors, whereas metastases were present in only 2 of 9 mice after sc implantation. Tumorigenesis and metastasis were also 100% after subserosal implantation of PC-3 cells within the wall of the urinary bladder. Subserosal implantation of PC-3 cells into the stomach wall also resulted in tumor formation and metastasis as well to regional lymph nodes in 100% of mice. In all experiments, regional lymph nodes were the most frequent site of metastasis, regardless of implantation site. The loss of organ specificity may have been due to use of cell suspensions instead of tumor fragments for orthotopic implantation (78, 111).

The invasive and metastatic behavior of metalloproteinase matrilysin transfected DU-145 cell lines injected into the dorsal lateral lobe of the prostate in SCID mice was compared to that observed when they are injected intraperitoneally. The results demonstrate that the level of mRNA expression of the matrilysin, stromelysin, TIMP-1, and TIMP-2 genes was similar at the two sites of injection. The invasive properties of DU-145 cells following orthotopic implantation were comparable to that observed on the diaphragm following intraperitoneal injection (112). Again this loss of host tissue specificity may have been due to use of cell suspensions instead of intact tissue fragments for orthotopic implantation. Further comparative experiments are necessary using the two techniques.

The use of GFP and now RFP allow unprecedented visualization of tumor growth *in vivo* including prostate cancer (74, 110). New techniques of *in vivo* imaging with these multicolor fluorescent reporters will enable important insight into the mechanisms of prostate cancer metastasis (110).

Recently transgenic models of prostate cancer have been developed, Gupta et al. (113) described the transgenic adenocarcinoma of the mouse prostate (TRAMP). In this model, expression of the SV40 early genes (T and t antigen, Tag) are driven by the prostate-specific promoter probasin which leads to cell transformation within the prostate. TRAMP mice develop prostate cancer without any chemical or hormonal treatment and metastasis to lymph nodes, lungs, liver, and bone occur over 12-28 weeks with median survival of 42 weeks. The potential question with these models is "what do they represent" since all cells express as an artifical transgene such as the SV40 T-antigens in the TRAMP model which is not the case in human prostate cancer.

REFERENCES

1. Jemal A, Thomas A, Murray T, Thun M. Cancer statistics, 2002. CA Cancer J Clin 2002, 52:23–47.
2. Huggins C, Hodges CV. Studies on prostatic cancer. I. The effcts of castration, of estrogen and of androgen injections on serum phosphatases in metastatic carcinoma of the prostate. Cancer Res 1941, 1:293–7.

3. Fu X, Herrera H, Hoffman RM. Orthotopic growth and metastasis of human prostate carcinoma in nude mice after transplantation of histologically intact tissue. Int J Cancer 1992, 52:987–0.
4. Crawford ED, Eisenberger MA, McLeod DG, Spaulding JT, Benson R, Dorr FA. A controlled trial of leuprolide with and without flutamide in prostate carcinoma. N Engl J Med 1989, 321:419–24.
5. Stamey TA, McNeal JE. Adenocarcinoma of the prostate, In: *Campbell's Urology, 6th Ed.* Walsh PC, Retik AB, Stamey TA, Vaughn ED Jr., eds, Philadelphia: W.B. Saunders, 1992.
6. An Z, Wang X, Geller J, Moossa AR, Hoffman RM. Surgical orthotopic implantation allows high lung and lymph node metastatic expression of human prostate carcinoma cell line PC-3 in nude mice. Prostate 1998, 34:169–74.
7. Nakamuto T, Chang C, Li A, Chokak G. Basic fibroblast growth factor in human prostate cancer cells. Cancer Res 1992, 52:571–7.
8. Ware JL. Prostate tumor progression and metastasis. Biochem Biophys Acta Rev Cancer 1987, 907:279–98.
9. Arnold W, Kopf-Maier P, Micheel B, eds, *Immunodeficient Animals: Models for Cancer Research.* Basel: Karger, 1996.
10. Rygaard J, Povlsen CO. Heterotransplantation of a human malignant tumour to "nude" mice. Acta Pathol Microbiol Scand 1969, 77:758–60.
11. Horoszewicz J, Leong S, Kawinski E, Karr J, Rosenthal H, Chu T *et al.* LNCap model of human prostatic carcinoma. Cancer Res 1983, 43:1809–11.
12. Stone KR, Mickey D, Wunderli H, Mickey G, Paulson D. Isolation of a human prostate carcinoma cell line (DU-145). Int J Cancer 1978, 21:274–81.
13. Kaighn M, Narayan K, Ohnuki Y, Lechner J, Jones LW. Establishment and characterization of a human prostatic carcinoma cell line (PC-3). Invest Urol 1979, 17:1623.
14. Kozlowski J, McEwan L, Keer H, Sensibar J, Sherwood ER, Lee C *et al.* Prostate cancer, the invasive phenotype: Application of new in vivo, in vitro approaches, pp. 189–231. In: *Tumor Progression, Metastasis.* Fidler IJ, Nicholson G, eds, New York: Alan R. Liss, 1988.
15. Dunning WF. Prostate cancer in the rat. Nat Cancer Inst Monogr 1963, 12:351–69.
16. Ware JJ, Paulson DF, Mickey GH, Webb KS. Spontaneous metastasis of cells of the human prostate carcinoma cell line PC-3 in athymic nude mice. J Urol 1982, 128:1064–7.
17. Ware JL, Lieberman AP, Webb KS, Vollmer RT. Factors influencing phenotypic diversity of human prostate carcinoma cells metastasizing in athymic nude mice. Exp Cell Biol 1985, 53:163–9.
18. Sherwood E, Ford J, Lee C, Kozlowski J. Therapeutic efficacy of recombinant tumor necrosis factor alpha in an experimental model of human prostatic carcinoma. J Biol Resp Mod 1990, 9:44–52.
19. Shevrin Kukreja D, Ghosh S, Lad LT. Development of skeletal metastasis by human prostate cancer in athymic nude mice. Clin Exp Metastasis 1988, 6:401–9.
20. Shevrin D, Gorny K, Kukreja S. Patterns of metastasis by the human prostate cancer cell line PC-3 in athymic nude mice. Prostate 1989, 15:187–94.
21. Wu TT, Sike RA, Cui Q, Thalmann GN, Kao C, Murphy CF *et al.* Establishing human prostate cancer cell xenografts in bone: Induction of osteoblastic reaction by prostate-specific antigen-producing tumors in athymic and SCID/bg mice using LNCaP and lineage-derived metastatic sublines. Int J Cancer 1998, 77:887–94.

22. Lim DJ, Liu X, Sutkowski DM, Braun EJ, Lee C, Kozlowski JM. Growth of an androgen-sensitive human prostate cancer cell line, LNCaP, in nude mice. Prostate 1993, 22:109–1.
23. Wang WR, Sordat B, Piguet D, Sordat M. Human colon tumors in nude mice: Implantation site, expression of the invasive phenotype, pp. 239–45. In: *Immune-Deficient Animals. 4th Int. Workshop on Immune-Deficient Animals in Experimental Research*. Sordat B, ed., Basel: Karger, 1984.
24. Naito S, von Eschenbach AC, Glavazzi R, Fidler IJ. Growth and metastasis of tumor cells isolated from a human renal cell carcinoma implanted into different organs of nude mice. Cancer Res 1986, 46:4109–15.
25. Naito S, von Eschenbach AC, Fidler IJ. Different growth pattern and biologic behavior of human renal cell carcinoma implanted into different organs of nude mice. J Natl Cancer Inst 1987, 78:377–85.
26. Morikawa K, Walker SM, Jessup JM, Fidler IJ. *In vivo* selection of highly metastatic cells from surgical spcimens of different primary human colon carcinoma implanted into nude mice. Cancer Res 1988, 48:1943–8.
27. Ahlering TE, Dubeau L, Jones PA. A new *in vivo* model to study invasion and metastasis of human bladder carcinoma. Cancer Res 1987, 47:6660–5.
28. Nakajima M, Morkawa K, Fabra A, Bucana CD, Fidler IJ. Infuence of organ microenvironment on extracellular matrix degradative activity and metastasis of human colon carcinoma cells. J Natl Cancer Inst 1990, 82:1890–8.
29. Price JE, Polyzos A, Zhang RD, Daniels LM. Tumorigenicity and metastasis of human breast carcinoma cell line in nude mice. Cancer Res 1990, 50:717–21.
30. Giavazzi R, Campbell DE, Jessup JM, Cleary K, Fidler IJ. Metastatic behavior of tumor cells isolated from primary and metastatic human colorectal carcinomas implanted into different sites in nude mice. Cancer Res 1986, 46:1928–33.
31. Stephenson RA, Dinney CPN, Gohji K, Ordonez NG, Killion JJ, Fidler IJ. Metastatic model for human prostate cancer using orthotopic implantation in nude mice. J Natl Cancer Inst 1992, 84:951–7.
32. Vieweg J, Heston WDW, Gilboa E, Fair WR. An experimental model simulating local recurrence and pelvic lymph node metastasis following orthotopic induction of prostate cancer. Prostate 1994, 24:291–8.
33. Pettaway CA, Pathak S, Greene G, Ramirez E, Wilson MR, Killion JJ, Fidler IJ. Selection of highly metastatic variants of different human prostatic carcinomas using orthotopic implantation in nude mice. Clin Cancer Res 1996, 2:1627–36.
34. Rembrink K, Romijn JC, van der Kwast TH, Rubben H, Schroder FH. Orthotopic implantation of human prostate cancer cell lines: A clinically relevant animal model for metastatic prostate cancer. Prostate 1997, 31:168–74.
35. Sato N, Gleave ME, Bruchovsky N, Rennie PS, Beraldi E, Sullivan LD. A metastatic and androgen-sensitive human prostate cancer model using intraprostatic inoculation of LNCaP cells in SCID mice. Cancer Res 1997, 57:1584–9.
36. Thalmann GN, Anezinis PE, Chang SM, Zhau HE, Kim EE, Hopwood VL *et al*. Androgen-independent cancer progression and bone metastasis in the LNCaP model of human cancer. Cancer Res 1994, 54:2577–81.
37. Kusaka N, Nasu Y, Arata R, Saika T, Tsushima T, Kraaij R *et al*. Transrectal ultrasound for monitoring murine orthotopic prostate tumor. Prostate 2001, 47:118–24.
38. Meyvisch C. Influence of implantation site on formation of metastasis. Cancer Metastasis Rev 1983, 2:295–306.

39. White DC, DeCosse JJ. Experimental arterial dissemination of tumor cells. Cancer 1968, 21:9–15.
40. Stackpole CW. Distant lung-colonizing and lung-metastasizing cell populations in B16 mouse melanoma. Nature 1981, 289:798–800.
41. Fisher B, Fisher ER. Transmigration of lymph nodes by tumor cells. Science 1966, 152:1397–8.
42. Ishibashi T, Yamada H, Harada S, Harada Y, Miyazaki N, Takamoto M, Watanabe K. Distant metastasis facilitated by BCG: Spread of tumor cells injected in the BCG-primed site. Br J Cancer 1980, 41:553–61.
43. Kopf-Maier P. Dying and regeneration of human tumor cells after heterotransplantation to athymic mice. Histol Histopathol 1986, 1:383–90.
44. Kopf-Maier P, Jackel M. Proliferation behavior of xenografted human tumors: A flow cytometric study. Anticancer Res 1988, 8:1355–60.
45. Wilson EL, Gartner M, Campbell JAH, Dowdle EB. Growth and behavior of human melanomas in nude mice.Effect of fibroblasts, pp. 357–61. In: *Immuno-Deficient Animals.*, Sordat B, ed., Karger, 1984.
46. Picard O, Rolland Y, Poupon MF. Fibroblast-dependent tumorigenicity of cells in nude mice: Implication for implantation of metastasis. Cancer Res 1986, 46:3290–4.
47. Horgan K, Jones DL, Mansel RE. Mitogenicity of human fibroblasts *in vivo* for human breast cancer cells. Br J Surg 1987, 74:227–9.
48. Fridman R, Giaccone G, Kanemoto T, Martin GR, Gazdar AF, Mulshine JL. Reconstituted basement membrane (matrigel) and laminin can enhance the tumorigenicity and the drug resistance of small cell lung cancer cell lines. Proc Natl Acad Sci USA 1990, 87:6689–702.
49. Pretlow TG, Delmoro CM, Dilley GG, Spadafora CG, Pretlow TP. Transplantation of human prostate carcinoma into nude mice in matrigel. Cancer Res 1991, 51:3814–7.
50. Fridman R, Kibbey MC, Royce LS, Zain M, Sweeney TM, Jicha DL *et al.* Enhanced tumor growth of both primary and established human and murine tumor cells in athymic mice after coinjection with matrigel. J Natl Cancer Inst 1991, 83:769–4.
51. Noel A, Borcy V, Bracke M, Gilles C, Bernard J, Birembaut P *et al.* Heterotransplantation of primary and established human tumor cells in nude mice. Anticancer Res 1995, 15:1–8.
52. Kleinman HK. Basement membrane complexes with biological activity. Biochemistry 1986, 25:312–8.
53. Liotta LA, Steeg PS, Stetler-Stevenson WG. Metastasis and angiogenesis: An imbalance of positive and negative regulation. Cancer 1991, 64:327–6.
54. Passaniti A, Isaacs JT, Haney JA, Adler SW, Cujdik TJ, Long PV, Kleinman HK. Stimulation of human prostate carcinoma tumor growh in athymic mice and control of migration in culture by extracellular matrix. Int J Cancer 1992, 51:318–24.
55. Fu X, Besterman JM, Monosov A, Hoffman RM. Models of human metastatic colon cancer in nude mice orthotopically constructed by using histologically-intact patient specimens. Proc Natl Acad Sci USA 1991, 88:9345–9.
56. Fu X, Herrera H, Kubota T, Hoffman RM. Extensive liver metastasis from human colon cancer in nude and scid mice after orthotopic onplantation of histologically-intact human colon carcinoma tissue. Anticancer Res 1992, 12:1395–8.
57. Fu X, Theodorescu D, Kerbel RS, Hoffman RM. Extensive multi-organ metastasis following orthotopic onplantation of histologically-intact human bladder carcinoma tissue in nude mice. Int J Cancer 1991, 49:938–9.

58. Fu X, Hoffman RM. Human RT-4 bladder carcinoma is highly metastatic in nude mice, comparable to rash-transformed RT-4 when orthotopically onplanted as histologically-intact tissue. Int J Cancer 1992, 51:989–1.
59. Wang X, Fu X, Hoffman RM. A new patient-like metastatic model of human lung cancer constructed orthotopically with intact tissue via thoracotomy in immunodeficient mice. Int J Cancer 1992, 51:992–5.
60. Wang X, Fu X, Hoffman RM. A patient-like metastasizing model of human lung adenocarcinoma constructed via thoracotomy in nude mice. Anticancer Res 1992, 12:1399–402.
61. Wang X, Fu X, Kubota T, Hoffman RM. A new patient-like metastatic model of human small-cell lung cancer constructed orthotopically with intact tissue via thoracotomy in nude mice. Anticancer Res 1992, 12:1403–6.
62. Kuo T-H, Kubota T, Watanabe M, Furukawa T, Kase S, Tanino H et al. Orthotopic reconstitution of human small-cell lung carcinoma after intravenous transplantation in SCID mice. Anticancer Res 1992, 12:1407–0.
63. Fu X, Guadagni F, Hoffman RM. A metastatic nude-mouse model of human pancreatic cancer constructed orthotopically from histologically intact patient specimens. Proc Natl Acad Sci USA 1992, 89:5645–9.
64. Furukawa T, Fu X, Kubota T, Watanabe M, Kitajima M, Hoffman RM. Nude mouse metastatic models of human stomach cancer constructed using orthotopic implantation of histologically intact tissue. Cancer Res 1993, 53:1204–8.
65. An Z, Jiang P, Wang X, Moossa AR, Hoffman RM. Development of a high metastatic orthotopic model of human renal cell carcinoma in nude mice: Benefits of fragment implantation compared to cell-suspension injection. Clin Exp Metastasis 1999, 17:265–70.
66. Fu X, Le P, Hoffman RM. A metastatic orthotopic-transplant nude-mouse model of human patient breast cancer. Anticancer Res 1993, 13:901–4.
67. Fu X, Hoffman RM. Human ovarian carcinoma metastatic models constructed in nude mice by orthotopic transplantation of histologically-intact patient specimens. Anticancer Res 1993, 13:283–6.
68. Chishima T, Miyagi Y, Wang X, Tan Y, Shimada H, Moossa AR, Hoffman RM. Visualization of the metastatic process by green fluorescent protein expression. Anticancer Res 1997, 17:2377–84.
69. Chishima T, Miyagi Y, Wang X, Baranov E, Tan Y, Shimada H et al. Metastatic patterns of lung cancer visualized live and in process by green fluorescence protein expression. Clin Exp Metastasis 1997, 15:547–2.
70. Chishima T, Miyagi Y, Li L, Tan Y, Baranov E, Yang M et al. Use of histoculture and green fluorescent protein to visualize tumor cell host interaction. In Vitro Cell Dev Biol Animal 1997, 33:745–7.
71. Chishima T, Yang M, Miyagi Y, Li L, Tan Y, Baranov E et al. Governing step of metastasis visualized in vitro. Proc Natl Acad Sci USA 1997, 94:11573–6.
72. Yang M, Hasegawa S, Jiang P, Wang X, Tan Y, Chishima T et al. Widespread skeletal metastatic potential of human lung cancer revealed by green fluorescent protein expression. Cancer Res 1998, 58:4217–21.
73. Dolman CS, Mueller BM, Lode HN, Xiang R, Gillies SD, Reisfeld RA. Suppression of human prostate carcinoma metastases in severe combined immunodeficient mice by interleukin 2 immunocytokine therapy. Clin Cancer Res 1998, 4:2551–7.

74. Yang M, Jiang P, Sun FX, Hasegawa S, Baranov E, Chishima T *et al*. A fluorescent orthotopic bone metastasis model of human prostate cancer. Cancer Res 1999, 59:781–6.
75. Fidler IJ. Critical factors in the biology of human cancer metastasis: Twenty-eigth G.H.A. clows memorial award lecture. Cancer Res 1990, 50:6130–8.
76. Poste G, Fidler IJ. The pathogenesis of cancer metastasis. Nature 1980, 283:139–45.
77. Feldman M, Eisenbach L. What makes a tumor cell metastatic. Sci Am 1988, 259: 60–5, 68, 85.
78. Waters DJ, Janovitz EB, Chan TCK. Spontaneous metastasis of PC-3 cells in athymic mice after implantaion in orthotopic or ectopic microenvironments. Prostate 1995, 26:227–34.
79. Ozen M, Multani AS, Kuniyasu H, Chung LW, von Eschenbach AC, Pathak S. Specific histologic and cytogenetic evidence for in vivo malignant transformation of murine host cells by three human prostate cancer cell lines. Oncol Res 1997, 9:433–8.
80. Hall SJ, Thompson TC. Spontaneous but not experimental metastatic activities differentiate primary tumor-derived vs metastasis-derived mouse prostate cancer cell lines. Clin Exp Metastasis 1997, 15:630–8.
81. Chang XH, Fu YW, Na WL, Wang J, Sun H, Cai L. Improved metastatic animal model of human prostate carcinoma using surgical orthotopic implantation (SOI). Anticancer Res 1999, 19(5B):4199–202.
82. Wang X, An Z, Geller J, Hoffman RM. High malignancy orthotopic nude mouse model of human prostate cancer LNCaP. Prostate 1999, 39:182–6.
83. Mundy GR. Mechanisms of bone metastasis. Cancer 1997, 80:1546–56.
84. Maeda H, Segawa T, Kamoto T, Yoshida H, Kakizuka A, Ogawa O, Kakehi Y. Rapid detection of candidate metastatic foci in the orthotopic inoculation model of androgen-sensitive prostate cancer cells introduced with green fluorescent protein. Prostate 2000, 45:335–40.
85. Patel S, Turner PR, Stubberfield C, Barry E, Rohlff CR, Stamps A *et al*. Hyaluronidase gene profiling and role of hyal-1 overexpression in an orthotopic model of prostate cancer. Int J Cancer 2002, 97:416–24.
86. Cao G, Su J, Lu W, Zhang F, Zhao G, Marteralli D, Dong Z. Adenovirus-mediated interferon-beta gene therapy suppresses growth and metastasis of human prostate cancer in nude mice. Cancer Gene Ther 2001, 8:497–505.
87. Chu LW, Pettaway CA, Liang JC. Genetic abnormalities specifically associated with varying metastatic potential of prostate cancer cell lines as detected by comparative genomic hybridization. Cancer Genet Cytogenet 2001, 127:161–7.
88. Bex A, Wullich B, Endris V, Otto T, Rembrink K, Stockle M, Rubben H. Comparison of the malignant phenotype and genotype of the human androgen-independent cell line DU-145 and a subline derived from metastasis after orthotopic implantation in nude mice. Cancer Genet Cytogenet 2001, 124:98–104.
89. Timár J, Rásó E, Döme B, Li L, Grignon D, Nie D *et al*. Expression, subcellular localization and putative function of platelet-type 12-lipoxygenase in human prostate cancer cell lines of different metastatic potential. Int J Cancer 2000, 87:37–43.
90. Inoue K, Slaton JW, Eve BY, Kim SJ, Perrotte P, Balbay MD *et al*. Interleukin 8 expression regulates tumorigenicity, metastases in androgen-independent prostate cancer. Clin Cancer Res 2000, 6:2104–19.

91. Stearns ME, Wang M. Antimestatic and antitumor activities of interleukin 10 in transfected human prostate PC-3 ML clones: Orthotopic growth in severe combined immunodeficient mice. Clin Cancer Res 1998, 4:2257–63.
92. Stearns ME, Garcia FU, Fudge K, Rhim J, Wang M. Role of interleukin 10 and transforming growth factor BETA1 in the angiogenesis and metastasis of human prostate primary tumor lines from orthotopic implants in severe combined immunodeficiency mice. Clin Cancer Res 1999, 5:711–20.
93. Trikha M, Raso E, Cai Y, Fazakas Z, Paku S, Porter AT et al. Role of alphaii(b)BETA3 integrin in prostate cancer metastasis. Prostate 1998, 35:185–92.
94. Marengo SR, Sikes RA, Anezinis P, Chang SM, Chung LW. Metastasis induced by overexpression of P185NEU-T after orthotopic injection into a prostatic epithelial cell line (nbe). Mol Carcinog 1997, 19:165–75.
95. Greene GF, Kitadai Y, Pettaway CA, von Eschenbach AC, Bucana CD, Fidler IJ. Correlation of metastasis-related gene expression with metastatic potential in human prostate carcinoma cells implanted in nude mice using an in situ messenger RNA hybridization technique. Am J Pathol 1997, 150:1571–82.
96. Olson KA, Byers HR, Key ME, Fett JW. Prevention of human prostate tumor metastasis in athymic mice by antisense targeting of human angiogenin. Clin Cancer Res 2001, 7:3598–605.
97. Dong Z, Greene G, Pettaway C, Dinney CP, Eue I, Lu W et al. Suppression of angiogenesis, tumorigenicity, and metastasis by human prostate cancer cells engineered to produce interferon-beta. Cancer Res 1999, 59:872–9.
98. Nasu Y, Bangma CH, Hull GW, Lee HM, Hu J, Wang J et al. Adenovirus-mediated interleukin-12 gene therapy for prostate cancer: Suppression of orthotopic tumor growth and pre-established lung metastases in an orthotopic model. Gene Ther 1999, 6:338–49.
99. Hull GW, Mccurdy MA, Nasu Y, Bangma CH, Yang G, Shimura S et al. Prostate cancer gene therapy: Comparison of adenovirus-mediated expression of interleukin 12 with interleukin 12 plus B7-1 for in situ gene therapy and gene-modified, cell-based vaccines. Clin Cancer Res 2000, 6:4101–9.
100. Eastham JA, Grafton W, Martin CM, Williams BJ. Suppression of primary tumor growth and the progression to metastasis with P53 adenovirus in human prostate cancer. J Urol 2000, 164(3 Pt 1):814–9.
101. Hall SJ, Mutchnik SE, Chen SH, Woo SL, Thompson TC. Adenovirus-mediated herpes simplex virus thymidine kinase gene and ganciclovir therapy leads to systemic activity against spontaneous and induced metastasis in an orthotopic mouse model of prostate cancer. Int J Cancer 1997, 70:183–7.
102. Hall SJ, Sanford MA, Atkinson G, Chen SH. Induction of potent antitumor natural killer cell activity by herpes simplex virus-thymidine kinase and ganciclovir therapy in an orthotopic mouse model of prostate cancer. Cancer Res 1998, 58:3221–5.
103. Maeda H, Hori S, Nishitoh H, Ichijo H, Ogawa O, Kakehi Y, Kakizuka A. Tumor growth inhibition by arsenic trioxide (AS2O3) in the orthotopic metastasis model of androgen-independent prostate cancer. Cancer Res 2001, 61:5432–40.
104. Tahir SA, Yang G, Ebara S, Timme TL, Satoh T, Li L et al. Secreted caveolin-1 stimulates cell survival/clonal growth and contributes to metastasis in androgen-insensitive prostate cancer. Cancer Res 2001, 61:3882–5.

105. Saffran DC, Raitano AB, Hubert RS, Witte ON, Reiter RE, Jakobovits A. Anti-PSCA mAbs inhibit tumor growth and metastasis formation and prolong the survival of mice bearing human prostate cancer xenografts. Proc Natl Acad Sci USA 2001, 98:2658–63.
106. Anidjar M, Villette JM, Devauchelle P, Delisle F, Cotard JP, Billotey C et al. In vivo model mimicking natural history of dog prostate cancer using DPC-1, a new canine prostate carcinoma cell line. Prostate 2001, 46:2–10.
107. Yang M, Baranov E, Jiang P, Sun F-X, Li X-M, Li L et al. Whole-body optical imaging of green fluorescent protein-expressing tumors and metastases. Proc Natl Acad Sci USA 2000, 97:1206–1.
108. Yang M, Baranov E, Li X-M, Wang J-W, Jiang P, Li L et al. Whole-ody and intravital optical imaging of angiogenesis in orthotopically implanted tumors. Proc Natl Acad Sci USA 2001, 98:2616–1.
109. Yang, Baranov ME, Moossa AR, Penman S, Hoffman RM. Visualizing gene expression by whole-body fluorescence imaging. Proc Natl Acad Sci USA 2000, 97:12278–82.
110. Yang M, Baranov E, Wang J-W, Jiang P, Wang X, Sun F-X et al. Direct external imaging of nascent cancer, tumor progression, angiogenesis, and metastasis on internal organs in the fluorescent orthotopic model. Proc Natl Acad Sci USA 2002, 99:3824–9.
111. Hoffman RM. Orthotopic metastatic mouse models for anticancer drug discovery and evaluation: A bridge to the clinic. Invest New Drugs 1999, 17:343–59.
112. Knox JD, Mack CF, Powell WC, Bowden GT, Nagle RB. Prostate tumor cell invasion: A comparison of orthotopic and ectopic models. Invasion Metastasis 1993, 13:325–1.
113. Gupta S, Hastek K, Ahmad N, Lewin JS, Mukhtar H. Inhibhtion of prostate carcinogenesis in TRAMP mice by oral infusion of green tea polyphenols. Proc Natl Acad Sci USA 2001, 98:10350–55.

Chapter 9

ß-CATENIN, ITS BINDING PARTNERS AND SIGNALLING MECHANISMS: IMPLICATIONS IN PROSTATE CANCER

Gaynor Davies[1], Gregory M. Harrison[1] and Malcolm D. Mason[2]
[1]*Metastasis Research Group, University Department of Surgery, University of Wales College of Medicine, Heath Park, Cardiff, Wales, UK*
[2]*Department of Medicine, Section of Clinical Oncology, Velindre Hospital, Cardiff, Wales, UK*

Abstract: ß-catenin is a cytoplasmic protein that has been well documented in recent years by a number of investigators. It is now firmly established that ß-catenin plays a dual role through its function in facilitating intercellular adhesion by binding to E-cadherin, and also for its key role as a mediator of the Wnt signal transduction pathway. This chapter summarises some of the scientific and clinical advances made during the last decade on the molecular and cellular functions of ß-catenin, including its role in Wnt signalling, adherence junction assembly and its impact on prostate cancer progression.

Key words: ß-catenin, signalling, cell adhesion and prostate cancer

1. INTRODUCTION

The ß-catenin protein was originally identified as a component of the adherens junction, a multi-protein complex supporting tight cell-cell contacts in the presence of extracellular calcium (1–4). However, ß-catenin is now known to be a key player in the *Wnt* signalling transduction pathway. Cell-cell adhesion is mediated by ß-catenin as well as plakoglobin (i.e., γ-catenin), by their direct association with the highly conserved cytoplasmic domain of classical (i.e., N-, P- and E-cadherins) cadherins (1). The cadherin/catenin complex is linked either directly to the cytoskeleton through interaction with α-catenin (5), or indirectly to the actin filament network via association with the actin binding proteins α-actinin or vinculin (6). The architectural integrity of adherens junctions appears to be dynamically regulated by tyrosine phosphorylation of ß-catenin. Previous studies have shown ß-catenin to be phosphorylated by the multi-functional cytokine hepatocyte growth factor/scatter factor (HGF/SF), resulting in the dismantling of cadherin/catenin complexes and the increased invasiveness of bladder cancer cells (7). ß-catenin is regulated by components of the axin complex, including *APC* (adenomatous polyposis coli) and GSK-3ß (glycogen synthase kinase-3ß), that process ß-catenin for subsequent ubiquitination and proteosomal de-radation. Stabilisation of cytosomal ß-catenin arises from deregulated ß-catenin signalling, that has been observed in many human tumors and is thought to a play a pivotal role in the genesis of a variety of malignancies (8–9). Mutational inactivation of *APC* has been detected in a majority of colorectal cancers (10), this ultimately contributes to the accumulation of intracellular ß-catenin, and deregulated expression of its downstream target genes, some of which have been implicated in a variety of human cancers (11–13). These mechanisms will be discussed in greater detail in later sections of this chapter.

2. THE CADHERIN/CATENIN COMPLEX AND SIGNALLING EVENTS

Cadherins, together with their associated catenin proteins, were initially thought to function solely as cell adhesion molecules initiating firm cell-cell adhesion contacts, an essential requirement for the architectural maintenance of epithelial derived cells. However, recent studies in this field have indicated that their role is much more diverse than originally envisaged. Much of the evidence to date is reflected by the increasing number of molecules mediated by the complex and the increased number of cellular events that occurs as a result of the adhesion complex.

2.1 Key Components of the Cadherin/Catenin Complex

The cadherin adhesion complex is composed of the following components: cadherin (such as E-cadherin), intracellular components associated with cadherin (such as catenins) and the cytoskeleton (such as actin) as shown in Figure 1. Catenins are a group of cytoplasmic proteins that

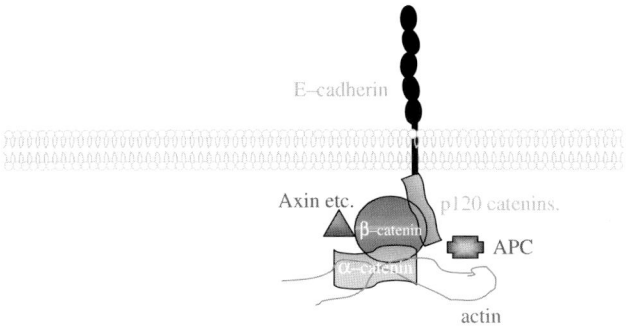

Figure 1. The E-cadherin/ß-catenin complex and its associated cytoplasmic members involved in the mediation of adherence junction assembly (52).

interact with the intracellular domain of the cadherin molecule, providing anchorage to the microfilament cytoskeleton and serve to regulate cadherin function (1–4, 14). The three main catenin types identified according to their electrophoretic mobility on SDS-PAGE are α-, ß- and γ-catenins (1–2, 15–17). α-catenin has been reported to provide direct mechanical linkage to the actin cytoskeleton, as it shares partial homology with the actin-binding protein vinculin (18–19). Another protein molecule called p120^{cas} has also been identified as a family member belonging to this catenin group (20–22). Furthermore, this cadherin-associated src (Rous Sarcoma virus gene family) substrate (p120^{cas}) has been implicated to serve as a tyrosine kinase substrate, after phosphorylation by several receptor tyrosine kinases, such as: epidermal growth factor, platelet-derived growth factor and colony stimulating factor-1 (23–24). In addition, p120^{cas} shares partial homology with: ß-catenin, plakoglobin (γ-catenin) and the *Drosophila* segment polarity gene product *armadillo* (25–28).

2.2 Catenins

Both ß-catenin and plakoglobin associate directly with cadherin, and can be substituted for each other within the cadherin-catenin complex (29–32). Plakoglobin, ß-catenin, and *armadillo* also share partial homology with *APC*, a tumor suppressor gene frequently mutated in colon cancers (33–36). *APC* forms a complex with GSK-3ß, which in turn, leads to the stabilisation of both ß-catenin and plakoglobin levels (37). Such complexes form part of the signalling pathway driven by the secreted glycoprotein wingless (Wg/Wnt) in *Drosophila* (38). Alterations in the expression of catenin proteins *in vivo* may play an important role in the initiation of metastatic tumor spread (39). A reduced level, or loss of α-catenin expression is likely to result in an impairment of E-cadherin function (40–41). Furthermore, deletion of the α-catenin gene *in vitro*, results in the inactivation of E-cadherin-mediated cell-cell adhesion in prostate cancer cells (42). Consequently a mutation or dysfunctional ß-catenin molecule may also result in both cell-cell disengagement, and to a more invasive phenotype (43). Tyrosine phosphorylation of ß-catenin has also been shown to affect the cadherin/catenin complex in both metastatic fibroblasts (44) and breast cancer cells (45) respectively. Interestingly, ß-catenin has been identified as a proto-oncogene (46), while its homolgue γ-catenin (plakoglobin) appears to function as a tumor suppressor gene (47).

2.2.1 p120 Catenin Family Members, Another Expanding Family of Cadherin Associated Molecules

The p120 catenin protein has been defined as an onco-protein and is found to be associated with the intracellular domain of cadherin (20, 22). However, the precise role of this molecule within the cadherin complex was not established until recently (48). A large number of molecules have been identified as p120 catenin family members, including $p120^{cas}$ (cadherin-associated src, or $p120^{ctn}$, p120 catenin), ARVCF (Armadillo repeat gene deleted in velo-cardio-facial syndrome) δ-catenin/NPRAP/neurojungin, armadillo proteins plakophilin 1, plakophilin 2, plakophilin 3 and plakophilin 4 (i.e., also known as p0071) (48–50). ARVCF and δ-catenin/NPRAP/neurojungin share over 40% homology with $p120^{cas}$, and all three bind to classical cadherins. The plakophilins share 30% homology with $p120^{cas}$ and possibly interact with desmosomal cadherins. In contrast, β-catenin binds to the catenin-binding domain (CBD), while $p120^{cas}$ binds to the juxtamembrane domain of cadherins. The juxtamembrane domain of cadherins has also been implicated in the regulation (suppression) of the invasive and motile behaviour of cancer cells (51)

The exact role of $p120^{cas}$ in cadherin mediated cell adhesion has yet to be clarified. However, Reynolds and colleagues (20) have proposed that $p120^{cas}$ may be involved in both 'positive' (activation) and 'negative' (inhibition) regulation of cell adhesion, possibly depending on the function status of the protein. Interestingly, $p120^{cas}$ is found to be able to mediate nuclear signalling, similar to that of β-catenin. This is perhaps achieved by direct interaction with a transcription factor known as Kaiso (49–50).

3. ß-CATENIN PLAYS A KEY ROLE IN INTRACELLULAR SIGNALLING

3.1 ß-Catenin Binds to a Number of Intracellular Signalling Molecules

ß-catenin was initially discovered as an associated cytoskeletal protein of the cadherin complex, whose main role was to facilitate cell-cell adhesion. However, it was soon realised to be a central player in a chain of complex signalling events. This was manifested by the presence of binding domains, and by its interactions with an array of other molecules important in signalling and gene expression including cadherin, α-catenin, axin, conductin, GSK-3β and *APC*. The association of cytoplasmic ß-catenin with such molecules is a tightly regulated event that is determined by the other intra- or extra-cellular signals. This complex not only decides the fate of ß-catenin, but also directly influences a number of cellular events and initiates gene transcription.

3.1.1 ß-Catenin and its Interaction with GSK3ß

It is now well established that GSK-3ß binds to ß-catenin and upon engagement phosphorylates ß-catenin on specific serine and threonine residues in its amino-terminal region (37, 52). The unique processing of ß-catenin by GSK-3ß and other molecules including Axin, and *APC* results in the targeting of ß-catenin for ubiquitnation by an E3 ubiquitin ligase containg the F-box protein ß-TRCP (46, 53). Consequently this results in the rapid degradation of ß-catenin within the proteosome in the absence of *Wnt* signalling (54–55). However, it was soon realised that the cytoplasmic interactions of ß-catenin occurs in a more complex pattern than originally thought. Such interactions involve molecules that were seemingly unrelated to the complex such as TCF/LEF-1 (T cell factor/lymphoid enhancer factor-1), NLK (NEMO-like kinase), Pontin52 and Duplin. The association of these molecules with cytoplasmic ß-catenin will be discussed in greater detail in a later section of this chapter.

3.1.2 ß-Catenin and its Interaction with APC

The *APC* gene product encodes a 2843 amino acid polypeptide that has been shown to participate in a number of cellular processes including the regulation of intracellular ß-catenin (56). *APC* is frequently mutated in colorectal cancers, a condition resulting in an autosomal dominant disorder referred to as familial adenomatous polyposis (FAP) (57). In the central domain of *APC* a 15-amino-acid motif is repeated three times, plus seven 20-amino-acid repeats (58). The existence of these amino acid repeats form the basis of *APC's* interaction with intracellular ß-catenin by binding to ß-catenin, and down-regulating its levels (33–36, 59). Furthermore, within the central domain of *APC* exists another 4-amino-acid motif repeated three times. These polypeptide motifs are known as the SAMP (Ser-Ala-Met-Pro) repeats and they provide critical binding sites for both conductin and axin to associate with this *APC*/ß-catenin/GSK-3ß complex, that in turn aids in the regulation of intracellular ß-catenin (60–62).

3.1.3   ß-Catenin and its Interaction with Axin/Conductin

Axin, encoded by AXIN1 was cloned from a mouse mutant with body-axis duplication and was found to have a direct interaction site with ß-catenin (63). Axin serves as a scaffold protein, due to its multiple binding sites for interaction with many of the proteins involved in *Wnt* signalling, including *APC*, GSK-3ß, ß-catenin, the catalytic subunit of the serine/threonine protein phosphatase PP2A (PP2Ac), the cytoplamic phosphoprotein Dishevelled and in fact, for axin itself (61, 64–68). Axin1 homologues include conductin (60), axin2 (69) or an axin-like protein known as Axil (70) that play key roles in ß-catenin regulation. However, although axin2 is functionally similar to axin1, it has not been has extensively characterised as its orthologue. Axin1 is an important component of *Wnt* signalling as it is constitutively expressed during ß-catenin degradation by the proteosome. Furthermore, axin1 increases ß-catenin phosphorylation via its association with GSK-3ß, which in turn accelerates the down-regulation of ß-catenin (60, 63). Axin2 also acts as a scaffold protein on which the phosphorylation of ß-catenin by GSK-3ß is assembled and negatively regulated in the absence of *Wnt* signalling (68). However, unlike axin1, axin2 is mutated in a sub-set of colorectal cancers (71–72). In addition, axin2 expression is only up-regulated in response to increased levels of ß-catenin within the cytosol, thereby limiting the duration and intensity of the *Wnt*/ß-catenin signal (73–74).

3.2   GSK-3ß Regulates Intracellular ß-Catenin Levels

GSK-3ß is able to phosphorylate *APC* and the subsequent binding of axin/conductin to *APC* further enhances this phosphorylation. The single most interesting feature of *APC* in cancers, particularly in colon cancer, is its frequent mutation especially in regions including the binding domains for ß-catenin and GSK-3ß. These mutations eventually lead to damage of the ß-catenin complex preventing effective phosphorylation of ß-catenin and finally to the targeted destruction of ß-catenin by the proteosome (46). This would ultimately lead to the accumulation of ß-catenin within the nucleus, a common feature frequently observed in cancer cells. Recently, another *APC* like protein was identified known as *APCL* or *APC2* (75). The overall structure of *APC2* is similar to that of *APC*. This polypeptide is much smaller in size (approximately 550 amino acids shorter than *APC*) compared to *APC*, however, it still retains the seven 20-amino-acid repeats necessary for the down-regulation of cytoplasmic ß-catenin (75). Therefore, mutations occurring within the ß-catenin and GSK-3ß binding sites of *APC2*, particularly in cancer cells, will require extensive investigations in the future.

4. ß-CATENIN DESTRUCTION IS CONTROLLED BY *WNT* SIGNALLING

As previously mentioned the fate of cytoplasmic ß-catenin is decided by its interaction with a group of other intracellular proteins including *APC*, axin and GSK-3ß. However, the degradation of ß-catenin by this complex is a tightly regulated event controlled via the *Wnt* signalling cascade. *Wnt* proteins are a family of cystein-rich secreted ligands that control embryonic development. These molecules are known to participate in the regulation of cell growth, proliferation, morphology, motility and organ development (37, 76, 77). *Wnt* proteins are now known to bind to another group of transmembrane proteins, referred to as Frizzled or the Wg receptor. The *Wnt* signalling pathway is an important component of cell-cell adhesion since it regulates ß-catenin degradation as shown in Figure 2.

In the absence of *Wnt* signalling (i.e., *Wnt* is switched off), *APC* and axin family members form a complex, bind to and activate GSK-3ß. Upon activation GSK-3ß interacts with *APC* and phosphorylates it. The phosphorylated *APC* has an increased affinity to ß-catenin, and allows the addition of phosphate groups to ß-catenin (phosphorylated). Phosphorylated ß-catenin is then able to bind to a F-box protein known as ß-TRCP. As a consequence of its interaction with ß-TRCP, ß-catenin acquires the ability to interact with an E3 ubiquitin ligase. The ß-catenin-ubiquitin complex is subsequently degraded via processing through the proteosome (i.e., cell protein recycling centre) (53).

Conversely, in the presence of *Wnt* signalling (i.e., *Wnt* is switched on), Wnt proteins interact, firstly with serpentine receptors Wg (i.e., the Frizzled families), and secondly, this interaction activates another protein known as Dishevelled. The activation of Dishevelled results in the dephosphorylation

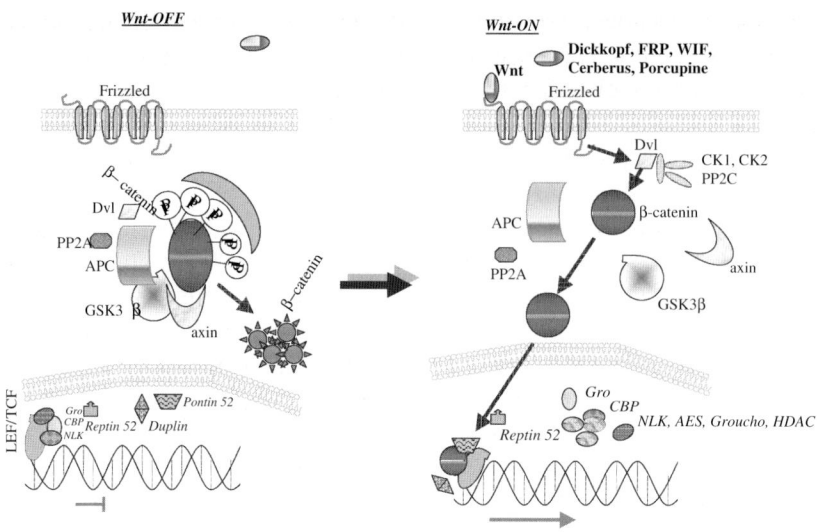

Figure 2. The key role played by ß-catenin in the Wnt signalling transduction pathway (52).

of GSK-3ß, and this in turn, antagonises the action of the *APC*/axin/GSK-3ß complex on the phosphorylation of ß-catenin. This deactivation prevents the ubiquitn-mediated degradation of ß-catenin and ultimately leads to the accumulation of ß-catenin within the cytosol. Cytoplasmic ß-catenin eventually translocates to the nucleus and participates in the regulation of gene expression via its interaction with transcription factors TCF/LEF-1 (referred to in a later section).

Other molecules may also play a role in the degradation process of ß-catenin. Casein kinase1ε (CK1ε), is a seriene/threonin kinase, downstream of Dishevelled, and upstream of GSK3ß, and has been shown to stabilise ß-catenin (78–79). However, new evidence has recently emerged showing the converse (80–82). CK1ε was originally thought to be a positive transducer of the *Wnt* signal, thereby stabilising ß-catenin levels in order to engage transcription factors of the LEF/TCF family to activate various target genes (1, 46, 83). In fact, three recent publications report CK1ε to prime ß-catenin for its subsequent phosphorylation by GSK-3ß, thereby negatively regulating its level within the cytoplasm (80–82). In addition, PP2A, a protein phosphatase, has been shown to dephosphorylate axin, and thus regulate ß-catenin stability (84). ß-catenin/LEF-1 signalling by *Wnt*-1, or over expression of ß-catenin itself, is also inhibited by caveolin-1 expression (85). Recombinant expression of caveolin-1, in caveolin-1 negative cells is sufficient to recruit ß-catenin to caveolar membranes, thereby blocking ß-catenin-mediated transactivation. Thus caveolin-1 expression can modulate *Wnt*/ß-catenin/LEF-1 signalling by regulating the intracellular localisation of ß-catenin (85).

4.1   ß-Catenin and its Role in Gene Expression

Perhaps one of most exciting discoveries made regarding the function of ß-catenin is that, in addition to acting as an adhesion regulator, it plays an essential role in the transcription of a number of target genes (1, 83). Cytoplasmic ß-catenin, once dissociated from the axin complex and upon entering the nucleus, interacts with TCF and LEF-1 (i.e., members belonging to the HMG box transcription factors of T-cell factor/lymphoid enhancing factor-1 family). Both TCF and LEF differ quite considerably from all other classical transcription factors, as they are unable to activate gene transcription alone. Instead, intracellular ß-catenin engages with TCF/LEF, thus enabling TCF/LEF to bind to DNA and initiate the transcription process. The following genes are traditional targets of TCF: *c-myc, c-jun, fra-1, PPARδ, uPA* and *cyclins* (11, 13, 86–88). Fibronectin and matrix metalloproteinase-7 (MMP-7) are new targets of ß-catenin that have been identified during the last few years (89–90). Interestingly, activation of ß-catenin has been found to suppress the expression of monocyte chemotactic protein-3 (MCP-3), a chemokine known to reduce tumorigenicity (91–93).

TCF negatively regulates ß-catenin by interacting with TCF binding proteins including NLK, co-activators, CBP (Cre-element binding protein (CREB)-binding protein) and the transcription repressor Groucho (94–96). In the absence of *Wnt* signalling, TCF is associated with Groucho/TLE (transducin-like enhancer-of-split) and maintains an inactive state of target genes (94, 97–98). The ß-catenin/TCF interaction may be further enhanced by its involvement with other nuclear proteins such as Pontin52 and Duplin (11, 13, 87). It is also interesting to note that Pontin52 and its interacting partner Reptin52, associate with the TATA-box binding protein (TBP) and as such, antagonise the trans-activation potential of the ß-catenin/TCF complex (99). Furthermore, p300/CBP histone acetyltransferase (HAT) has been shown to function as a transcriptional co-activator of ß-catenin by alleviating Groucho-mediated repression (100), hence regulating ß-catenin/TCF transcription via its interaction with ß-catenin's N-terminus (88). This interaction and the subsequent activation of this complex have also been implicated in the neoplastic transformation of ß-catenin. Taken together, ß-catenin-mediated neoplastic transformation and tumor progression involve not only the activation of oncogenes and tumor enhancer genes, but also suppression of tumor inhibitor genes, such as MCPs (91–93).

4.2 Mutations in ß-Catenin and its Associated Binding Partners

Genetic alterations in a number of genes involved in the down–regulation of ß-catenin include *APC*, AXIN1, AXIN2 and ß-catenin itself. These mutations have been reported in a number of cancer cell types, and lead to the stabilisation of ß-catenin by inhibiting phosphorylation of ß-catenin via GSK-3ß and subsequent proteasomal degradation (9, 71,101–102). Most mutations occur within the ß-catenin gene (CTNNB1) at highly conserved amino acids sites encoded by exon 3, and have revealed disruption to serine/threonine phosphorylation residues that are critical regions for ß-catenin phosphorylation by GSK-3ß (101). CTNNB1 mutations result in the accumulation of ß-catenin within the cytosol, its binding with transcription factors TCF/LEF, its subsequent translocation to the nucleus, and the activation of oncogenic target genes that regulate cellular growth, differentiation and apoptosis (103–104). Voeller *et al.* (101) examined 104 prostate cancer tissues to determine whether mutations in exon 3 of the ß-catenin gene play an important role in the malignant transformation of prostate cancer. They detected 5 mutations in prostate cancer tissues out of a total of 104 specimens screened. Four out of the five mutations detected involved alteration to serine or threonine residues implicated in ß-catenin degradation, while the fifth tumor had a mutation at codon 32, changing a highly conserved aspartic acid to a tyrosine. They concluded that mutational analysis of multiple regions from several tumor samples showed that ß-catenin mutations were present focally and therefore may occur during tumor progression.

In a separate study conducted by Taniguchi *et al.* (68), the mutational status and expression of the CTNNB1, AXIN1 and AXIN2 genes were assessed to determine their roles in liver carcinogenesis. This group assessed 73 hepatocellular carcinomas (HCC), and 27 hepatoblastomas (HB) and reported the following mutational frequencies in liver cancer: 14 out of 73 (19.2%) cases were reported to have ß-catenin mutations in HCC's, and 19 out of 27 (70.4%) cases had ß-catenin mutations in HB's; AXIN1 mutations occurred in 7 (9.6%) cases of HCC's and 2 (7.4%) cases of HB's; whereas AXIN 2 mutations were found in 2 (2.7%) cases of HCC's but not in HB's. Perhaps the most interesting discovery made by this group is that 2 HCC's tumors had mutations in both the ß-catenin and AXIN1 genes, and in contrast, 1 HCC tumor had mutations in both the ß-catenin and AXIN2 genes. They concluded that AXIN1 mutations in HB and AXIN2 mutations in HCC might contribute to ß-catenin dysregulation in a sub-set of these tumor types.

APC is a large protein comprising multiple functional domains, and in particular it possesses two motifs that have been reported to associate directly with ß-catenin (33, 53). Wild type *APC* protein also contains two functional nuclear export signals (NES) that can shuttle ß-catenin out of the nucleus for subsequent ubiquitination and degradation (105–107). *APC* gene mutations are characterised by the development of multiple colorectal adenomas, some of which progress to carcinoma (108). Furthermore, mutational inactivation of *APC* initiates nuclear accumulation and stabilisation of cytoplasmic ß-catenin in cancer cells, including colorectal (109) and breast cancers (110–111). *APC* is a component of the canonical *Wnt* signal transduction pathway, of which one target is TCF-1. Recently, mutations in both *APC* and TCF-1 genes in mice have been implicated in mammary tumorigenesis, blocking normal mammary gland development and directly initiating acanthoma (112). ß-catenin and TCF-4 have been shown to form a transcription complex that plays a key role in the maintenance of normal epithelium, and in the development of colorectal tumors. Ruckert *et al*. (113) has recently reported a frameshift mutation to frequently occur in the TCF-4 A(9) monorepeat, located in exon 17 of the TCF-4 gene. However, upon further investigation by this group they concluded that mutations found in the TCF-4 gene did not contribute to colorectal tumorigenesis.

5. FACTORS AFFECTING THE SUBCELLULAR LOCALISATION OF ß-CATENIN

As previously mentioned, truncated *APC* protein, resulting from most *APC* mutations, ultimately leads to elevated ß-catenin levels in a variety of cancer cell types. *APC*, GSK-3ß and axin thus form a large protein complex that facilitates ß-catenin regulation within the cytoplasm. Anderson *et al*. (114) recently examined the localisation and level of endogenous ß-catenin/*APC*/axin protein complexes using laser scanning confocal microscopy, and immunofluorescence staining in both normal, and neoplastic colon tissues obtained from more than 50 patients. They found *APC* and axin to be co-localised within the nucleus and at lateral cell borders, whereas, levels of axin2 were found to be limited in the nucleus only. Furthermore, they observed nuclear ß-catenin in fewer than half of the carcinomas screened, and upon further examination was rarely found to be observed in adenomatous polyps, thereby indicating that nuclear translocation of ß-catenin may not be an immediate consequence of *APC* loss.

Subcellular localisation of ß-catenin has also been assessed in both normal and malignant (cell lines SCC15 and SCC25) oral keratinocytes, and in 24 frozen samples of oral squamous cell carcinomas (OSSC) (115). Gasparoni *et al.* (115) used a double-staining technique for assessing the level of ß-catenin expression, and found ß-catenin to be localised at the plasma membrane in normal oral keratinocytes and SCC15 cells, but not in SCC25 cells. In the SCC25 cell line, they observed ß-catenin staining to be localised mainly within the perinuclear and nuclear areas, whereas in OSSC sections, nuclear ß-catenin staining was localised only within the invading islands of two carcinomas deep in the underlying connective tissue. Their findings indicated that intranuclear ß-catenin did not appear to be a common phenomenon in OSSC, and that a no clear association *in vivo* could be established between intranuclear ß-catenin, histopathological grade and malignancy index.

HGF/SF has also been reported to induce the phosphorylation of GSK-3ß, a potential target for ß-catenin ubiquitination and degradation. Recent studies conducted by Liu *et al.* (116), have demonstrated HGF/SF to mediate the phosphorylation of GSK-3ß, which in turn, has been shown to correlate strongly with enhanced ß-catenin immunoreactivity in endothelial cell-cell junctions. This group concluded that HGF/SF mediated phosphorylation of GSK-3ß, increases the availability of cytoplasmic ß-catenin, thereby enhancing endothelial junctional integrity and vascular barrier function. Previously, we have demonstrated that cytoplasmic pools of ß-catenin associate more directly with components of the axin complex in the absence of E-cadherin, whereas in its presence, the subcellular localisation of ß-catenin is stabilised by its interaction with E-cadherin that in turn, facilitates tight cell-cell contacts in prostate cancer cells. Using immunofluorescence, we found the level of co-localised cytoplasmic staining between ß-catenin and GSK-3ß to be enhanced in prostate cancer cells by HGF/SF, irrespective of E-cadherin status (117). In contrast, co-localised cytoplasmic staining between *APC* and ß-catenin was increased by HGF/SF, and detected only in E-cadherin negative cells (i.e., PC-3 cells) thus indicating a regulatory role for E-cadherin in the stabilisation of both ß-catenin and in the maintenance of epithelial architecture.

Previous studies from our group have shown HGF/SF to be implicated in the mediation of E-cadherin/β-catenin dissociation in prostate cancer cells, as demonstrated by immunoprecipitation and co-precipitation experiments shown in Figure 3 (118). We found dissociation of the cadherin/catenin complex to be affected by the choice of lysis buffer used to extract the protein components as previously described by Hinck *et al.* (30). In this study we

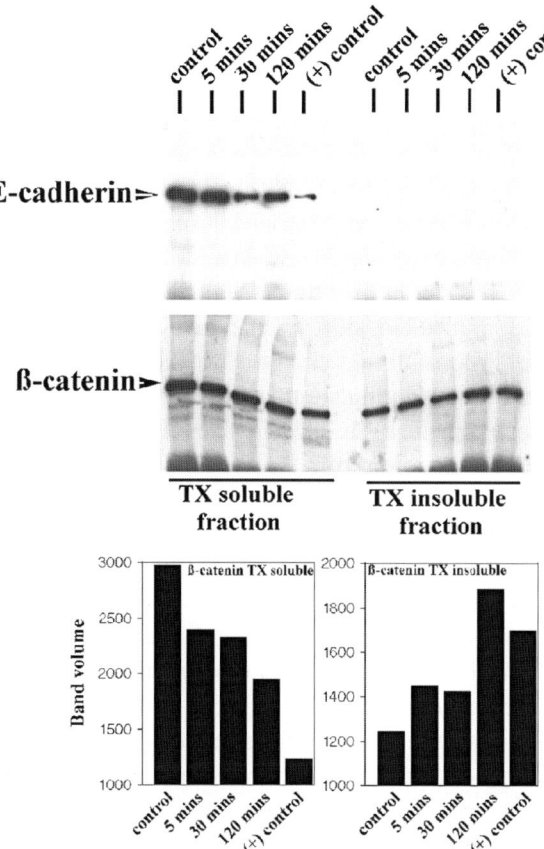

Figure 3. Changes in co-precipitated E-cadherin/β-catenin and immunoprecipitated β-catenin levels from Triton soluble, and insoluble fractions. LNCapFGC cells were stimulated with HGF/SF (40ng/ml) for the times indicated, and immunoprecipitated β-catenin protein was first extracted using a buffer containing 1.5% Triton X-100. This fraction was referred to as the Triton soluble fraction (left). Immunoprecipitated β-catenin protein from the insoluble pellets, were further extracted using a buffer containing 0.5% SDS. This fraction was referred to as the Triton insoluble fraction (right). Both fractions were then separated on an 8% SDS PAGE gel and probed separately with either an anti-E-cadherin (top), or an anti-β-catenin (middle) antibody. Co-precipitated E-cadherin/β-catenin levels were reduced by HGF/SF in the Triton soluble fraction only (top left). HGF/SF also induced a reduction in the level of immunoprecipitated β-catenin protein from the Triton soluble fraction (middle and bottom left). However, this level was seen to increase in the Triton insoluble fraction (middle and bottom right) (118).

have shown that the majority of co-precipitated E-cadherin/β-catenin was extracted from LNCapFGC cells using a lysis buffer containing 1.5% Triton. In addition, we also observed a reduction in this adhesion complex (Triton soluble fraction) after treatment by HGF/SF. However, there was no detection of co-precipitated E-cadherin/β-catenin in the Triton insoluble fraction. Interestingly, the same lysis buffer only extracted part of immunoprecipitated β-catenin (Triton- soluble fraction), and again there was a reduction in the level of immunoprecipitated β-catenin (Figure 3, middle and bottom, left hand sides), after treatment by HGF/SF. This reduction in the level of immunoprecipitated β-catenin from the Triton soluble fraction was subsequently observed as an increase in the Triton insoluble fraction (SDS containing buffer) (Figure 3, middle and bottom, right hand sides). Thus suggesting that HGF/SF had induced a shift in the level of immunoprecipitated β-catenin from the Triton soluble fraction, to the Triton insoluble fraction. Furthermore, this may also indicate that free pools of cytoplasmic β-catenin had increased after exposure to HGF/SF, as a result of tyrosine phosphorylation and its subsequent dissociation from the E-cadherin/catenin complex (118).

We have previously shown prostate cancer cells to exhibit a diverse range of molecules associated with cell-cell adhesion and *Wnt* signalling (119). Using immunocytochemistry, the localisation of signalling intermediates including *APC*, ß-catenin, GSK-3α, GSK-3ß and *Wnt-1* were assessed in DU-145, LNCapFGC, PC-3 (i.e., three cell lines of high invasive potential), CA-HPV-10 and PZ-HPV-7 (i.e., two cell lines of low invasive potential) prostate cancer cell lines. ß-catenin and GSK-3ß were expressed by all five prostate cancer cell lines and were confined to areas of cell-cell contact in four of the cell lines screened. PC-3 cells were found to be the only exception; the staining characteristics for ß-catenin and GSK-3ß in this cell line were located within the nucleus. We also observed the cell lines of high invasive potential to express *APC*, GSK-3α and *Wnt-1*, while the two cell lines of low invasive potential were found to lack expression of these protein molecules. We concluded that the expression of these adhesion molecules may have an important relationship with the invasive phenotype of prostate cancer cells.

6. THE CADHERIN/CATENIN COMPLEX AND CLINICAL PERSPECTIVES

The importance of the biological function of the cadherin/catenin complex has prompted extensive clinical studies on the precise role that these molecules play in cancer development. The most extensively studied cancers to date include some of the neurological tumors, breast, colorectal, oesophageal, lung and liver cancers. Although studies on prostate cancer are rather limited in number, there is strong evidence indicating a pivotal role of E-cadherin and catenins in the development and progression of human prostate cancer.

Numerous clinical studies have demonstrated that down regulation of the cadherin/catenin complex contributes to the invasive behaviour of urological cancers, and therefore, may be related to clinicopathological data (120–124). The conclusions drawn from such studies were that E-cadherin was a prognostic factor for determining the extent of cancer development. Mialhe *et al.* (125) assessed the level of E-cadherin and its full catenin compliment in 99 bladder tumors using immunohistochemistry in an effort to evaluate their prognostic value. They reported high levels of expression for the E-cadherin/catenin complex in normal urothelium. However, upon examination of tumor tissue, histopathological data revealed disrupted expression of E-cadherin, α-catenin and ß-catenin respectively. This study clearly demonstrated a statistically significant association between abnormal α-catenin expression, and poor survival for patients with carcinoma of the bladder, thereby indicating that α-catenin does have a prognostic value.

Immunohistochemical detection of the E-cadherin/catenin complex has also been assessed in 45 prostate tumor tissues obtained by radical prostatectomy (126). This study demonstrated that aberrant expression of each adhesion molecule was associated with high tumor grade and lower survival. Therefore, these findings suggest that all three catenin types (α-, ß- and γ-catenins) may be useful in the prognosis of biologically aggressive cancers of the prostate. In contrast, a study by Aaltomaa *et al.* (127) revealed α-catenin to be the only biological indicator to have any prognostic value in assessing the degree of both local, and locally advanced prostate cancer. In this study, the E-cadherin/catenin complex was examined using immunohistochemistry in 215 males with cancer of the prostate. Their results revealed α-catenin to be down regulated in 19% of the cases examined, with a further 3% of patient's tumors lacking α-catenin expression altogether. Furthermore, the abnormality in α-catenin expression was found to be associated with high Gleason score, perineural growth and poor survival outcome.

A later study conducted by Aaltomaa *et al.* (128), demonstrated α-catenin levels to have no relationship with seminal vesicle invasion and Gleason score, in 87 patients with prostate cancer who had been previously treated by radical prostatectomy. In the same year, Wang *et al.* (129) used mutiplex real time quantitative RT-PCR on both paired prostate tumors, and on non-neoplastic primary prostate cultures to assess the level of cadherins and associated catenins. Prostate tumor tissues were shown to express moderately-to-markedly decreased levels of E-cadherin, P-cadherin, α-catenin and ß-catenin respectively.

The analysis of E-cadherin and α-catenin may have some clinical use in detecting prostate cancer, since abnormal expression of the E-cadherin/α-catenin complex has been reported to significantly correlate with Gleason score and poor survival outcome (130) thus indicating that down regulation of the cadherin/catenin complex causes disruption to cell-cell adhesion mechanisms and to a gain in the metastatic potential of prostate cancer spread. Therefore, it seems likely that the analysis of both E-cadherin and α-catenin expression may be of clinical use in the detection of prostate cancer. However, it is important to stress that E-cadherin, α-catenin or ß-catein are unlikely to be used individually as prognostic markers in prostate cancer. It is more feasible that a combination of these proteins might be used as they may provide a better marker, as reported for other tumor types including colorectal and liver cancers (131–134).

Kallakury *et al.* (135–136) assessed a wide variety of cell adhesion molecules and associated proteins as a means of achieving more reliable prognostic value in prostate cancer patients. Using immunohistochemistry to screen the level of these protein molecules in 118 prostatic adenocarcinomas, they found that decreased expression of α-catenin, ß-catenin, p120CNT, E-cadherin and CD44 (range 5–49%) were correlated with high tumor grade. Reduced E-cadherin and p120CNT levels were also correlated with tumor stage and ploidy. Down-regulation of α-catenin correlated with both aneuploidy and decreased expression of E-cadherin, whereas reduced expression of CD44s correlated with ploidy, serum prostate-specific antigen (PSA) and post-operative disease recurrence in prostate cancer patients. However, pre-operative serum PSA levels were correlated with loss of P120CNT. Interestingly, N-cadherin was present in 5% of the samples screened, but did not correlate with any of the prognostic parameters used in this study. They concluded that decreased expression of the cadherin/catenin complex is strongly correlated with an aggressive phenotyope in prostatic adenocarcinoma. Therefore, altered expression within these protein molecules may provide a prognostic value to patients with prostate cancer.

ß-catenin has also been reported to affect both the androgen receptor (AR) transcriptional activity, and the ligand specificity of prostate cancer cells (137). This was demonstrated in a study by Truica *et al.* (137) who showed ß-catenin to increase the AR transcriptional activation by androstenedione, and by estradiol through diminishing the antagonistic action of bicalutamide. This group further demonstrated, using co-precipitation studies of ß-catenin with AR on prostate cancer cells LNCap, that these two molecules were in fact, identified as components of the same complex. They also found that the amount of ß-catenin in this complex with AR to be increased upon exposure to androgen stimulation. Therefore, these findings implicate ß-catenin in the regulation of AR function, and support a role for ß-catenin mutations in the pathogenesis of prostate cancer (137).

In a more recent study conducted by Yang *et al.* (138), the ligand binding site of AR plus the NH(2) terminal domain of ß-catenin, combined with its first six armadillo repeats were shown to be critical locations for binding between these two molecules. It is through this specific interaction that ß-catenin is able to increase the ligand-dependent activity of AR in prostate cancer cells. The same group also demonstrated that transfection of E-cadherin cDNA into E-cadherin negative prostate cancer cells, causes the relocation of cytoplasmic ß-catenin to collect at peripheral zones and this in turn reduces AR-mediated transcription. This suggests that loss of E-cadherin can elevate the cytoplasmic levels of ß-catenin in prostate cancer cells, contributing to a more invasive phenotype by increasing the AR transcriptional activity during prostate cancer progression (138). Finally, these two latter studies also indicate a tantalising possibility of regulating E-cadherin/catenin function and its expression via a therapeutic means.

7. CONCLUSIONS

The cadherin/catenin complex plays a vital role in facilitating tight cell-cell adhesion contacts thereby regulating the architectural integrity of epithelial tissue. The establishment of intercellular adhesion mediated by this intact protein complex is therefore a pre-requisite for differentiation and morphogenesis. A mutation or dysfunction within the ß-catenin gene can affect the functioning of cadherin/catenin complexes, irrespective of E-cadherin status, resulting in subsequent cell-cell disengagement that may contribute to the invasive potential of cancer cells (43). Intracelluar ß-catenin levels are tightly regulated and processed by *Wnt* signalling components including axin, *APC* and GSK-3ß, a multi-protein complex that facilitates the rapid degradation of ß-catenin by the proteosome. However, signalling from *Wnt*, or mutations arising within components of the axin complex, ultimately leads to ß-catenin stabilisation through its association with transcription factors TCF/LEF, that in turn, activate target genes controlling a number of biological processes. Kim *et al.* (139) recently reported that LEF-1 induces epithelial-mesenchymal transformation (EMT) directly in epithelial tumors (DLD-1 cells) when stable levels of nuclear ß-catenin activate its transcription activity. In contrast, they found normal adult epithelial cells to use *APC* to shuttle ß-catenin out of the nucleus, thereby avoiding pathologies such as metastases due to LEF-1/ß-catenin-induced EMT (139). Thus ß-catenin is a multi-functional protein that binds to a variety of other intracellular proteins that controls the cellular processes of cancer cells including its pathogenesis.

ACKNOWLEDGEMENTS

We thank Cancer Research Wales for funding our work.

REFERENCES

1. Ozawa M, Baribault H, Kemler R. The cytoplasmic domain of the cell adhesion molecule uvomorulin associates with three independent proteins structurally related in different species. EMBO J 1989, 8:1711–17.
2. Wheelock MJ, Knudsen KA. Cadherins and associated proteins. In Vivo 1991, 5: 505–13.
3. Tsukita S, Tsukita S, Nagafuchi A, Yonemura S. Molecular linkage between cadherins and actin filaments in cell-cell adherens junctions. Curr Opin Cell Biol 1992, 4:834–9.
4. Kemler R. From cadherins to catenins: Cytoplasmic protein interactions and regulation of cell adhesion. Trends Genet 1993, 9:317–21.
5. Rimm DL, Koslov ER, Kebriaei P, Cianci CD, Morrow JS. Alpha 1(E)-catenin is an actin-binding, -bundling protein mediating the attachment of F-actin to the membrane adhesion complex. Proc Natl Acad Sci USA 1995, 92:8813–17.
6. Knudsen KA, Soler AP, Johnson KR, Wheelock MJ. Interaction of alpha-actinin with the cadherin/catenin cell-cell adhesion complex via alpha-catenin. J Cell Biol 1995, 130:67–77.
7. Davies G, Jiang WG, Mason MD. Cell-cell adhesion molecules and their associated proteins in bladder cancer cells and their role in mitogen induced cell-cell dissociation and invasion. Anticancer Res 1999, 19:547–52.
8. Bienz M, Clevers H. Linking colorectal cancer to wnt signalling. Cell 2000, 103: 311–20.
9. Polakis P. Wnt signaling and cancer. Genes Dev 2000, 14:1837–51.
10. Kinzler KW, Vogelstein B. Lessons from hereditary colorectal cancer. Cell 1996, 87:159–70.
11. He TC, Sparks AB, Rago C, Hermeking H, Zawel L, da Costa LT et al. Identification of c-MYC as a target of the APC pathway. Science 1998, 281:1509–12.
12. Pennica D, Swanson TA, Welsh JW, Roy MA, Lawrence DA, Lee J et al. WISP genes are members of the connective tissue growth factor family that are up-regulated in wnt-1-transformed cells and aberrantly expressed in human colon tumors. Proc Natl Acad Sci USA 1998, 95:14717–22.
13. Tetsu O, McCormick F. Beta-catenin regulates expression of cyclin D1 in colon carcinoma cells. Nature 1999, 398:422–6.
14. Jiang WG. E-cadherin and its associated protein catenins, cancer invasion and metastasis. Br J Surg 1996, 83:437–46.
15. Nagafuchi A, Takeichi M. Cell binding function of E-cadherin is regulated by the cytoplasmic domain. EMBO J 1988, 7:3679–84.

16. McCrea PD, Gumbiner BM. Purification of a 92-kDa cytoplasmic protein tightly associated with the cell-cell adhesion molecule E-cadherin (uvomorulin) characterization and extractability of the protein complex from the cell cytostructure. J Biol Chem 1991, 266:4514–20.
17. McCrea PD, Turck CW, Gumbiner B. A homolog of the armadillo protein in drosophila (plakoglobin) associated with E-cadherin. Science 1991, 254:1359–61.
18. Herrenknecht K, Ozawa M, Eckerskorn C, Lottspeich F, Lenter M, Kemler R. The uvomorulin-anchorage protein alpha catenin is a vinculin homologue. Proc Natl Acad Sci USA 1991, 88:9156–60.
19. Nagafuchi A, Takeichi M, Tsukita S. The 102 kd cadherin-associated protein: Similarity to vinculin and posttranscriptional regulation of expression. Cell 1991, 65:849–57.
20. Reynolds AB, Daniel J, McCrea PD, Wheelock MJ, Wu J, Zhang Z. Identification of a new catenin: The tyrosine kinase substrate P120CAS associates with E-cadherin complexes. Mol Cell Biol 1994, 14:8333–42.
21. Aghib, DF, McCrea. PD. The E-cadherin complex contains the src substrate P120. Exp Cell Res 1995, 218:359–69.
22. Shibamoto S, Hayakawa M, Takeuchi K, Hori T, Miyazawa K, Kitamura N et al. Association of P120, a tyrosine kinase substrate, with E-cadherin/catenin complexes. J Cell Biol 1995, 128:949–57.
23. Downing JR, Reynolds AB. PDGF, CSF-1, and EGF induce tyrosine phosphorylation of P120, a PP60SRC transformation-associated substrate. Oncogene 1991, 6:607–13.
24. Kanner SB, Reynolds AB, Parsons JT. Tyrosine phosphorylation of a 120-kilodalton PP60SRC substrate upon epidermal growth factor and platelet-derived growth factor receptor stimulation and in polyomavirus middle-T-antigen-transformed cells. Mol Cell Biol 1991, 11:713–20.
25. Riggleman B, Wieschaus E, Schedl P. Molecular analysis of the armadillo locus: Uniformly distributed transcripts and a protein with novel internal repeats are associated with a drosophila segment polarity gene. Genes Dev 1989, 3:96–113.
26. Peifer M, Wieschaus E. The segment polarity gene armadillo encodes a functionally modular protein that is the drosophila homolog of human plakoglobin. Cell 1990, 63:1167–76.
27. Reynolds AB, Herbert L, Cleveland JL, Berg ST, Gaut JR. P120, a novel substrate of protein tyrosine kinase receptors and of P60V-src, is related to cadherin-binding factors beta-catenin, plakoglobin and armadillo. Oncogene 1992, 7:2439–45.
28. Peifer M, Berg S, Reynolds AB. A repeating amino acid motif shared by proteins with diverse cellular roles. Cell 1994, 76:789–91.
29. Butz S, Kemler R. Distinct cadherin-catenin complexes in ca(2+)-dependent cell-cell adhesion. FEBS Lett 1994, 355:195–200.
30. Hinck L, Nathke IS, Papkoff J, Nelson WJ. Dynamics of cadherin/catenin complex formation: Novel protein interactions and pathways of complex assembly. J Cell Biol 1994, 125:1327–40.
31. Nathke IS, Hinck L, Swedlow JR, Papkoff J, Nelson WJ. Defining interactions and distributions of cadherin and catenin complexes in polarized epithelial cells. J Cell Biol 1994, 125:1341–52.
32. Sacco PA, McGranahan TM, Wheelock MJ, Johnson KR. Identification of plakoglobin domains required for association with N-cadherin and alpha-catenin. J Biol Chem 1995, 270:20201–6.

33. Rubinfeld B, Souza B, Albert I, Muller O, Chamberlain SH, Masiarz FR *et al.* Association of the APC gene product with beta-catenin. Science 1993, 262:1731–4.
34. Su LK, Vogelstein B, Kinzler KW. Association of the APC tumor suppressor protein with catenins. Science 1993, 262:1734–7.
35. Hulsken J, Birchmeier W, Behrens J. E-cadherin, APC compete for the interaction with beta-catenin, the cytoskeleton. J Cell Biol 1994, 127:2061–9.
36. Shibata T, Gotoh M, Ochiai, A, Hirohashi. S. Association of plakoglobin with APC, a tumor suppressor gene product, its regulation by tyrosine phosphorylation. Biochem Biophys Res Commun 1994, 203:519–22.
37. Cox RT, Peifer M. Wingless signaling: The inconvenient complexities of life. Curr Biol 1998, 8:R140– R144.
38. Peifer M, Sweeton D, Casey M, Wieschaus E. Wingless signal and zeste-white 3 kinase trigger opposing changes in the intracellular distribution of armadillo. Development 1994, 120:369–80.
39. Hiscox, S, Jiang. WG. Expression of E-cadherin, alpha, beta and gamma-catenin in human colorectal cancer. Anticancer Res 1997, 17:1349–54.
40. Shimoyama Y, Nagafuchi A, Fujita S, Gotoh M, Takeichi M, Tsukita S, Hirohashi S. Cadherin dysfunction in a human cancer cell line: Possible involvement of loss of alpha-catenin expression in reduced cell-cell adhesiveness. Cancer Res 1992, 52: 5770–4.
41. Breen E, Clarke A, Steele G Jr, Mercurio AM. Poorly differentiated colon carcinoma cell lines deficient in alpha-catenin expression express high levels of surface E-cadherin but lack ca(2+)-dependent cell-cell adhesion. Cell Adhes Commun 1993, 1:239–50.
42. Morton RA, Ewing CM, Nagafuchi A, Tsukita S, Isaacs WB. Reduction of E-cadherin levels and deletion of the alpha-catenin gene in human prostate cancer cells. Cancer Res 1993, 53:3585–90.
43. Kawanishi J, Kato J, Sasaki K, Fujii S, Watanabe N, Niitsu Y. Loss of E-cadherin-dependent cell-cell adhesion Due To mutation of the beta-catenin gene in a human cancer cell line, HSC-39. Mol Cell Biol 1995, 15:1175–81.
44. Matsuyoshi N, Hamaguchi M, Taniguchi S, Nagafuchi A, Tsukita S, Takeichi M. Cadherin-mediated cell-cell adhesion is perturbed by v-src tyrosine phosphorylation in metastatic fibroblasts. J Cell Biol 1992, 118:703–14.
45. Sommers CL, Gelmann EP, Kemler R, Cowin P, Byers SW. Alterations in beta-catenin phosphorylation and plakoglobin expression in human breast cancer cells. Cancer Res 1994, 54:3544–52.
46. Polarkis P. Casein kinase 1: A wnt'er of disconnect. Curr Biol 2002, 12:R499–501.
47. Lipschutz JH, Kissil JL. Expression of beta-catenin and gamma-catenin in epithelial tumor cell lines and characterization of a unique cell line. Cancer Lett 1998, 126: 33–41.
48. Anastasiadis PZ, Reynolds AB. The P120 catenin family: Complex roles in adhesion, signaling and cancer. J Cell Sci 2000, 113:1319–34.
49. van Hengel J, Vanhoenacker P, Staes K, van Roy F. Nuclear localization of the P120(ctn) armadillo-like catenin is counteracted by a nuclear export signal and by E-cadherin expression. Proc Natl Acad Sci USA 1999, 96:7980–5.
50. Mariner DJ, Wang J, Reynolds AB. ARVCF localizes to the nucleus and adherens junction and is mutually exclusive with P120(ctn) in E-cadherin complexes. J Cell Sci 2000, 113:1481–90.

51. Chen H, Paradies NE, Fedor-Chaiken M, Brackenbury R. E-cadherin mediates adhesion, suppresses cell motility via distinct mechanisms. J Cell Sci 1997, 110:345–56.
52. Mason MD, Davies G, Jiang WG. Cell adhesion molecules and adhesion abnormalities in prostate cancer. Crit Rev Oncol Hematol 2002, 41:11–28.
53. Rubinfeld B, Albert I, Porfiri E, Fiol C, Munemitsu S, Polakis P. Binding of GSK3BETA to the APC-beta-catenin complex and regulation of complex assembly. Science 1996, 272:1023–6.
54. Aberle H, Bauer A, Stappert J, Kispert A, Kemler R. Beta-catenin is a target for the ubiquitin-proteasome pathway. EMBO J 1997, 16:3797–804.
55. Orford K, Crockett C, Jensen JP, Weissman AM, Byers SW. Serine phosphorylation-regulated ubiquitination and degradation of beta-catenin. J Biol Chem 1997, 272:24735–8.
56. Rubinfeld B, Souza B, Albert I, Munemitsu S, Polakis P. The APC protein and E-cadherin form similar but independent complexes with alpha-catenin, beta-catenin, and plakoglobin. J Biol Chem 1995, 270:5549–55.
57. Groden J, Thliveris A, Samowitz W, Carlson M, Gelbert L, Albertsen H et al. Identification and characterization of the familial adenomatous polyposis coli gene. Cell 1991, 66:589–600.
58. Smits R, Kielman MF, Breukel C, Zurcher C, Neufeld K, Jagmohan-Changur S et al. APC1638T: A mouse model delineating critical domains of the adenomatous polyposis coli protein involved in tumorigenesis and development. Genes Dev 1999, 13:1309–21.
59. Munemitsu S, Albert I, Souza B, Rubinfeld B, Polakis P. Regulation of intracellular beta-catenin levels by the adenomatous polyposis coli (APC) tumor-suppressor protein. Proc Natl Acad Sci USA 1995, 92:3046–50.
60. Behrens J, Jerchow BA, Wurtele M, Grimm J, Asbrand C, Wirtz R et al. Functional interaction of an axin homolog, conductin, with beta-catenin, APC, and GSK3BETA. Science 1998, 280:596–9.
61. Hart MJ, de los Santos R, Albert IN, Rubinfeld B, Polakis P. Downregulation of beta-catenin by human axin and its association with the APC tumor suppressor, beta-catenin and GSK3 beta. Curr Biol 1998, 8:573–81.
62. Nakamura T, Hamada F, Ishidate T, Anai K, Kawahara K, Toyoshima K, Akiyama T. Axin, an inhibitor of the wnt signalling pathway, interacts with beta-catenin, GSK-3beta and APC and reduces the beta-catenin level. Genes Cells 1998, 3:395–403.
63. Sakanaka C, Weiss JB, Williams LT. Bridging of beta-catenin and glycogen synthase kinase-3beta by axin and inhibition of beta-catenin-mediated transcription. Proc Natl Acad Sci USA 1998, 95:3020–3.
64. Fagotto F, Jho E, Zeng L, Kurth T, Joos T, Kaufmann C, Costantini F. Domains of axin involved in protein-protein interactions, wnt pathway inhibition, and intracellular localization. J Cell Biol 1999, 145:741–56.
65. Hsu W, Zeng L, Costantini F. Identification of a domain of axin that binds to the serine/threonine protein phosphatase 2a and a self-binding domain. J Biol Chem 1999, 274:3439–45.
66. Julius MA, Schelbert B, Hsu W, Fitzpatrick E, Jho E, Fagotto F et al. Domains of axin and disheveled required for interaction and function in wnt signaling. Biochem Biophys Res Commun 2000, 276:1162–9.

67. Jho EH, Zhang T, Domon C, Joo CK, Freund JN, Costantini F. Wnt/beta-catenin/tcf signaling induces the transcription of AXIN2, a negative regulator of the signaling pathway. Mol Cell Biol 2002, 22:1172–83.
68. Taniguchi K, Roberts LR, Aderca IN, Dong X, Qian C, Murphy LM et al. Mutational spectrum of beta-catenin, AXIN1, and AXIN2 in hepatocellular carcinomas and hepatoblastomas. Oncogene 2002, 21:4863–71.
69. Mai M, Qian C, Yokomizo A, Smith DI, Liu W. Cloning of the human homolog of conductin (AXIN2), a gene mapping to chromosome 17Q23-Q24. Genomics 1999, 55:341–4.
70. Yamamoto H, Kishida S, Uochi T, Ikeda S, Koyama S, Asashima M, Kikuchi A. Axil, a member of the axin family, interacts with both glycogen synthase kinase 3ß and ß-catenin and inhibits axis formation of *Xenopus* embryos. Mol Cell Biol 1998, 18:2867–75.
71. Liu W, Dong X, Mai M, Seelan RS, Taniguchi K, Krishnadath KK et al. Mutations in AXIN2 cause colorectal cancer with defective mismatch repair by activating beta-catenin/TCF signalling. Nat Genet 2000, 26:146–7.
72. Dong X, Seelan RS, Qian C, Mai M, Liu W. Genomic structure, chromosome mapping and expression analysis of the human AXIN2 gene. Cytogenet Cell Genet 2001, 93:26–8.
73. Lustig B, Jerchow B, Sachs M, Weiler S, Pietsch T, Karsten U et al. Negative feedback loop of wnt signalling through upregulation of conductin/AXIN2 in colorectal and liver tumors. Mol Cell Biol 2001, 22:1184–93.
74. Yan D, Wallingford JB, Sun TQ, Nelson AM, Sakanaka C, Reinhard C et al. Cell autonomous regulation of multiple dishevelled-dependent pathways by mammalian nkd. Proc Natl Acad Sci USA 2001, 98:3802–7.
75. Nakagawa H, Murata Y, Koyama K, Fujiyama A, Miyoshi Y, Monden M et al. Identification of a brain-specific APC homologue, APCL, and its interaction with beta-catenin. Cancer Res 1998, 58:5176–81.
76. Aoki M, Hecht A, Kruse U, Kemler R, Vogt PK. Nuclear endpoint of wnt signaling: Neoplastic transformation induced by transactivating lymphoid-enhancing factor 1. Proc Natl Acad Sci USA 1999, 96:139–44.
77. Seidensticker MJ, Behrens J. Biochemical interactions in the wnt pathway. Biochim Biophys Acta 2000, 1495:168–82.
78. Peters JM, McKay RM, McKay JP, Graff JM. Casein kinase I transduces wnt signals. Nature 1999, 401:345–50.
79. Sakanaka C, Leong P, Xu L, Harrison SD, Williams LT. Casein kinase iepsilon in the wnt pathway: Regulation of beta-catenin function. Proc Natl Acad Sci USA 1999, 96:12548–52.
80. Amit S, Hatzubai A, Birman Y, Andersen JS, Ben-Shushan E, Mann M et al. Axin-mediated CKI phosphorylation of beta-catenin at ser 45: A molecular switch for the wnt pathway. Genes Dev 2002, 16:1066–76.
81. Liu C, Li Y, Semenov M, Han C, Baeg GH, Tan Y et al. Control of beta-catenin phosphorylation/degradation by a dual-kinase mechanism. Cell 2002, 108:837–47.
82. Yanagawa S, Matsuda Y, Lee JS, Matsubayashi H, Sese S, Kadowaki T, Ishimoto A. Casein kinase I phosphorylates the armadillo protein and induces its degradation in drosophila. EMBO J 2002, 21:1733–42.
83. Ozawa M, Engel J, Kemler R. Single amino acid substitutions in one CA2+ binding site of uvomorulin abolish the adhesive function. Cell 1990, 63:1033–8.

84. Willert K, Shibamoto S, Nusse R. Wnt-induced dephosphorylation of axin releases beta-catenin from the axin complex. Genes Dev 1999, 13:1768–73.
85. Galbiati F, Volonte D, Brown AM, Weinstein DE, Ben-Ze'ev A, Pestell RG, Lisanti MP. Caveolin-1 expression inhibits wnt/beta-catenin/lef-1 signaling by recruiting beta-catenin to caveolae membrane domains. J Biol Chem 2000, 275:23368–77.
86. Gradl D, Kuhl M, Wedlich D. The wnt/wg signal transducer beta-catenin controls fibronectin expression. Mol Cell Biol 1999, 19:5576–87.
87. Mann B, Gelos M, Siedow A, Hanski ML, Gratchev A, Ilyas M *et al*. Target genes of beta-catenin-T cell-factor/lymphoid-enhancer-factor signaling in human colorectal carcinomas. Proc Natl Acad Sci USA 1999, 96:1603–8.
88. Sun Y, Kolligs FT, Hottiger MO, Mosavin R, Fearon ER, Nabel GJ. Regulation of beta-catenin transformation by the P300 transcriptional coactivator. Proc Natl Acad Sci USA 2000, 97:12613–18.
89. Brabletz T, Jung A, Dag S, Hlubek F, Kirchner T. Beta-catenin regulates the expression of the matrix metalloproteinase-7 in human colorectal cancer. Am J Pathol 1999, 155:1033–8.
90. Crawford HC, Fingleton BM, Rudolph-Owen LA, Goss KJ, Rubinfeld B, Polakis P, Matrisian LM. The metalloproteinase matrilysin is a target of beta-catenin transactivation in intestinal tumors. Oncogene 1999, 18:2883–91.
91. van Damme J, Proost P, Lenaerts JP, Opdenakker G. Structural and functional identification of two human, tumor-derived monocyte chemotactic proteins (MCP-2 and MCP-3) belonging to the chemokine family. J Exp Med 1992, 176:59–65.
92. Fioretti F, Fradelizi D, Stoppacciaro A, Ramponi S, Ruco L, Minty A *et al*. Reduced tumorigenicity and augmented leukocyte infiltration after monocyte chemotactic protein-3 (MCP-3) gene transfer: Perivascular accumulation of dendritic cells in peritumoral tissue and neutrophil recruitment within the tumor. J Immunol 1998, 161:342–6.
93. Fujita M, Furukawa Y, Nagasawa Y, Ogawa M, Nakamura Y. Down-regulation of monocyte chemotactic protein-3 by activated beta-catenin. Cancer Res 2000, 60:6683–7.
94. Cavallo RA, Cox RT, Moline MM, Roose J, Polevoy GA, Clevers H *et al*. Drosophila tcf and groucho interact to repress wingless signalling activity. Nature 1998, 395:604–8.
95. Chen G, Fernandez J, Mische S, Courey AJ. A functional interaction between the histone deacetylase RPD3 and the corepressor groucho in drosophila development. Genes Dev 1999, 13:2218–30.
96. Ishitani T, Ninomiya-Tsuji J, Nagai S, Nishita M, Meneghini M, Barker N *et al*. The TAK1-NLK-MAPK-related pathway antagonizes signalling between beta-catenin and transcription factor TCF. Nature 1999, 399:798–802.
97. Levanon D, Goldstein RE, Bernstein Y, Tang H, Goldenberg D, Stifani S *et al*. Transcriptional repression by AML1 and LEF-1 is mediated by the TLE/groucho corepressors. Proc Natl Acad Sci USA 1998, 95:11590–5.
98. Roose J, Molenaar M, Peterson J, Hurenkamp J, Brantjes H, Moerer P *et al*. The xenopus wnt effector xtcf-3 interacts with groucho-related transcriptional repressors. Nature 1998, 395:608–12.
99. Bauer A, Chauvet S, Huber O, Usseglio F, Rothbacher U, Aragnol D *et al*. PONTIN52 and REPTIN52 function as antagonistic regulators of beta-catenin signalling activity. EMBO J 2000, 19:6121–30.

100. Hecht A, Vleminckx K, Stemmler MP, van Roy F, Kemler R. The P300/CBP acetyltransferases function as transcriptional coactivators of beta-catenin in vertebrates. EMBO J 2000, 19:1839–50.
101. Voeller HJ, Truica CI, Gelmann EP. Beta-catenin mutations in human prostate cancer. Cancer Res 1998, 58:2520–3.
102. Satoh S, Daigo Y, Furukawa Y, Kato T, Miwa N, Nishiwaki T et al. AXIN1 mutations in hepatocellular carcinomas, and growth suppression in cancer cells by virus-mediated transfer of AXIN1. Nat Genet 2000, 24:245–50.
103. Behrens J, von Kries JP, Kuhl M, Bruhn L, Wedlich D, Grosschedl R, Birchmeier W. Functional interaction of beta-catenin with the transcription factor LEF-1. Nature 1996, 382:638–42.
104. Peifer M. Beta-catenin as oncogene: The smoking gun. Science 1997, 275:1752–3.
105. Henderson BR. Nuclear-cytoplasmic shuttling of APC regulates beta-catenin subcellular localization and turnover. Nat Cell Biol 2000, 2:653–60.
106. Neufeld KL, Nix DA, Bogerd H, Kang Y, Beckerle MC, Cullen BR, White RL. Adenomatous polyposis coli protein contains two nuclear export signals and shuttles between the nucleus and cytoplasm. Proc Natl Acad Sci USA 2000, 97:12085–90.
107. Rosin-Arbesfeld R, Townsley F, Bienz M. The APC tumour suppressor has a nuclear export function. Nature 2000, 406:1009–12.
108. Fearnhead NS, Britton, MP, Bodmer. WF. The abc of apc. Hum Mol Genet 2001, 10:721–33.
109. Sparks AB, Morin PJ, Vogelstein B, Kinzler KW. Mutational analysis of the APC/beta-catenin/tcf pathway in colorectal cancer. Cancer Res 1998, 58:1130–4.
110. Thompson AM, Morris RG, Wallace M, Wyllie AH, Steel CM, Carter DC. Allele loss from 5Q21 (APC/MCC) and 18Q21 (DCC) and DCC mRNA expression in breast cancer. Br J Cancer 1993, 68:64–8.
111. Kashiwaba M, Tamura G, Ishida M. Aberrations of the APC gene in primary breast carcinoma. J Cancer Res Clin Oncol 1994, 120:727–31.
112. Gallagher RC, Hay T, Meniel V, Naughton C, Anderson TJ, Shibata H et al. Inactivation of apc perturbs mammary development, but only directly results in acanthoma in the context of tcf-1 deficiency. Oncogene 2002, 21:6446–57.
113. Ruckert S, Hiendlmeyer E, Brueckl WM, Oswald U, Beyser K, Dietmaier W et al. T-cell factor-4 frameshift mutations occur frequently in human microsatellite instability-high colorectal carcinomas but do not contribute to carcinogenesis. Cancer Res 2002, 62:3009–13.
114. Anderson CB, Neufeld KL, White RL. Subcellular distribution of wnt pathway proteins in normal and neoplastic colon. Proc Natl Acad Sci USA 2002, 99:8683–8.
115. Gasparoni A, Chaves A, Fonzi L, Johnson GK, Schneider GB, Squier CA. Subcellular localization of beta-catenin in malignant cell lines and squamous cell carcinomas of the oral cavity. J Oral Pathol Med 2002, 31:385–94.
116. Liu F, Schaphorst KL, Verin AD, Jacobs K, Birukova A, Day RM et al. Hepatocyte growth factor enhances endothelial cell barrier function and cortical cytoskeletal rearrangement: Potential role of glycogen synthase kinase-3beta. FASEB J 2002, 16:950–62.
117. Davies G, Jiang WG, Mason MD. The interaction between beta-catenin, GSK3BETA and APC after motogen induced cell-cell dissociation, and their involvement in signal transduction pathways in prostate cancer. Int J Oncol 2001, 18:843–7.

118. Davies G, Jiang WG, Mason MD. Matrilysin mediates extracellular cleavage of E-cadherin from prostate cancer cells: A key mechanism in hepatocyte growth factor/scatter factor-induced cell-cell dissociation and in vitro invasion. Clin Cancer Res 2001, 7:3289–97.
119. Davies G, Jiang WG, Mason MD. Cell-cell adhesion molecules and signaling intermediates and their role in the invasive potential of prostate cancer cells. J Urol 2000, 163:985–92.
120. Umbas R, Schalken JA, Aalders TW, Carter BS, Karthaus HF, Schaafsma HE et al. Expression of the cellular adhesion molecule E-cadherin is reduced or absent in high-grade prostate cancer. Cancer Res 1992, 52:5104–9.
121. Otto T, Rembrink K, Goepel M, Meyer-Schwickerath M, Rubben H. E-cadherin: A marker for differentiation, invasiveness in prostatic carcinoma. Urol Res 1993, 21:359–62.
122. Ross JS, Figge HL, Bui HX, del Rosario AD, Fisher HA, Nazeer T et al. E-cadherin expression in prostatic carcinoma biopsies: Correlation with tumor grade, DNA content, pathologic stage, and clinical outcome. Mod Pathol 1994, 7:835–41.
123. Umbas R, Isaacs WB, Bringuier PP, Schaafsma HE, Karthaus HF, Oosterhof GO et al. Decreased E-cadherin expression is associated with poor prognosis in patients with prostate cancer. Cancer Res 1994, 54:3929–33.
124. Cheng L, Nagabhushan M, Pretlow TP, Amini SB, Pretlow TG. Expression of E-cadherin in primary and metastatic prostate cancer. Am J Pathol 1996, 148:1375–80.
125. Mialhe A, Louis J, Montlevier S, Peoch M, Pasquier D, Bosson JL et al. Expression of E-cadherin and alpha-, beta- and gamma-catenins in human bladder carcinomas: Are they good prognostic factors. Invasion Metastasis 1997, 17:124–37.
126. Morita, N, Uemura, H, Tsumatani, K, Cho, M, Hirao, Y, Okajima, E et al. E-cadherin, alpha-, beta-, gamma-catenin expression in prostate cancers: Correlation with tumor invasion. Br J Cancer 1999, 79:1879–83.
127. Aaltomaa S, Lipponen P, Ala-Opas M, Eskelinen M, Kosma VM. Alpha-catenin expression has prognostic value in local and locally advanced prostate cancer. Br J Cancer 1999, 80:477–82.
128. Aaltomaa S, Lipponen P, Viitanen J, Kankkunen JP, Ala-Opas M, Kosma VM. Prognostic value of CD44 standard, variant isoforms 3 and 6 and -catenin expression in local prostate cancer treated by radical prostatectomy. Eur Urol 2000, 38:555–62.
129. Wang J, Krill D, Torbenson M, Wang Q, Bisceglia M, Stoner J et al. Expression of cadherins and catenins in paired tumor and non-neoplastic primary prostate cultures and corresponding prostatectomy specimens. Urol Res 2000, 28:308–15.
130. Richmond, PJ, Karayiannakis, AJ, Nagafuchi, A, Kaisary, AV, Pignatelli. M. Aberrant E-cadherin, alpha-catenin expression in prostate cancer: Correlation with patient survival. Cancer Res 1997, 57:3189–93.
131. Miyata M, Shiozaki H, Iihara K, Shimaya K, Oka H, Kadowaki T et al. Relationship between E-cadherin expression and lymph-node metastasis in human esophageal cancer. Int J Oncol 1994, 4:61–5.
132. Garcia S, Martini F, De Micco C, Andrac L, Hardwigsen J, Sappa P et al. Immuno-expression of E-cadherin and beta-catenin correlates to survival of patients with hepatocellular carcinomas. Int J Oncol 1998, 12:443–7.
133. Ghadimi BM, Behrens J, Hoffmann I, Haensch W, Birchmeier W, Schlag PM. Immunohistological analysis of E-cadherin, alpha-, beta- and gamma-catenin

expression in colorectal cancer: Implications for cell adhesion and signaling. Eur J Cancer 1999, 35:60–5.
134. Zheng Z, Pan J, Chu B, Wong YC, Cheung AL, Tsao SW. Downregulation and abnormal expression of E-cadherin and beta-catenin in nasopharyngeal carcinoma: Close association with advanced disease stage and lymph node metastasis. Hum Pathol 1999, 30:458–66.
135. Kallakury BV, Sheehan CE, Winn-Deen E, Oliver J, Fisher HA, Kaufman RP Jr, Ross JS. Decreased expression of catenins (alpha and beta), P120 CTN, and E-cadherin cell adhesion proteins and E-cadherin gene promoter methylation in prostatic adenocarcinomas. Cancer 2001, 92:2786–95.
136. Kallakury BV, Sheehan CE, Ross JS. Co-downregulation of cell adhesion proteins alpha- and beta-catenins, P120CTN, E-cadherin, and CD44 in prostatic adenocarcinomas. Hum Pathol 2001, 32:849–55.
137. Truica CI, Byers S, Gelmann EP. Beta-catenin affects androgen receptor transcriptional activity and ligand specificity. Cancer Res 2000, 60:4709–13.
138. Yang F, Li X, Sharma M, Sasaki CY, Longo DL, Lim B, Sun Z. Linking beta-catenin to androgen-signaling pathway. J Biol Chem 2002, 277:11336–44.
139. Kim K, Lu Z, Hay ED. Direct evidence for a role of ß-catenin/LEF-1 signaling pathway in induction of EMT. Cell Biol Int 2002, 26:463–76.

Chapter 10

HEPATOCYTE GROWTH FACTOR/SCATTER FACTOR AND PROSTATE CANCER METASTASIS

Gaynor Davies[1], Wen G. Jiang[1] and Malcolm D. Mason[2]
[1]*Metastasis Research Group, University Department of Surgery, University of Wales College of Medicine, Heath Park, Cardiff, Wales, UK*
[2]*Department of Medicine, Section of Clinical Oncology, Velindre Hospital, Cardiff, Wales, UK*

Abstract: Metastasis is a life-threatening event in tumor bearing patients resulting in total organ failure and to subsequent death. Understanding the fundamental processes involved in how cancer cells detach from the primary tumor in order to enter the metastatic cascade is a key factor in delivering therapeutic starategies to prevent metatasis from occuring. Hepatocyte Growth Factor/Scatter Factor (HGF/SF) is an unique growth factor capable of inducing a number of biological responses in a wide variety of normal and neoplastic cells, including invasion, cell spreading, scattering, motility and shedding of cell-cell adhesion molecules. This review is intended to highlight some of the more recent discoveries made in scientific and clinical research, with particular emphasis on the effect of HGF/SF on protsate cancer metastasis and invasion.

Key words: prostate cancer, HGF/SF, invasion and metastasis

1. PREFACE TO TUMOR PROGRESSION AND METASTASIS IN THE DEVELOPMENT OF PROSTATE CANCER

Metastasis is perhaps the single, most important rate-limiting factor affecting the survival outcome of patients with cancer. In particular, prostate cancer remains one of the leading male cancers diagnosed in Western countries (1). The incidence and mortality rate for prostate cancer has increased dramatically during the last decade. It was estimated that the incidence alone for prostate cancer increased to 126% in the early 1990's, compared that that observed in the 1970's. During the same time period, the mortality rate for prostate cancer was also estimated to have increased at a rate of more than 1% per year. As a consequence, this has given rise to more than 15.6 deaths per 100,000 per year in the UK alone. Tumor metastasis to distant organs is dependent on the detachment of cancer cells from their primary location and their subsequent invasion to the surrounding tissues. There are a number of key factors known to play definitive roles in tumor metastasis including hepatocyte growth factor/scatter factor (HGF/SF), and this motogen has been shown to influence the development of prostate cancer. The mechanisms involving HGF/SF mediated responses in prostate cancer progression will be explained in greater detail at a later stage in this review. Finally, there remains very little knowledge concerning the underlying influences that contribute to the incidence of prostate cancer, such as tumor biology, the mechanisms of disease progression and its prognosis. Therefore, this article will attempt to address some of the more recent discoveries made in these areas.

2. HISTORICAL BACKGROUND CHRONICALING THE DISCOVERY OF HGF/SF

HGF was originally identified as a powerful stimulant for hepatocyte growth *in vitro* (2–4). However, subsequent cloning and sequencing of this molecule revealed that it was homologous to both hepatopoietin A and a tumor toxic factor (5–8). Previously, a fibroblast-derived protein was reported to scatter tightly-packed colonies of epithelial cells and this was subsequently termed scatter factor (SF) (9). In addition, partial amino acid sequencing of SF revealed that it was over 90% homologous to both rat and human variants of HGF (10–13). Therefore, it was generally accepted that the term HGF/SF should be used to describe this multi-functional cytokine (14–15).

2.1 Biological Activity and Structure of HGF/SF

HGF/SF is synthesised and secreted as a single peptide chain of 728 amino acid residues, containing a signal sequence of 29 amino acid residues and a pro-sequence of 25 amino acid residues (16–17). Furthermore, the single chain pro-form of HGF/SF needs to be converted to its mature active heterodimeric form, by extracellular cleavage of a pro-sequence Arg^{494}-Val^{495} bond via an unique serine protease (6, 16–19). HGF/SF in its mature form is composed of one heavy peptide α-chain (69 kDa), and one light peptide β-chain (34 kDa), which are linked together by a disulfide bridge forming a heterodimer (16–17). The α-subunit of HGF/SF is composed of four triple-disulphide structures called kringle domains and a putative N-terminal hairpin loop domain (20), homologous to plasminogen preactivation peptide (PAP), and responsible for both heparin and *c-Met* receptor binding (21–23). The first and second of these kringle domains have been reported to be necessary for the correct biological functioning of HGF/SF (24). These kringle domains are also known to be involved in protein-protein binding and as such, mediate receptor-ligand binding on plasminogen activator (25–26). The β-subunit has a domain similar to that of a serine protease, although no protease activity occurs due to amino acid substitution within the catalytic site (27). The complete lack of protease activity within the β-subunit of HGF/SF results in the absence of highly conserved triad residues present within active serine proteases (5, 16).

HGF-converting enzyme has been implicated in the conversion of pro-HGF/SF into its active heterodimeric form via proteolytic cleavge of the single chain precursor form of HGF/SF (23). Similarly, urokinase-type plasminogen activator (uPA) and tissue-type plasminogen activator (tPA) have also been shown (*in vitro*) to convert pro-HGF/SF into a mature active form of HGF/SF (19, 28). Another mechanism of activation exists which occurs in response to tissue injury (Figure 1), where a precursor of an HGF/SF activator (HGFA) is produced by epithelial cells and is then activated by thrombin (a component of the blood coagulation cascade), which in turn goes on to process pro-HGF/SF into its bioactive form (29). HGF/SF is regulated by an injurin like factor (humoral type factor) produced in non-injured distant organs following hepatic or renal injury and where it has been found to induce the expression of HGF/SF mRNA in rat lungs (30–32). Injurin is a small non-protein factor (8–15kDa) that is located in a number of tissue extracts (liver, kidney, brain and lung) and has been shown to translationally enhance HGF/SF production (33). A possible role for injurin in the activation of pro-HGF/SF is shown in Figure 1.

2.2 Structure and Function of the HGF/SF Receptor C-Met

There are various biological responses following stimulation by HGF/SF which are mediated by its mature proto-oncogene receptor *c-Met* (34–35). The HGF/SF receptor was first identified as an activated oncogene in an

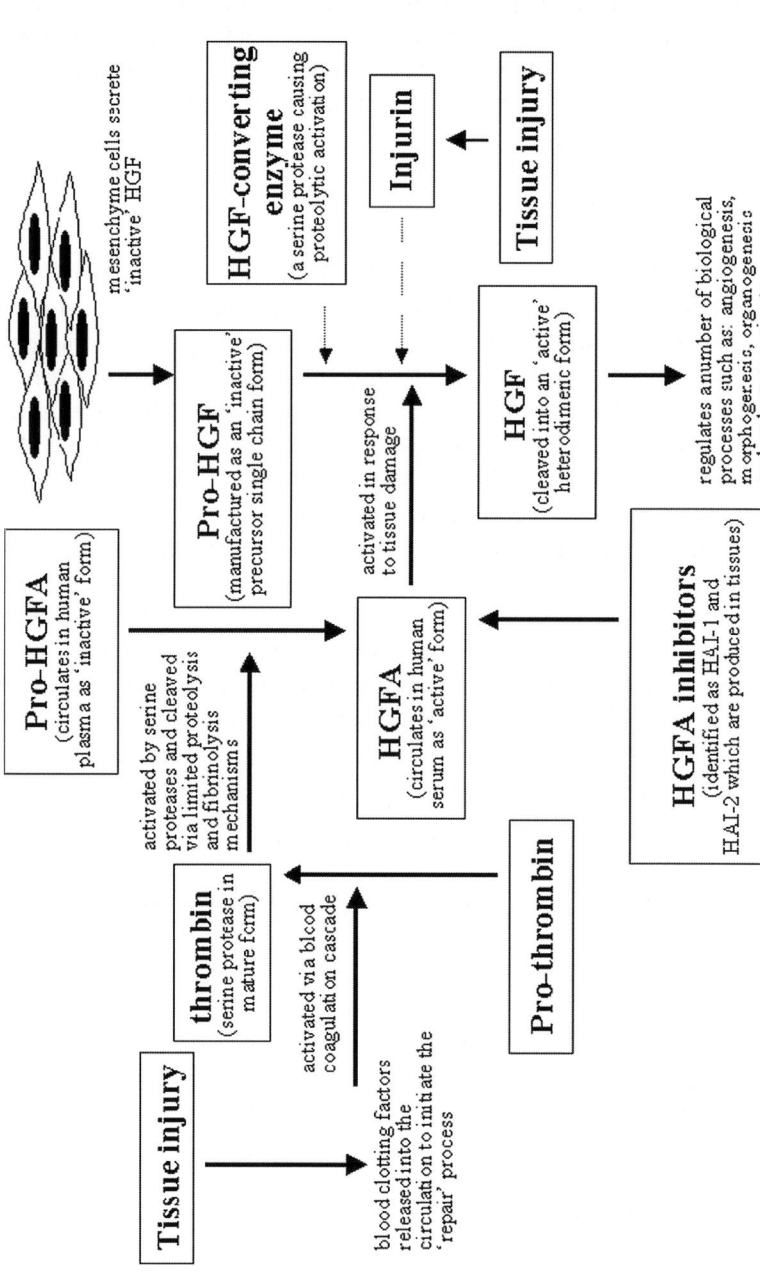

Figure 1. A pathway showing the secretion, activation and regulation of HGF/SF. The broken arrows indicate unknown mechanisms of HGF/SF activation involving injurin.

N-methyl-N'-nitrosoguanidine-treated human osteogenic sarcoma cell Line (MNNG-HOS), by its ability to transform NIH 3T3 mouse fibroblasts (36–37). The receptor encoded by the *c-Met* proto-oncogene is a two chain protein composed of an α-subunit (50 kDa), linked to a membrane-spanning β-subunit (145 kDa) joined together (producing an αβ complex of 190 kDa) by disulphide bonding (34–35, 38). The intracellular portion of the *c-Met* β-chain possesses a tyrosine kinase domain that identifies the HGF/SF receptor as a member of the receptor tyrosine kinase (RTK) family of cell surface molecules (34–35, 38–39).

HGF/SF binds to its receptor and induces tyrosine phosphorylation in the intracellular domain located on the β-chain of mature *c-Met*, causing ligand-dependent receptor homodimerisation and cross-phosphorylation within the tyrosine kinase domain (40). Such events are thought to promote binding of intracellular signalling proteins containing *src* homology (SH) regions, such as: phospholipse-C-γ (PLC-γ), Ras, GTPase-activating protein (GAP), phosphatidylinositol 3-kinase (PI3K), $pp^{60c-src}$ and the Grb2-SOS complex, to the activated HGF/SF receptor (41–44). A schematic representation of intracellular signal transducers that are associated with tyrosine phosphorylation of *c-Met*, have been described elsewhere (45). HGF/SF has also been shown to stimulate the *ras*-guanine nucleotide exchanger, thus promoting the GTP-bound active state of the Ras protein (46). This association implicates the Ras pathway in the mediation of HGF/SF-induced cell motility, via its interaction with components of the cell's cytoskeleton (47).

3. BIOLOGICAL EFFECTS OF HGF/SF ON TUMOR INVASION AND METASTASIS

The most significant factor affecting the survival outcome in cancer patients is metastatic spread. The process is referred to as the 'metastatic cascade' and it is controlled by a number of essential rate-limiting steps including: (i) the loss of cell-cell contact from the primary tumor site; (ii) enzymatic degradation of both basement and extracellular matrix components, resulting in adhesion to the matrix and to subsequent invasion through these components; (iii) intravasation; (iv) survival within the circulation; (v) adhesion to the endothelium followed by extravasation, and (vi) establishment of a secondary tumor and angiogenesis (48–49). HGF/SF has been shown to cause a number of biological responses, such as increased cell motility (50), cell growth (51–52), invasion (53), angiogenesis (54–55), morphogenesis (56) and embryogenesis (57). The profound stimulatory effects induced by HGF/SF upon tumor cell function are central to the process of metastasis *in vitro*, and as such this motogen has now been implicated as a mediator of metastatic spread *in vivo* (14). An increase in HGF/SF-induced cell motility and cellular scattering been demonstrated in a variety of cell types including tumor-derived cells (58–61). Furthermore, HGF/SF promotes the growth of hepatopoietic and hematopietic cells in culture (51–52), since the removal of this growth factor induces apoptosis (62–63). Exposure to HGF/SF has also been shown to reverse the effects of TGF-β1 (transforming growth factor-β1) induced growth arrest in epithelial and endothelial cells (64). Therefore, regulation of cell growth by HGF/SF may represent part of a co-ordinated cell growth control state (14).

HGF/SF causes the disassembly of cadherin/catenin complexes in a number of epithelial derived cells, resulting in a more invasive phenotype through the dissociation of β-catenin from E-cadherin (65–66). This has been demonstrated in our laboratory using co-precipitation experiments on prostate cancer cells LNCaPFGC (67). Stimulation with HGF/SF over a 2h incubation period induced the dissociation of co-precipitated E-cadherin/β-catenin using a lysis buffer containing the detergent Triton X-100 (also known as the Triton soluble fraction). Previous studies by our group have also indicated that HGF/SF promotes the invasion of a number of cell types into collagen gels and artificial basement membranes (59, 68–69). Such studies have revealed quite conclusively that HGF/SF affects the functioning of cellular adhesion molecules such as E-cadherin, promoting the *in vitro* invasiveness of both bladder and prostate cancer cells through Matrigel, via the neutralisation of E-cadherin with an anti-E-cadherin antibody (66, 70). Cellular-matrix adhesion (mediated through cell-matrix receptors called integrins) of cancer cells is known to play a key role in the process of metastasis and is necessary for both tumor cell matrix degradation, and for subsequent invasion through components of the ECM. A study by Parr *et al.* (71) demonstrates quite clearly that HGF/SF enhances cell-matrix adhesion, membrane ruffling, cellular spreading and invasiveness in prostate cancer cells, thus implicating HGF/SF as an inducer of cancer spread *in vitro* (14).

3.1 Induction of Motogen Induced Cell-Cell Dissociation and Migration

HGF/SF inhibits cadherin function by altering the phosphorylation status of cadherin-associated catenin proteins, thus affecting their binding to the intracellular portion of E-cadherin (65–66). In addition, HGF/SF induces tyrosine phosphorylation of β-catenin causing down-regulation of cadherin-mediated cell-cell adhesion (66, 72–73). HGF/SF has also been shown to promote dissociation in epithelial cells through the dismantling of cell-cell adhesion complexes, resulting in an increase in cell motility/migration (14, 66). Cell motility may be initiated through a number of steps including: (i) the assembly and disassembly of focal adhesion; (ii) as integrin attachment to, and detachment from, the extracellular matrix, and (iii) through actomyosin cytoskeleton reorganisation (74). We have recently shown that HGF/SF influences both cell motility and migration in prostate cancer (DU-145) cells *in vitro*, events necessary for metastatic spread *in vivo*. The biological effects of HGF/SF and its antagonist NK4, on cell motility/migration in prostate cancer were assessed using a computerised motion analysis technique (71). Addition of HGF/SF was found to increase both cell motility (Figure 2A) and migration (Figure 2B) in DU-145 cells, but its effect was inhibited by incubation with NK4, thus indicating HGF/SF's ability to enhance the metastatic potential of DU-145 cells *in vitro*.

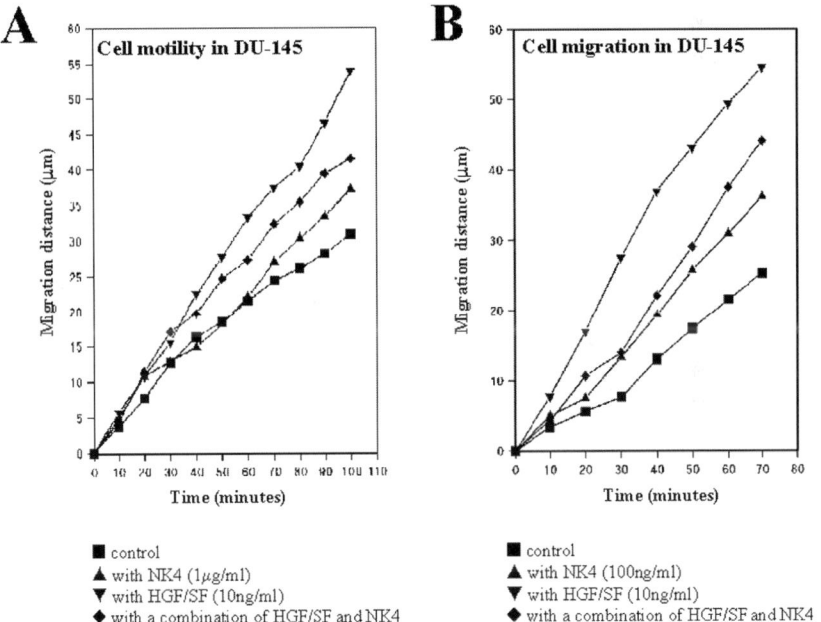

Figure 2. (A). Effect of NK4 on HGF/SF-induced cell motility in DU-145 cells using a motion analysis software package. The results indicate that HGF/SF (10ng/ml) induced tumor cell migration. However, NK4 (1 μg/ml) was able to antagonise the influence of HGF/SF. (B). NK4 suppressed HGF/SF action during migration of DU-145 cells in wound closure, using a wounding assay and motion analysis technique. HGF/SF dramatically increased migration of the cell fronts to close the wound; however, the addition of NK4 significantly ($p < 0.05$) reduced the biological influence of HGF/SF elicited in DU-145 cells (ref 71).

An enhanced metastatic phenotype after stimulation by HGF/SF has been demonstrated by Rong *et al.* (75), after transfecting *c-Met* cDNA into a cell line lacking the HGF/SF receptor. The *c-Met* receptor has been reported to be primarily located at intracellular junctions together with E-cadherin in normal epithelium. However, it remains unclear whether their peripheral localisation facilitates their physical interactions, or allows the regulation of cell adhesion (76, 77). Presumably the latter holds true, since we have shown that HGF/SF increases the co-precipitation level between the E-cadherin/catenin complex and the HGF/SF receptor *c-Met*, thereby regulating intercellular adhesion in prostate cancer cells following stimulation by this motogen (78). Miura *et al.* (79) have shown that exposure to HGF/SF demonstrates an induced cellular scattering in DU-145 cells, by decreasing the expression of E-cadherin and causing its subsequent translocation into the cytoplasm. Similarly, we also report that HGF/SF promotes the loss of cell-cell contact in LNCaPFGC cells due to a reduction in the level of co-localised peripheral staining (using immunofluoresecence) between E-cadherin and *c-Met*, and to an increase in the level of cytoplasmic staining (78). Cell scattering in prostate cancer via HGF/SF stimulation is thought to occur as a result of cellular regulation through the endocytosis and degradation of E-cadherin (79). Furthermore, the translocation of E-cadherin into the cytoplasm may help to either regulate, or redistribute protein levels within the cell's microenvironment. The most likely mode of mediation is via proteolytic degradation of endocytosed E-cadherin within lysosomes, or by the transportation of E-cadherin in recycling vesicles to the plasma membrane for future reuse (80–81). Therefore, it would appear that HGF/SF mediates the recycling of E-cadherin levels in prostate cancer cells, thus providing a potential mechanism for regulating cadherin dynamics within the cell's microenvironment.

4. ENHANCEMENT OF CELL MOTILITY VIA THE DEGRADATION OF EXTRACELLULAR MATRIX PROTEINS

Components of the extracellular matrix (ECM) including basement membranes, are critical entities in providing both structure, and maintenance to tissue architecture (82–84). The loss of tissue integrity involves both the degradation of ECM proteins, and the coordinated synthesis of newly processed matrix components, essential metabolic steps governing the cell's microenvironment (85–86). Enzymatic digestion of components of the ECM occurs during inflammatory responses, cell migration, tumor invasion, cell motility and metastasis (86). Matrix metalloproteinases (MMPs) are a family of zinc-dependent enzymes (comprising of more than 20 family members) implicated in the degradation of connective tissue and basement membranes, thereby playing pivotal roles during both tumor development and progression (85–88). HGF/SF can bind to a variety of ECM components (such as thrombospondin-1, fibronectin and heparan sulfate proteoglycan), thereby creating a pool of HGF/SF located within the ECM serving to localise the release of matrix-degrading proteolytic enzymes, which in turn enhances the metastatic potential and motile behaviour of cancer cells, thus allowing invasion to occur through the ECM (15).

4.1 The Release of Soluble Forms of Cell Adhesion Molecules by Matrix-Degrading Enzymes

Activated forms of MMPs are believed to be responsible for both tumor invasion and metastasis because of their ability to degrade extracellular matrix, and basement membrane components respectively (87). HGF/SF has been implicated in the upregulation of MMP-1, MMP-9 and MMP-14 production in mesothelioma cells in a dose-dependent manner (89). Similarly, Dunsmore et al. (90) has shown that HGF/SF stimulates the production of MMP-1 and MMP-3 in keratinocytes, in a dose-dependent and matrix-dependent manner. In another study by Bennett et al. (91), HGF/SF was shown to regulate the production of MMPs by oral carcinoma cells. We have shown in Figure 3 the release of matrilysin (otherwise known as MMP-7; the smallest known family member of MMPs) mediated by HGF/SF, causing cleavage to the ectodomain of E-cadherin (producing a soluble 80kDa fragment into the cell supernatant fraction) which in turn, causes an increase in both cellular scattering (Figure 4A) and invasion (Figure 4B) in prostate cancer (67). Furthermore, we have also demonstrated how we may effectively block this mechanism with an antisense-oligonucleotide specifically directed towards matrilysin.

Activation of MMPs are subject to regulation by their association with TIMPs (tissue inhibitors of metalloproteinases) and once activated, may be inactivated by the presence of TIMPs. However, other modes of metalloproteinase activation involving the shedding of cell-cell adhesion molecules are thought to exist. One such mechanism may include the involvement of HGF/SF in the activation of urokinase-type plasminogen, thereby converting the pro-active form (28kDa) of matrilysin into its active (19kD) form, in order to release a soluble 80kDa fragment of E-cadherin within the cell's supernatant fraction (67). A schematic representation of this possible mode

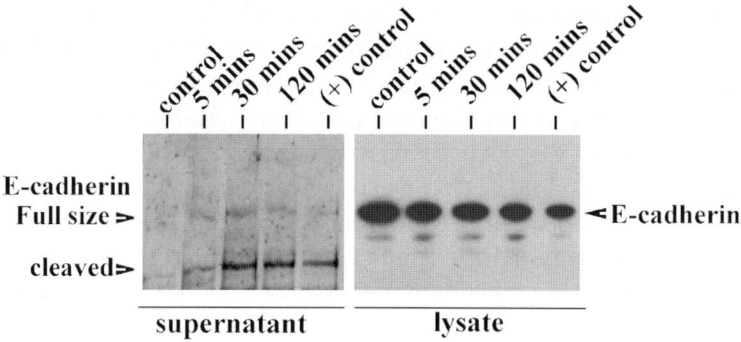

Figure 3. HGF/SF induced a loss of E-cadherin from LNCaPFGC cells. Cells were stimulated with HGF/SF (40ng/ml) for the times indicated. The supernatant fractions were collected and the cells lysed. The level of E-cadherin in the cell lysate fraction was reduced after HGF/SF stimulation (right). Consequently, a small fragment of approximately 80kDa appeared in the supernatant fractions (left), after challenging with HGF/SF. This fragment was recognised upon probing with an anti-E-cadherin antibody (ref 67).

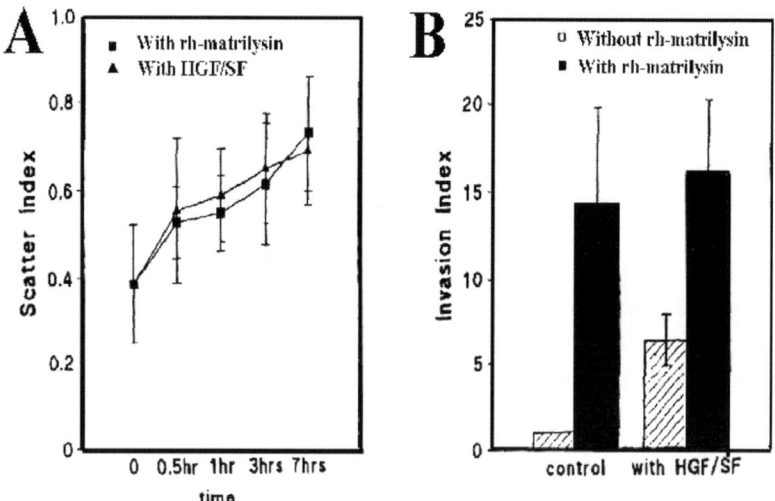

Figure 4. (A). The effect of rh-matrilysin (100units/ml), or HGF/SF (60ng/ml) on colony scattering in LNCaPFGC cells after incubation at 37oC for upto 7 hours. There was a significant difference in scattering index as determined by area morphometry after 30 mins exposure to either rh-matrilysin ($p = 0.008$), or HGF/SF ($p = 0.021$) respectively, using the mean + sem from 10 colonies per time point. (B). The invasive capacity of LNCaPFGC cells through basement membrane matrigel was significantly enhanced by inclusion of either; 100Units/ml of rh-matrilysin ($p = 0.0037$), or 40ng/insert of HGF/SF ($p = 0.0004$) respectively, after 96 hours of culture at 37oC (67).

of activation is demonstrated in Figure 5. MMPs-3 and -7 have also been reported to cleave the extracellular portion of E-cadherin from both MCF-7 and MDCKts.*src*Cl2 cells, releasing a circulating (80kDa) fragment into the culture medium of cells after stimulation with phorbol-12-myristate-13-acetate (92). This effect was inhibited by over-expression of TIMP-2, suggesting that MMPs were indeed responsible for E-cadherin cleavage in these cell types (92). Furthermore, forced expression of an activated form of MMP-3 has been reported to cleave and degrade E-cadherin levels, thus contributing to an invasive mesenchymal transformation in mammary epithelial cells (85). MMPs have also been implicated in the proteolytic cleavage of VE-cadherin producing a soluble 90kDa fragment after growth factor deprivation-induced apoptosis (93). It would appear that MMPs play definitive roles in enhancing the metastatic potential of cancer cells by firstly, degrading components of the ECM and secondly, disrupting cell-cell adhesion mechanisms giving rise to a more invasive phenotype.

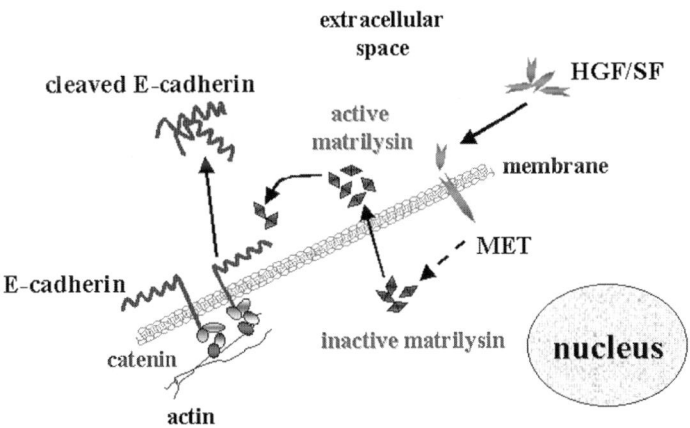

Figure 5. A schematic representation of the possible pathway involved in HGF/SF activation of its receptor c-Met, which in turn activates 'pro-active' matrilysin into its 'active' form (i.e. the pathway for this mechanism is not known as indicated by the broken arrow head). The subsequent release of activated matrilysin into cell supernatant fraction results in the cleavage of the extracellular domain of E-cadherin, producing an 80 kDa soluble fragment. Full length E-cadherin (120 kDa) associates with a group of cytoplasmic proteins called catenins (i.e. α-, β- and γ-catenins) which aid in homophilic interactions in the presence of extracellular calcium, forming tight cell-cell adhesion complexes.

5. HGF/SF, ITS RECEPTOR AND CLINICAL ASPECTS IN PROSTATE CANCER

A correlation between the level of HGF/SF and disease progression in prostate cancer has recently become established. For instance, immunoreactive HGF/SF in the serum of patients with prostate cancer has been detected. Naughton *et al.* (94) have shown a stepwise increase in the level of HGF/SF in serum from patients with adenocarcinoma of the prostate (i.e., 700 pg/ml in normal controls; 974 pg/ml in patients with localised prostate cancer; and 2117 pg/ml in patients with metastatic disease). It is interesting to note that in this study when the level of prostate-specific antigen (PSA) and tumor grade were known, the level of HGF/SF was the most significant predictor for the presence of metastatic disease. Interestingly, a similar pattern of increase for HGF/SF receptor staining has been observed. Furthermore, staining for the HGF/SF receptor was detected in 18% of benign prostate lesions; 84% of primary prostate cancers; and 100% of metastatic bone marrow, and lymph node lesions respectively (95). In addition, the same study showed a significant correlation between the intensity of staining for the HGF/SF receptor and grade of prostate cancer (i.e., 20% in Grade I; 88% in Grade II; 93% Grade III; and 100% in Grade IV). In an independent study conducted by Watanabe *et al.* (96), a stepwise increase in the expression of the HGF/SF receptor; prostatic intraepithelial neoplasia (PIN) (36%); latent prostate cancer (33%); clinical prostate cancer (71%); and metastatic prostate cancer (100%) has been demonstrated. These clinical observations are supported by laboratory studies showing that the HGF/SF receptor is expressed in prostate cancer cell lines (78, 97); that HGF/SF is expressed; and that bioactive HGF/SF is produced by both prostate stromal fibroblasts, and myofibroblastic cells (97–99). *In vitro*, HGF/SF has been shown to increase the migration, invasiveness, and growth of prostate cancer cells (56, 78, 97, 99). Interestingly, HGF/SF has also been shown to activate the androgen receptor, and may thus be involved in androgen-dependent, and independent growth of prostate cancer cells (98, 100, 101).

The role of HGF/SF and its receptor in the interplay between prostate cancer cells and stromal cells has been well documented. Stromal fibroblasts from prostate tissues have been shown to express and produce bioactive HGF/SF. Furthermore, the amount of bioactive HGF/SF produced by prostate stromal fibroblasts was found to be significantly higher than the amount secreted from skin and bone marrow fibroblasts respectively (98–99). In addition, prostate fibroblasts have been shown to significantly increase the growth of prostate cancer cells *in vitro* and *in vivo* (98, 102–104). The importance of HGF/SF in the development of prostate cancer is further reinforced by a more recent study showing that normal prostate epithelial cells respond differently to prostate cancer cells (99). In this study, Gmyrek *et al.* (99) demonstrated that both normal prostate epithelial, and prostate cancer cells express the HGF/SF receptor and respond to HGF/SF stimulation with increased migration. However, prostate cancer cells were found to exhibit a significant increase in proliferation to HGF/SF stimulation, while prostate epithelial cells had a reduced proliferation response to HGF/SF. Therefore, it would appear that the induction of invasiveness in response to HGF/SF is most likely to occur as a result of an increase in the amount of bioactive HGF/SF secreted by stromal cells, and by the presence of the HGF/SF receptor on cancer cells (105).

Another report implicating the level of HGF/SF and its receptor on the behaviour of prostate cancer has been clearly demonstrated in a study comparing the incidence of prostate cancer between African American and white Americans (i.e., the incidence of prostate cancer was found to be 2–3 times higher in African Americans than white Americans). In addition, this study has shown that African Americans have a 4-fold increase in the level of HGF/SF receptor expression present in prostate cancer tissues, compared with samples taken from matched Caucasian populations (106).

6. THE THERAPEUTIC ASPECT OF HGF/SF IN PROSTATE CANCER, STUDIES ON THE HGF/SF ANTAGONIST, NK4

Given the pivotal roles of HGF/SF and its receptor in cancer, considerable effort has been made to identify possible therapeutic targets to inhibit the actions of HGF/SF and its receptor in a variety of cancer cell types, including prostate cancer. A number of agents have now been shown to suppress the functions of HGF/SF in cancer cells, including retinoic acid and its derivatives (15); inhibitory factors to invasiveness (107); and gamma linolenic acid (69). Although the action of these products are not specific to HGF/SF; a more recently identified antagonist known as NK4, has been reported to specifically inhibit HGF/SF mediated responses.

6.1 Biological Structure of the HGF/SF Antagonist NK4

There have been a number of studies performed to date, examining the biological effects induced by HGF/SF and their consequences on cancer development and progression. This has, therefore, prompted attempts to minimise the pleiotrophic actions of HGF/SF both *in vitro* and *in vivo*. The idea of using part of the HGF/SF molecule as a specific antagonist to this motogen through competitive binding to *c-Met* has been postulated at great length (71, 108–110). Date *et al.* (108) constructed a protein called NK4 (50kDa) through enzymatic (elastase-digested HGF/SF) cleavage of mature HGF/SF, which retained the N-terminal hairpin loop (i.e., *c-Met* receptor binding domain) plus all four kringle domains; but was completely devoid of the HGF/SF β-chain and amino acid residues responsible for dimerisation on the C-terminus of the α-chain, thus allowing NK4 to completely inhibit the biological responses driven by HGF/SF through *c-Met* receptor coupling; by competing for binding to the *c-Met*-HGF/SF receptor tyrosine kinase, but without causing the activation of *c-Met* (108, 111–112).

6.2 Inhibitory Effects of NK4 and Clinical Perspectives

NK4 has been shown to display complete antagonism towards HGF/SF mediated responses in hepatocytes and MDCK cells (108, 112) respectively. Furthermore, NK4 has been shown to inhibit tumor invasion through the basement membrane using a co-culture system mimicking tumor-stroma interactions (111, 113). NK4 has also been shown to inhibit the effects of HGF/SF on *in vitro* angiogenesis in human vascular endothelial cells (114). The HGF/SF antagonist NK4, also inhibits cell migration and *in vitro* invasion in a variety of cancer cell types including prostate, colon and breast cancer cells (71, 109, 115). Date *et al.* (111) also reported that local administration of NK4 into mice inhibited tumor growth, invasion and metastasis. Similarly, in a more recent study conducted by Kuba *et al.* (116), NK4 was reported to suppress both tumor growth and metastasis in nude mice by inhibiting HGF/SF mediated angiogenesis. Furthermore, in a separate study carried out by Kuba *et al.* (117) the four kringle domains of HGF/SF known as K1-4 (63kDa) have also been shown to have an anti-angiogenic effect on cultured endothelial cells, however, this variant was found to lack antagonistic activity to HGF/SF-induced responses. Therefore, NK4, reputed to be a specific antagonist to HGF/SF, may offer both unique and strong opportunities in the treatment of cancer, where abnormal expression of HGF/SF and/or its receptor are associated with the disease progression, and prognosis in tumor bearing patients (15, 110).

7. CONCLUSIONS

There is now abundant evidence demonstrating the diverse biological effects displayed by HGF/SF on cells *in vitro* and *in vivo*. HGF/SF has been implicated in the regulation of mitogenesis, motogenesis and morhogenesis; playing pivotal roles in a number of regulatory responses including physiological and pathological processes. In addition, HGF/SF is now known to be widely involved in cellular migration, scattering, motility, matrix adhesion and its degradation, shedding of cell surface adhesion molecules and increased invasiveness of cancer cells. Furthermore, HGF/SF is a known potent factor of angiogenesis in both normal and neoplastic cells. This motogen has also been shown to play a key regulatory role in cancer development. Thus, identifying mechanisms of HGF/SF activation, and more importantly inhibitors and antagonists to this motogen, may help to address the more important clinical issues of cancer treatment such as the prevention of invasion, and metastasis in tumor bearing patients. Although most inhibitors to HGF/SF are still at a developmental stage, recent studies on cancer treatment using NK4 in experimental models look quite promising, and have demonstrated quite clearly the unique therapeutic potential of this HGF/SF antagonist (111, 116). However, the possibility that NK4 can be of therapeutic value to tumor bearing patients clearly warrants further investigation. Therefore, preventing the metastatic spread of cancer cells remains a long-term objective that may greatly benefit the overall management of cancer patients.

ACKNOWLEDGEMENTS

We thank Cancer Research Wales for providing financial support.

REFERENCES

1. Mason MD, Davies G, Jiang WG. Cell adhesion molecules and adhesion abnormalities in prostate cancer. Crit Rev Oncol Hematol 2002, 41:11–28.
2. Michalopoulos G, Houck KA, Dolan ML, Leutteke NC. Control of hepatocyte replication by two serum factors. Cancer Res 1984, 44:4414–19.
3. Nakamura T, Nawa K, Ichihara A. Partial purification and characterization of hepatocyte growth factor from serum of hepatomized rats. Biochem Biophys Res Commun 1984, 122:1450–9.
4. Russell WE, McGowan JA, Bucher NLR. Partial characterisation of a hepatocyte growth factor from rat platelets. J Cell Physiol 1984, 119:183–92.

5. Miyazawa K, Tsubouchi H, Naka D, Takahashi K, Okigaki M, Arakaki N et al. Molecular cloning and sequence analysis of cDNA for human hepatocyte growth factor. Biochem Biophys Res Commun 1989, 163:967–73.
6. Zarnegar R, Muga S, Enghild J, Michalopoulos G. NH2-terminal amino acid sequence of rabbit hepatopoitin A, a heparin bindinding polypeptide growth factor for hepatocytes. Biochem Biophys Res Commun 1989, 163:1370–6.
7. Higashio K, Shima N, Goto M, Itagaki Y, Nagao M, Yasuda H, Morinaga T. Identity of a tumor cytotoxic factor from human fibroblasts and hepatocyte growth factor. Biochem Biophys Res Commun 1990, 170:397–404.
8. Zarnegar R, DeFrances MC, Oliver L, Michalopoulos GK. Identification and partial characterisation of receptor binding sites for HGF on rat hepatocytes. Biochem Biophys Res Commun 1990, 173:1179–85.
9. Stoker M, Perryman M. An epithelial scatter factor released by embryo fibroblasts. J Cell Sci 1985, 77:209–23.
10. Gherardi E, Stoker M. Hepatocytes and scatter factor. Nature 1990, 346:228.
11. Weidner KM, Behrens J, Vandekerckhove J, Birchmeier W. Scatter factor: Molecular characteristics and effect on the invasiveness of epithelial cells. J Cell Biol 1990, 111:2097–108.
12. Furlong RA, Takehara T, Taylor WG, Nakamura T, Rubin JS. Comparison of biological and immunochemical properties indicates that scatter factor and hepatocyte growth factor are indistinguishable. J Cell Sci 1991, 100:173–7.
13. Gherardi E, Stoker M. Hepatocyte growth factor/scatter factor: Mitogen, motogen and met. Cancer Cells 1991, 3:227–32.
14. Jiang WG, Hiscox S. Hepatocyte growth factor/scatter factor, a cytokine playing multiple and converse roles. Histol Histopathol 1997, 12:537–55.
15. Jiang WG, Hiscox S, Matsumoto K, Nakamura T. Hepatocyte growth factor/scatter factor, its molecular, cellular and clinical implications in cancer. Crit Rev Oncol Hematol 1999, 29:209–48.
16. Nakamura T, Nishizawa T, Hagiya M, Seki T, Shimonishi M, Sugimura A et al. Molecular cloning and expression of human hepatocyte growth factor. Nature 1989, 342:440–3.
17. Nakamura T. Structure and function of hepatocyte growth factor. Prog Growth Factor Res 1991, 3:67–85.
18. Miyazawa K, Shimomura T, Naka D, Kitamura N. Proteolytic activation of hepatocyte growth factor in response to tissue injury. J Biol Chem 1994, 269:8966–70.
19. Naldini L, Vigna E, Bardelli A, Follenzi A, Galimi F, Comoglio PM. Biological activation of pro-HGF (hepatocyte growth factor) by urokinase is controlled by a stoichiometric reaction. J Biol Chem 1995, 270:603–11.
20. Patthy L, Trexler M, Vali Z, Banyai L, Varadi A. Kringles: Modules specialized for protein binding. Homology of the gelatin-binding region of fibronectin with the kringle structures of proteases. FEBS Lett 1984, 171:131–6.
21. Lokker NA, Godowski PJ. Generation and characterisation of a competitive antagonist of human hepatocyte growth factor, HGF/NK1. J Biol Chem 1993, 268:17145–50.
22. Lyon M, Deakin JA, Mizuno K, Nakamura T, Gallaher JT. Interaction of hepatocyte growth factor with heparin sulfate. Elucidation of the major heparin sulfate structural determinants. J Biol Chem 1994, 269:11216–23.

23. Mizuno K, Tanoue Y, Okano I, Harano T, Takada K, Nakamura T. Purification and characterisation of hepatocyte growth factor (HGF)-converting enzyme-activation of pro-HGF. Biochem Biophys Res Commun 1994, 198:1161–9.
24. Matsumoto K, Takehara T, Inoue H, Hagiya M, Shimizu S, Nakamura T. Deletion of kringle domains or the N-terminal hairpin structure in hepatocyte growth factor results in marked decreases in related biological activities. Biochem Biophys Res Commun 1991, 181:691–9.
25. Lerch PG, Rickli EE, Lergier W, Gillessen D. Localisation of individual lysine binding regions in human plasminogen and investigations on their complex forming properties. Eur J Biochem 1980, 107:7–13.
26. van Zonneveld AJ, Veerman H, Pannekoek H. On the interaction of the finger and the kringle-2 domain of tissue-type plasminogen activator with fibrin. Inhibition of kringle-2 binding to fibrin by epsilon-amino caproic acid. J Biol Chem 1986, 261:14214–18.
27. Strain AJ. Hepatocyte growth factor: Another ubiquitous cytokine. J Endocrinol 1993, 137:1–5.
28. Mars WM, Zarnegar R, Michalopoulos GK. Activation of hepatocyte growth factor by the plasminogen activators uPA and tPA. Am J Pathol 1993, 143:949–58.
29. Shimomura T, Kondo J, Ochiai M, Naka D, Miyazawa K, Morimoto Y, Kitamura N. Activation of the zymogen of hepatocyte growth factor activator by thrombin. J Biol Chem 1993, 268:22927–32.
30. Matsumoto K, Tajima H, Hamanoue M, Kohno S, Kinoshita T, Nakamura T. Identification and characterization of "injurin," an inducer of expression of the gene for hepatocyte growth factor. Proc Natl Acad Sci USA 1992, 89:3800–4.
31. Matsumoto K, Tajima H, Okazaki H, Nakamura T. Negative regulation of hepatocyte growth factor gene expression in human lung fibroblasts and leukemic cells by transforming growth factor β1 and glucocorticoids. J Biol Chem 1992, 267:24917–20.
32. Matsumoto K, Tajima H, Okazaki H, Nakamura T. Heparin as an inducer of hepatocyte growth-factor. J Biochem 1993, 114:820–6.
33. Okazaki H, Matsumoto K, Nakamura T. Partial-purifation and characterization of injurin-like factor which stimulates production of hepatocyte growth-factor. Biochim Biophys Acta 1994, 1220:1291–8.
34. Bottaro DP, Rubin JS, Faletto DL, Chan AML, Kmiecik TE, VandeWoude GF, Aaronson SA. Identification of the hepatocyte growth factor receptor as the *c-Met* protooncogene product. Science 1991, 258:802–4.
35. Naldini L, Weidner KM, Vigna E, Gaudino G, Bardelli A, Ponzetto C *et al*. Scatter factor and hepatocyte growth factor are indistinguishable ligands for the *Met* receptor. EMBO J 1991, 10:2867–78.
36. Cooper CS, Park M, Blair Tainsky DGMA, Heubner K, Croce CM, VandeWoude GF. Molecular cloning of a new transforming gene from a chemically transformed human cell line. Nature 1984, 311:29–33.
37. Cooper CS. The met oncogene: From detection by transfection to transmembrane receptor for hepatocyte growth factor. Oncogene 1992, 7:3–7.
38. Park M, Dean M, Kaul K, Braun MJ, Gonda MA, VandeWoude GF. Sequence of met proto-oncogene cDNA has features characteristic of the tyrosine family of growth factor receptors. Proc Natl Acad Sci USA 1987, 84:6379–83.

39. Giordano S, Zhen Z, Medico E, Galimi F, Comoglio PM. Transfer of motogenic and invasive response to scatter factor/hepatocyte growth factor by transfection of human met protooncogene. Proc Natl Acad Sci USA 1993, 90:649–53.
40. Faletto DL, Kaplan DR, Halverson DO, Rosen EM, Vande Woude GF. Signal transduction in c-met mediated motogenesis, pp. 107–30. In: *Hepatocyte Growth Factor-Scatter Factor (HGF-SF), the c-Met Receptor.* Goldberg ID, Rosen EM, eds, Basel: Birkhauser Verlag, 1993.
41. Koch CA, Anderson D, Moran MF, Ellis C, Pawson T. SH2 and SH3 domains, elements that control interactions of cytoplasmic signalling proteins. Science 1991, 252:668–74.
42. Pawson T, Gish CD. SH2 and SH3 domains: From structure to function. Cell 1992, 71:359–62.
43. Ponzetto C, Bardelli A, Maina F, Longati P, Panayotou G, Dhand R *et al.* A novel recognition motif for phosphatidylinositol 3-kinase binding mediates its association with the hepatocyte growth-factor scatter factor-receptor. Mol Cell Biol 1993, 13:4600–8.
44. Ponzetto C, Bardelli A, Zhen Z, Maina F, Dallazonca P, Giordano S *et al.* A multifunctional docking site mediates signalling and transformation by the hepatocyte growth-factor scatter factor-receptor family. Cell 1994, 77: 261–71.
45. Matsumoto K, Nakamura T. HGF-c-met receptor pathway in tumor invasion-metastasis and potential cancer treatment with NK4, pp. 277–90. In: *Cancer Metastasis: Biology and Treatment Volume 2: Growth Factors and Their Receptors in Cancer Metastasis.* Jiang WG, Matsumoto K, Nakamura T, eds, Dordrecht, The Netherlands: Kluwer Academic Publishers, 2001.
46. Graziani A, Gramaglia D, Dalla ZP, Comoglio PM. Hepatocyte growth factor/scatter factor stimulates the ras-guanine nucleotide exchanger. J Biol Chem 1993, 268:9165–8.
47. Hartmann G, Weidner KM, Schwarz H, Birchmeier W. The motility signal of scatter factor hepatocyte growth-factor mediated through the receptor tyrosine kinase met requires intracellular action of ras. J Biol Chem 1994, 269:21936–9.
48. Hart IR, Goode NT, Wilson RE. Molecular aspects of the metastatic cascade. Biochim Biophys Acta 1989, 989:65–84.
49. Jiang WG, Puntis MCA, Hallett MB. Molecular and cellular basis of cancer invasion and metastasis: Implications for treatment. Br J Surg 1994, 81:1576–90.
50. Pepper MS, Matsumoto K, Nakamura T, Orci L, Montesano R. Hepatocyte growth-factor increases urokinase-type plasminogen-activator (u-PA) and u-PA receptor expression in madin-darby canine kidney epithelial-cells. J Biol Chem 1992, 267:20493–6.
51. Nishino T, Hisha H, Nishino N, Adachi M, Ikehara S. Hepatocyte growth-factor as a hematopoietic regulator. Blood 1995, 85:3093–100.
52. Zarnegar R, Michalopoulos GK. The many faces of hepatocyte growth-factor from hepatopoiesis to hematopoiesis. J Cell Biol 1995, 129:1177–80.
53. Sunitha I, Meighen DL, Hartman DP, Thompson EW, Byers SW, Avigan MI. Hepatocyte growth-factor stimulates invasion across reconstituted basement-membranes by a new human small-intestinal cell line. Clin Exp Metastas 1994, 12: 143–54.

54. Grant DS, Kleinman HK, Goldberg ID, Bhargava MM, Nickoloff BJ, Kinsella JL et al. Scatter factor induces blood-vessel formation in vivo. Proc Natl Acad Sci USA 1993, 90:1937–41.
55. Naidu YM, Rosen EM, Zitnik R, Goldberg I, Park M, Naujokas M et al. Role of scatter factor in the pathogenesis of AIDS-related karposi's sarcoma. Proc Natl Acad Sci USA 1994, 91:5282–5.
56. Brinkmann V, Foroutan H, Sachs M, Weidner KM, Birchmeier W. Hepatocyte growth-factor scatter factor induces a variety of tissue-specific morphogenic programs in epithelial cells. J Cell Biol 1995, 131:1573–86.
57. Karp SL, Ortizarduan A, Li SR, Neilson EG. Epithelial differentiation of metanephric mesenchymal cells after stimulation with hepatocyte growth-factor or embryonic spinal-cord. Proc Natl Acad Sci USA 1994, 91:5286–90.
58. Jiang WG, Lloyds D, Puntis MCA, Nakamura T, Hallett MB. Regulation of spreading and growth of human colon cancer cells by hepatocyte growth factor. Clin Exp Metastas 1993, 11:235–42.
59. Jiang WG, Hallett MB, Puntis MCA. Hepatocyte growth factor/scatter factor, liver regeneration and cancer metastases. Br J Surg 1993, 80:1368–73.
60. Jiang WG, Puntis MCA, Hallett MB. Monocyte conditioned media possess a novel factor which increases motility of cancer cells. Int J Cancer 1993, 53:426–31.
61. Jiang WG, Hallett MB, Puntis MCA. Motility factors in cancer invasion and metastasis. Surg Res Commun 1994, 16:219–37.
62. Revoltella RP, Borney F, Dalcanto B, Durso CM. Apoptosis of serum-free c2.8 Mouse embryo hepatocyte cells caused by hepatocyte growth-factor deprivation. Cytotechnology 1993, 13:13–19.
63. Revoltella RP, Dalcanto B, Caracciolo L, Durso CM. L-carnitine and some of its analogs delay the onset of apoptotic cell-death initiated in murine c2.8 Hepatocytic cells after hepatocyte growth-factor deprivation. Biochim Biophys Acta 1994, 1224:333–41.
64. Taipale J, Keski-Oja J. Hepatocyte growth factor releases epithelial and endothelial cells from growth arrest induced by transforming growth factor beta 1. J Biol Chem 1996, 271:4342–6.
65. Hiscox S, Jiang WG. HGF/SF regulates the phosphorylation of β-catenin and cell-cell adhesion in cancer cells. Proc Am Assoc Cancer Res 1998, 39:500–1.
66. Davies G, Jiang WG, Mason MD. Cell-cell adhesion molecules and their associated proteins in bladder cancer cells and their role in mitogen induced cell-cell dissociation and invasion. Anticancer Res 1999, 19:547–52.
67. Davies G, Jiang WG, Mason MD. Matrilysin mediates extracellular cleavage of E-cadherin from prostate cancer cells: A key mechanism in hepatocyte growth factor/scatter factor-induced cell-cell dissociation and in vitro invasion. Clin Cancer Res 2001, 7:3289–97.
68. Jiang WG, Hiscox S, Hallett MB, Scott C, Horrobin DF, Puntis MCA. Inhibition of hepatocyte growth factor-induced motility and *in vitro* invasion of human colon cancer cells by gamma-linolenic acid. Br J Cancer 1995, 71:744–52.
69. Jiang WG, Hiscox S, Hallett MB, Horrobin DF, Mansel RE, Puntis MCA. Regulation of the expression of E-cadherin on human cancer-cells by gamma-linolenic acid. Cancer Res 1995, 55:5043–8.

70. Davies G, Jiang WG, Mason MD. Cell-cell adhesion molecules and signalling intermediates and their role in the invasive potential of prostate cancer cells. J Urol 2000, 163:985–92.
71. Parr C, Davies G, Nakamura T, Matsumoto K, Mason MD, Jiang WG. The HGF/SF-induced phosphorylation of paxillin, matrix adhesion, and invasion of prostate cancer cells were suppressed by NK4, an HGF/SF variant. Biochem Biophys Res Commun 2001, 285:1330–7.
72. Shibamoto S, Hayakawa M, Takeuchi K, Hori T, Oku N, Miyazawa K *et al.* Tyrosine phosphorylation of β-catenin and plakoglobin enhanced by hepatocyte growth factor and epidermal growth factor in human carcinoma cells. Cell Adhes Commun 1994, 1:295–305.
73. Tannapfel A, Yasui W, Yokozaki H, Wittekind C, Tahara E. Effect of hepatocyte growth factor on the expression of E- and P-cadherin in gastric carcinoma cell lines. Virchows Arch 1994, 425:139–44.
74. Burridge K, Chrzanowska-Wodnicka M. Focal adhesions, contractility, and signaling. Annu Rev Cell Dev Biol 1996, 12:463–518.
75. Rong S, Bodescot M, Blair D, Dunn J, Nakamura T, Mizuno K *et al.* Tumorigenicity of the met proto-oncogene and the gene for hepatocyte growth factor. Mol Cell Biol 1992, 12:5152–8.
76. Crepaldi T, Pollack AL, Prat M, Zborek A, Mostov K, Comoglio PM. Targeting of the SF/HGF receptor to the basolateral domain of polarized epithelial-cells. J Cell Biol 1994, 125:313–20.
77. Kamei T, Matozaki T, Sakisaka T, Kodama A, Yokoyama S, Peng Y-F *et al.* Co-endocytosis of cadherin and c-met coupled to disruption of cell-cell adhesion in MDCK cells, regulation by rho, rac and rab small G proteins. Oncogene 1999, 18:6776–84.
78. Davies G, Jiang WG, Mason MD. HGF/SF modifies the interaction between its receptor c-met, and the E-cadherin/catenin complex in prostate cancer cells. Int J Mol Med 2001, 7:385–8.
79. Miura H, Nishimura K, Tsujimura A, Matsumiya K, Matsumoto K, Nakamura T, Okuyama A. Effects of hepatocyte growth factor on E-cadherin-mediated cell-cell adhesion in DU145 prostate cancer cells. Urology 2001, 58:1064–9.
80. Seaman MN, Burd CG, Emr SD. Receptor signalling and the regulation of endocytic membrane transport. Curr Opin Cell Biol 1996, 8:549–56.
81. Le, TL, Yap, AS, Stow JL. Recycling of E-cadherin: A potential mechanism for regulating cadherin dynamics. J Cell Biol 1999, 146:219–32.
82. Adams JC, Watt FM. Regulation of development and differentiation by the extracellular matrix. Development 1993, 117:1183–98.
83. Lochter A, Bissell MJ. Involvement of extracellular matrix constituents in breast cancer. Semin Cancer Biol 1995, 6:165–73.
84. Ashkenas J, Muschler J, Bissell MJ. The extracellular matrix in epithelial biology: Shared molecules and common themes in distant phyla. Dev Biol 1996, 180: 433–44.
85. Lochter A, Galosy S, Muschler J, Freedman N, Werb Z, Bissell MJ. Matrix metalloproteinase stromelysin-1 triggers a cascade of molecular alterations that leads to stable epithelial-to-mesenchymal conversion and a premalignant phenotype in mammary epithelial cells. J Cell Biol 1997, 139:1861–72.

86. Mauch C. Regulation of connective tissue turnover by cell-matrix interactions. Arch Dermatol Res 1998, 290(Suppl):S30– S36.
87. Chambers AF, Matrisian LM. Changing views of the role of matrix metalloproteinases in metastasis. J Natl Cancer Inst 1997, 89:1260–70.
88. Nelson AR, Fingleton B, Rothenberg ML, Matrisian LM. Matrix metalloproteinases: Biologic activity and clinical implications. J Clin Oncol 2000, 18: 1135–49.
89. Harvey P, Clark IM, Jaurand MC, Warn RM, Edwards DR. Hepatocyte growth factor/scatter factor enhances the invasion of mesothelioma cell lines and the expression of matrix metalloproteinases. Br J Cancer 2000, 83: 1147–53.
90. Dunsmore SE, Rubin JS, Kovacs SO, Chedid M, Parks WC, Welgus HG. Mechanisms of hepatocyte growth factor stimulation of keratinocyte metalloproteinase production. J Biol Chem 1996, 271:24576–82.
91. Bennett JH, Furness J, Atkin P, Speight PM. Scatter factor (SF) regulation of matrix metalloproteinase production by oral carcinoma cells. J Dental Res 1997, 76:2140–2140.
92. Noe V, Fingleton B, Jacobs K, Crawford HC, Vermeulen S, Steelant W *et al.* Release of an invasion promoter E-cadherin fragment by matrilysin and stromelysin-1. J Cell Sci 2001, 114:111–18.
93. Herren B, Levkau B, Raines EW, Ross R. Cleavage of beta-catenin and plakoglobin and shedding of VE-cadherin during endothelial apoptosis: Evidence for a role for caspases and metalloproteinases. Mol Biol Cell 1998, 9:1589–601.
94. Naughton M, Picus J, Zhu XP, Catalona WJ, Vollmer RT, Humphrey PA. Scatter factor-hepatocyte growth factor elevation in the serum of patients with prostate cancer. J Urol 2001, 165:1325–8.
95. Pisters LL, Troncoso P, Zhau HE, Li W, Voneschenbach AC, Chung LWK. C-met proto-oncogene expression in benign and malignant human prostate tissues. J Urol 1995, 154:293–8.
96. Watanabe M, Fukutome K, Kato H, Murata M, Kawamura J, Shiraishi T, Yatani R. Progression linked over-expression of c-met in prostatic intraepithelial neoplasia and latent as well as clinical prostate cancers. Cancer Lett 1999, 141:173–8.
97. Humphrey PA, Zhu X, Zarnegar R, Swanson P, Ratliff TL, Vollmer RT, Day ML. Hepatocyte growth factor and its receptor (c-MET) in prostatic carcinoma. Am J Pathol 1995, 147:386–96.
98. Nakashiro K, Okamoto M, Hayashi Y, Oyasu R. Hepatocyte growth factor secreated by prostate derived stromal cells stimulates growth of androgen-independent human prostatic carcinoma cells. Am J Pathol 2000, 157:795–803.
99. Gmyrek GA, Walburg M, Webb CP, Yu HM, You X, Vaughan ED *et al.* Normal and malignant prostate epithelial cells differ in their response to hepatocyte growth factor/scatter factor. Am J Pathol 2001, 159:579–90.
100. Sasaki M, Enami J. Hepatocyte growth factor supports androgen stimulation of growth of mouse ventral prostate epithelial cells in collagen gel matrix culture. Cell Biol Int 2000, 23:373–7.
101. Presnell SC, Borchert K, Gregory C, Maygarden S, Mohler J. Increased expression of hepatocyte growth factor, c-met, and androgen receptor is associated with

the transition from androgen-dependent to androgen-independent prostate cancer. FASEB J 2001, 15:A239.
102. Lang SH, Clarke NW, George NJR, Testa NG. Scatter factor influences the formation of prostate epithelial cell colonies on bone marrow stroma in vitro. Clin Exp Metastasis 1999, 17:333–40.
103. Nishimura K, Kitamura M, Miura H, Nonomura N, Takada S, Takahara S et al. Prostate stromal cell derived hepatocyte growth factor induces invasion of prostate cancer cell line DU145 through tumor stromal interaction. Prostate 1999, 41:145–53.
104. Olumi AF, Grossfeld GD, Hayward SW, Carroll PR, Tlsty TD, Cunha GR. Carcinoma associated fibroblasts direct tumor progression of initiated human prostatic epithelium. Cancer Res 1999, 59:5002–11.
105. Michieli P, Basilico C, Pennaccietti S, Maffe A, Tamagnone L, Giordano S et al. Mutant met-mediated transformation is ligand dependent and can be inhibited by HGF antagonists. Oncogene 1999, 18:5221–31.
106. Presnell SC, Borchert K, Gregory C, Maygarden S, Smith G, Mohler J. Differential expression of hepatocyte growth factor and c-met in prostate cancer amongst caucasian american vs. African american. FASEB J 2001, 15:A239.
107. Jiang WG, Hiscox S, Singhrao SK, Hallett MB, Puntis MCA, Nakamura T et al. Inhibition of motility and invasion by invasion inhibiting factor 2 on human colon cancer cells. Surg Res Commun 1995, 17:67–78.
108. Date K, Matsumoto K, Shimura H, Tanaka M, Nakamura T. HGF/NK4 is a specific antagonist for pleiotrophic actions of hepatocyte growth factor. FEBS Lett 1997, 420:1–6.
109. Parr C, Hiscox S, Nakamura T, Matsumoto K, Jiang WG. NK4, a new HGF/SF variant, is an antagonist to the influence of HGF/SF on the motility and invasion of colon cancer cells. Int J Cancer 2000, 85:563–70.
110. Parr C, Jiang WG. Hepatocyte growth factor activators, inhibitors and antagonists and their implication in cancer intervention. Histol Histopathol 2001, 16:251–68.
111. Date K, Matsumoto K, Kuba K, Shimura H, Tanaka M, Nakamura T. Inhibition of tumor growth and invasion by a four-kringle antagonist (HGF/NK4) for hepatocyte growth factor. Oncogene 1998, 17:3045–54.
112. Matsumoto K, Kataoka H, Date K, Nakamura T. Cooperative interaction between alpha- and beta-chains of hepatocyte growth factor on c-met receptor confers ligand-induced receptor tyrosine phosphorylation and multiple biological responses. J Biol Chem 1998, 273:22913–20.
113. Matsumoto K, Nakamura T. Hepatocyte growth factor and met in tumor invasion-metastasis: From mechanisms to cancer prevention, pp. 143–93. In: *Cancer Metastasis: Biology and Treatment Volume 1: Cancer Metastasis, Molecular and Cellular Mechanisms and Clinical Intervention.* Jiang WG, Mansel RE, eds, Dordrecht, The Netherlands: Kluwer Academic Publishers, 2000.
114. Jiang WG, Hiscox SE, Parr C, Martin TA, Matsumoto 7K, Nakamura T, Mansel RE. Antagonistic effect of NK4, a novel hepatocyte growth factor variant, on in vitro angiogenesis of human vascular endothelial cells. Clin Cancer Res 1999, 5:3695–703.
115. Hiscox S, Parr C, Nakamura T, Matsumoto K, Mansel RE, Jiang WG. Inhibition of HGF/SF-induced breast cancer cell motility and invasion by the HGF/SF variant, NK4. Breast Cancer Res Treat 2000, 59:245–54.

116. Kuba K, Matsumoto K, Date K, Shimura H, Tanaka M, Nakamura T. HGF/NK4, a four-kringle antagonist of hepatocyte growth factor, is an angiogenesis inhibitor that suppresses tumor growth and metastasis in mice. Cancer Res 2000, 60:6737–43.
117. Kuba K, Matsumoto K, Ohnishi K, Shiratsuchi T, Tanaka M, Nakamura T. Kringle 1-4 of hepatocyte growth factor inhibits proliferation, migration of human microvascular endothelial cells. Biochem Biophys Res Commun 2000, 279:846–52.

Chapter 11

MATRIX DEGRADATION IN PROSTATE CANCER

Michael J. Wilson[1,2,4] and Akhouri A. Sinha[3,4]
[1]*VA Medical Center and Departments of Laboratory Medicine and Pathology, University of Minnesota, Minneapolis, MN, USA;*
[2]*Urologic Surgery and Genetics Minneapolis, University of Minnesota, Minneapolis, MN, USA;*
[3]*Cell Biology, & Development, University of Minnesota, Minneapolis, MN, USA;*
[4]*University of Minnesota Cancer Center, University of Minnesota, Minneapolis, MN, USA*

Abstract: Metastasis is the critical factor in the lethality of prostate cancer. Alterations in expression of cellular adhesion, cytoskeletal and cell motility proteins, and constituents of the extracellular matrix (ECM), are intimately involved in tumor cell invasion and metastasis. Proteolysis of ECM is a highly regulated process that has traditionally been considered fundamental to tumor cell invasion and metastasis, permitting physical passage of malignant cells. But proteolytic functions are now recognized as instrumental in tumor growth through release of growth factor and chemoattractant molecules, modification of cell surface receptors, and molecular processing of cytokines, other proteases, and ECM proteins. This chapter focuses on the control of proteolytic systems that cleave ECM proteins in studies of human prostate tissues.

Key words: Basement membrane, extracellular matrix, stroma, matrix metalloproteinases, tissue inhibitors of matrix metalloproteinases, cathepsin B, cathepsin D, stefin A, serine proteases, prostate specific antigen, kallikreins, plasminogen activators, hepsin, serpins, plasminogen activator inhibitor type I, maspin

1. INTRODUCTION

Metastasis is a critical aspect in the lethality of prostatic adenocarcinoma. The movement of prostatic cancer cells from the acinar epithelium through the basement membrane (BM) and interstitial stroma into blood or lymph vessels, with subsequent malignant cell migration and colonization of distant tissue sites, is facilitated by altered expression and degradation of cell adhesion and extracellular matrix (ECM) proteins. Although alteration in expression of cellular adhesion molecules, such as the integrins, and changes in cytoskeleton and of cell motility proteins are intimately involved in tumor cell invasion and metastasis, the focus of this chapter is the control of proteolytic systems that cleave BM and stromal ECM proteins, promoting growth of the tumor and passage of malignant cells in the prostate from one biological compartment to another. In addition, this review also focuses on studies of human prostate tissues. Our current understanding of the highly regulated process of ECM protein proteolysis is that, in addition to degradation of ECM proteins permitting physical passage of malignant prostatic cells through the BM and supporting stroma, proteases also influence prostatic tumor growth through the release of growth factor and chemoattractant molecules from the ECM, and by the proteolytic processing of cytokines, other proteases, and existing or newly formed ECM proteins.

2. BASEMENT MEMBRANE

The literature describing the BM and interstitial stroma of normal and cancerous human and animal tissues is extensive (1–6). At the ultrastructrual level the BM is resolved into the lamina rara (or lucida), lamina densa, and subjacent reticular lamina (Figure 1a). The BM controls the passage of macromolecules including proteins between the epithelium and subadjacent stroma (3). BMs are present not only around acini and ducts in the prostate, but also smooth muscle, nerve fibers, and endothelia of blood vessels and capillaries. BMs are attenuated in lymphatic vessels (1). Type IV collagen, entactin, laminin, fibronectin, and heparan sulfate proteoglycans are prominent proteins in the acinar BM. Type IV collagen is a triple helical molecule 400 nm in length comprised of 6 possible chains; the isoform of two $\alpha 1(IV)$ and one $\alpha 2(IV)$ chains being present in all BMs (5). The BM of fetal and normal prostate and prostatic intraepithelial neoplasia (PIN) contain the classical $\alpha 1(IV)$ and $\alpha 2(IV)$ chains of type IV collagen (1, 6, 7) as well as the more novel $\alpha 5(IV)$ and $\alpha 6(IV)$ chains, but not $\alpha 3(IV)$ chains (6). The prostatic acinar BM demonstrates entactin (8) and strong Type VI and XV and faint Type XIX collagen immunoreactivity, whereas all of these components are localized in vascular and smooth muscle BMs in the prostatic stroma (9, 10). Laminins are a heterotrimeric group of high molelcular weight glycoproteins comprised of α, β, and γ chains of which there are 11 genetic chain variant forms (11). Immunogold electron microscopy shows a distribution of laminin (gold particles) predominantly in the lamina rara, and some in the lamina densa layers of prostatic acinar

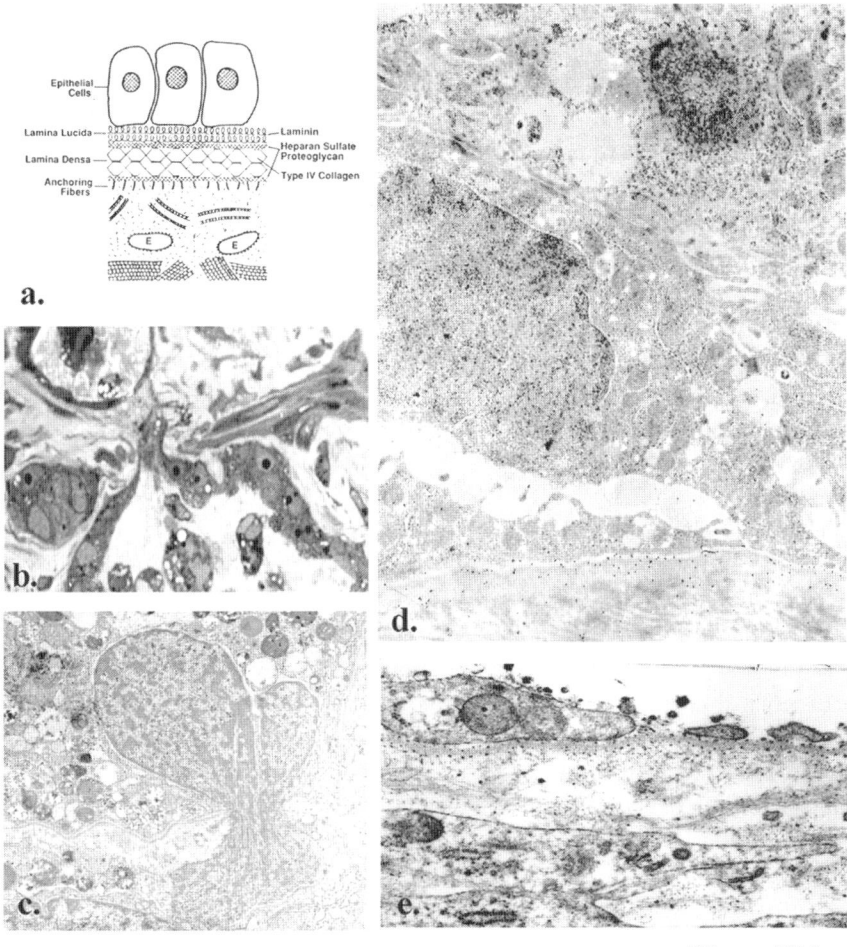

Figure 1. **A.** Diagrammatic representation of the relationship of epithelial cells with the underlying basement membrane and of its constituents in prostatic stroma. The basement membrane is distinguished cytolotically into the lamina lucida and densa layers. Laminin is subjacent to the epithelial cells whereas type IV collagen and heparan sulphate proteoglycan are intimately associated with the lamina densa. Anchoring fibers interface between the basement membrane and the subjacent connective tissue. The authors modified the figures of Martinez-Hernandez and Amenta (17) and Martin et al. (18). **B.** A micrograph of cancerous glands illustrates the migration of invasive cells from prostatic acini: some cells appear to be penetrating the basement membrane and invading the prostatic stroma, while other cells are still within acini. Also observe invasive cells and glands in the prostatic stroma. **C.** An electron micrograph of an invasive cell illustrates portions of the cell and nucleus within the acinus while the other portion protrudes into the prostatic stroma through a focally breached basement membrane. This invasive cell also illustrates well-developed Golgi complex, secretory and lysosomal granules (continued on page 224)

BMs (Figure 1d). Intense laminin localization is found in fetal prostate epithelial BMs, but BM areas locally thickened or non-reactive to laminin antibodies are also found (7). The $\alpha 3$, $\beta 3$, and $\gamma 2$ subchains of laminin 5, which is involved in hemidesmosome attachment of basal cells to the basal lamina, are present in the BM of normal prostate (11–13). Heparan sulfate proteglycans (7, 14), including perlecan, a multidomain heparan sulfate proteoglycan (15), are also components of BMs of prostatic acini and blood vessels, but not of smooth muscle (14). The distribution of heparan sulfate proteoglycans correspond to the distribution of heparan sulfate anionic charge sites in the acinar BM, which extend from the BM on bundles of collagen fibrils into the stromal interstitium and to fibroblasts. Anionic sites associated with the lamina rara and densa spanned over fenestrae of prostatic capillaries (Figure 1e), suggesting that these negatively charged sites may regulate passage of charged macromolecules through these fenestrae.

There are distinct disruptions to the BM of prostatic acini that permit physical passage of cancer cells into the stroma (Figures 1b, 1c). Breaching of the BM is accompanied by focal and wide spread diminished immunoreactivity for laminin, heparan sulfate proteoglycans and type IV collagen in prostatic acinar BMs in prostate cancers (1, 4, 14). However, distinct BM formations in contact with the stroma are still found in highly malignant prostatic lesions and metastases (4). Type IV collagen $\alpha 5$ and $\alpha 6$ chains are not detected in prostate cancers, whereas $\alpha 1$ and $\alpha 2$ type IV collagen chains continued to be expressed (6). Similarly, the message and not the protein of the $\beta 3$ and $\gamma 2$ chains of laminin 5 are detected in carcinoma cells (16). Changes in the production of BM constituent proteins, as well as degradation of BM proteins appears to be prerequisite for migration of prostate cancer cells through this structure (Figures 1b, 1c).

Figure 1. (continued) **D.** An electron micrograph illustrates localization of rabbit anti-laminin IgG in the basement membrane of a prostatic gland using goat anti-rabbit IgG complexed with 10–15 nm immunogold particles. Gold particles are distributed in both the lamina lucida and densa layers of the basement membrane. **E.** Micrograph illustrates localization of heparan sulphate-rich anionic sites using the cationic probe, polyethylenimine (PEI), in the basement membrane of prostatic endothelial cells. The presence of anionic sites over fenestrae indicates that negatively charged sites have the potential of regulating passage of charged macromolecules across the basement membrane of blood vessels, especially capillaries. Several studies have shown that heparan sulphate-rich anionic charge sites correspond with the distribution of HSPG in the BM (19–21).

3. INTERSTIAL STROMA

The ECM proteins of the prostatic interstitial stroma include collagens and non-collagenous proteins like fibronectin, elastin, and proteoglycans. Fibronectins are high molecular weight dimeric glycoproteins with binding sites for collagens, heparin/heparan glycoproteins, and cell surface receptors. Fibronectin is localized around glands and smooth muscle, whereas, collagen type III is distributed diffusely in the interstitial connective tissue of normal and benign prostatic hyperplasia (BPH) tissues (22, 23). Carcinoma is accompanied by an altered distribution (23) and increase in content (24) of fibronectin, due in part to a 3.5 fold increase in expression of the alternatively spliced fibronectin containing the ED-B segment. Expression of the ED-B domain is associated with fetal development, a variety of tumors, and wound healing (23). There is also an increased metabolism of collagen in prostate cancer, marked by an increase in collagen type I propeptides and collagen intermediate cross-linkage underscoring the increased synthesis of collagen, and increased matrix metalloproteinase (MMP)-2 activities correlated with collagen degradation (25). Galectin-1, a pleiotropic homodimer member of the β-galactoside-binding galectin family, and chondroitin sulfate containing proteoglycans, versican and decorin, are localized in the periglandular stroma of normal prostate and BPH, and are increased in prostatic carcinomas (26, 27). An increase in sialic acid (24), hyaluronan (28), and elastin (29) are also noted in prostate cancer.

In evaluating ECM components in prostatic carcinogenesis, it should be noted that changes in interstitial macromolecules also occur with formation of BPH. Gene expression by cDNA microarray analysis shows upregulation of ECM proteins laminin alpha 4 and beta 1, chondroitin sulfate proteoglycan 2, and lumican in BPH compared with normal prostate (30). There is a decreased amount of elastin message (31) and an increase in the ratio and size heterogeneity of the glycosaminoglycans chondroitin sulfate to dematan sulfate, with no quantitative change in hyaluronic acid and heparan sulfate content in BPH tissue (32).

Prostate adenocarcinoma, like several other solid organ cancers, demonstrates activation of the host stromal microenvironment or desmoplasia that features myofibroblasts and fibroblasts stimulated to express ECM components (33). Tenascin, a large ECM glycoprotein, is strongly expressed in the mesenchyme around developing prostatic glands, but is only weakly localized in periglandular matrix of normal or benign hyperplastic prostates, although it is consistently expressed in perivascular matrix of the same tissues (34, 35). In contrast to normal adult prostate and BPH, there is a broad and intense stromal distribution of tenascin in prostatic carcinomas (33–35).

In addition to tenascin, procollagen I and FAP (separase) are immunolocalized in stromal cells adjacent to PIN and carcinoma cells, indicating that these ECM changes occur early in carcinogenesis (33). Prostatic carcinogenesis is also accompanied by the down regulation of hevin, an acidic cysteine-rich ECM glycoprotein (36), and increased expression of osteopontin, an adhesive glycoprotein of the ECM containing a functional RGD cell binding domain (37).

4. PERICELLULAR PROTEOLYSIS

Proteolysis of ECM is fundamental to the invasion and metastasis of malignant cells in prostate cancer. MMPs, plasminogen activators, proteases of the coagulation system, and plasma membrane associated cathepsin B are representatives of diverse protease families that work in concert or in cascades to process ECM proteins (38). In general, regulation of expression of these protease groups occurs at the transcriptional, translational and post-translational levels. However, the specificity of control of extracellular proteolysis involves post-translation regulatory steps that include the production of these proteases in pro-enzyme inactive zymogens, activation of the zymogens commonly by proteolytic cleavage, specific subcellular localization through cell surface receptors or selective protein binding, and modulation of activity by endogenous inhibitor molecules.

4.1 Matrix Metalloproteinases

The MMP family is comprised of 25 or more structurally related enzymes that have been subclassified into 4 groups (collagenases, gelatinases, stromelysins, and matrilysins) based on ECM protein substrate specificity and into 8 groups based on their structure (5 secreted and 3 membrane-type sub-groups). Essentially any ECM protein can be cleaved by one or more of the MMP family (39–44). In many adenocarcinomas, matrilysin (MMP-7) is expressed in the epithelial compartment, whereas tumor cells induce (in part through EMMPRIN Extracellular matrix metalloproteinast inducer) other MMPs in adjacent host stromal cells. The stromal cell MMPs can subsequently be expressed in malignant epithelia of tumors that have undergone epithelial-to-mesenchymal transformation (42). The regulation of MMPs is complex and occurs at both transcriptional and post-translational levels. The MMPs are produced as latent zymogen molecules that must be proteolytically processed to become active. MMPs are localized to specific subcellular and extracellular sites since membrane-type MMPs (MT-MMPs) are in the plasma membrane and secreted MMPs associate with select cell surface and ECM proteins (39, 41, 42, 44–46). Complex formation with tissue inhibitors of matrix metalloproteinases (TIMPs), a group of 4 glycoproteins with reported molecular sizes of 21–36 kDa, inhibits the activity of MMPs (40, 41, 44, 47, 48). In addition MMP activity can be thwarted by α2-macroglobulin, thrombospondin, TFPI-2 (tissue factor pathway inhibitor-2), NC1 domain of type IV collagen, CT-PCPE (carboxy-terminal fragment of pro-collagen C-terminal proteinase enhancer protein), and membrane-bound RECK (reversion-inducing cysteine-rich protein with Kazal motifs) (42, 44, 46, 49). MMPs can also influence tumor growth and metastasis through cleavage of non matrix proteins that releases cell surface and matrix bound growth factors, exposes cryptic domains of ECM proteins that promote tumor cell migration, modifies growth factor receptors and adhesion molecules, regulates chemokine bioavailablity in chemokine directed cancer cell migration, and releases matrix-bound angiogenic factors and production of anti-angiogenic peptides from ECM proteins (42, 44–46).

Changes in expression of MMPs in the prostate is related to normal and pathological tissue organization changes (50). Morphogenesis in development and castration-induced regression of the prostate in the rat are marked by expression of the activated form of MMP-2 (51, 52). In the human prostate MMP-2 is upregulated in BPH compared with normal prostate (30), and MMP-2 has been localized by immunohistochemistry and *in situ* hybridization to basal cells, and to a lesser extent secretory epithelial cells, but not stromal cells of normal and BPH tissues (53–57). However, stromal cell MMP-2 immunoreactivity has also been reported (58). MMP-2 immunoreactivity is observed in PIN and is heterogeneous in intensity and location in prostatic adenocarinomas (Figure 2a) (54, 55, 57, 58), which express greater levels of MMP-2 protein and message (53, 59, 60). More intense MMP-2 staining in cribiform and solid/trabecular tumors is found in the cell layer adjacent to the stroma and in single or small clusters of tumor cells in the stroma (57, 61). MMP-2 mRNA transcripts, on the other hand, have been localized to stromal cells only (60, 62), or tumor but not stromal cells by others (54, 56). Increased expression of MMP-2, the ratio of MMP-2:TIMP-2 and particularly the active form of MMP-2, correlate with increasing Gleason score of prostatic cancers (56, 62, 63, 64). In addition, MT1-MMP, which has strong collagenolytic activity in its own right (46), and is involved in proMMP-2 activation (42, 44, 46), has a strong association of localizing with MMP-2 in prostatic tumors (58).

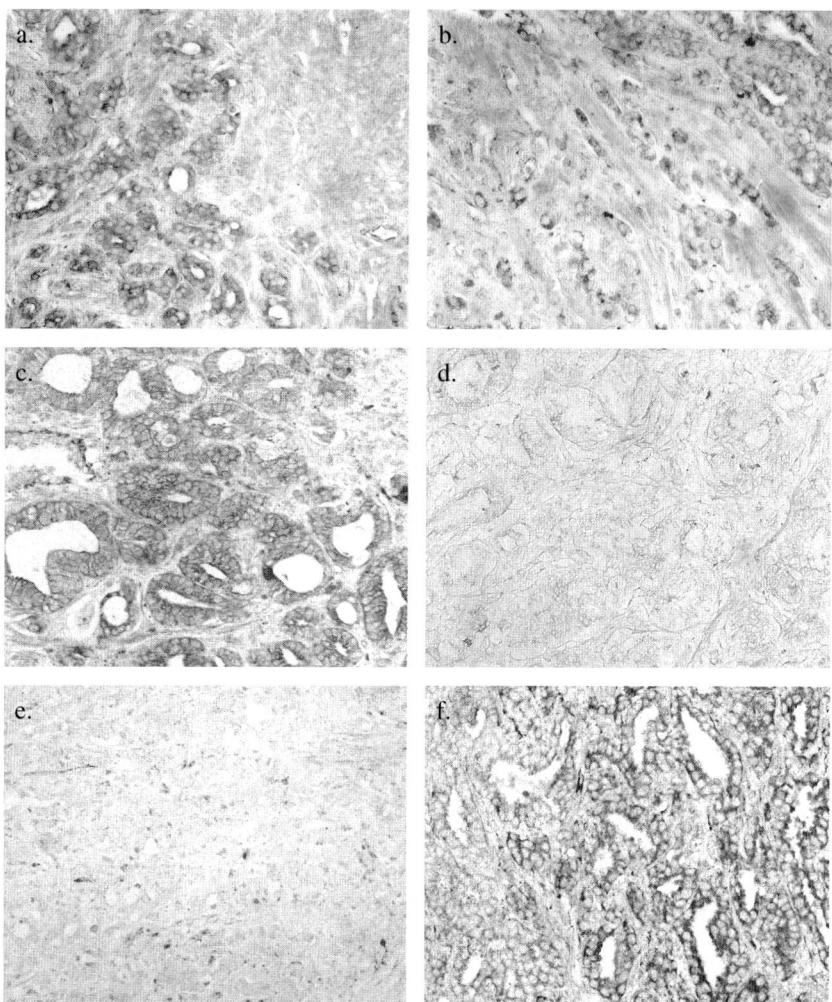

Figure 2. **A.** Immunohistochemical localization of MMP-2 in human prostate tumor cells (antibody from Dr. William Stetler-Stevenson). Tumor cells expressing MMP-2 are observed near the edge of this Gleason score 8 tumor, whereas, tumor cells more near the center of the did not show reaction products. **B.** Immunohistochemical localization of MMP-9 in human prostate tumor cells (antibody from William Stetler-Stevenson). MMP-9 expression is observed in prostate tumor cells (Gleason score 7), cells in the stroma, but only occasionally in acinar luminal cells. **C.** A micrograph illustrating strong tumor cell immunostaining for CB in a Gleason score 6 tumor. **D.** An adjacent section to that in Figure 2c illustrates markedly reduced immunostaining for stefin A. Comparison of Figures c and d shows a ratio of CB>stefin A in this Gleason score 6 tumor. **E.** This micrograph illustrates significantly reduced immunostaining for CB in a Gleason score 6 tumor. Compare with the CB immunostaining shown in Figure 2c. **F.** An adjacent section to that in Figure 2e illustrates strong immunostaining for stefin A. When compared to CB in Figure 2e, the ratio of CB<stefin A.

There are also discrepancies in reports of expression of MMP-9 in the prostate. MMP-9 immunolocalization has been reported as absent (57), or weak or absent in stroma but present in some prostatic cancers (Figure 2b), particularly those that are highly analplastic (65). MMP-9 is primarily in the pro-enzyme form (66). Likewise, expression of MMP-9 message was detected only in macrophages in areas of prostatic inflammation (60) and in the invasive edge of higher Gleason score tumors (64). The expression of MMP-9 in high grade prostate cancers may be indicative of mesenchymal-epithelial transformation that occurs with progression in tumors (67), particularly in view of the induction of MMP-2 and –9 in human epithelial cells in primary culture (68). Bombesin, a neuropeptide shown to stimulate MMP-9 secretion in human prostate tumor cell lines (69), is observed in the same cell populations expressing MMP-9 in higher grade prostatic tumors (70). A discrepancy between expression of bombesin and neuron-specific enolase indicates prostate cancer cells produce bombesin irrespective of neuroendocrine differentiation (70). The secretion of latent and active forms of MMP-2 and -9 has been observed in human prostatic secretions (71) and in experimental human prostatic organ and primary cell cultures (72, 73). However, Variani et al. (65) noted secretion of MMP-1, -2, and -9 in organ cultures of human prostate cancers in which the original tissues showed little or no immunohistochemical detection of these MMPs.

Epithelial cells in primary human prostate cancer also express greater levels of MMP-7 RNA and protein (59, 60). However the amount and proportion of the active and pro-enzyme forms of MMP-7 varied between cancers, and there was no correlation of extent of immunohistochemical MMP-7 expression with Gleason grade (60). Other studies show immunoreactivity of TIMP-2 (74) and MMP-3 and MMP-11 (57) in prostatic cancer stroma, the latter are particularly localized around blood vessels in the cancers. Messages for MT1 and MT3-MMP and TIMP-1 and –2 have been detected in both prostatic epithelial and stromal cells (75). There is also now data that show expression of members of the ADAMs (A Disintegrin And Metalloproteinase) and ADAMTS (ADAM with thrombospondin type I motifs) families in human prostate cancer cell lines (76). ADAMs are transmembrane proteins with disintegrin and metalloproteinase domains, however, only about half of the nearly 30 ADAMs have metalloproteinase activity and function in shedding of cell surface proteins, many of which function in growth regulation (42, 44).

Additional MMPs have been identified in the human prostate, but their role in prostate function or pathology have not been established. These enzymes include MMP-26, which has amino acid sequence similarity with MMP-7 (77).

4.2 Cathepsins

The cathepsins are a large group of primarily lysosomal cellular proteinases that are classified functionally as to their pH optima and inhibitor specificity, and according to the amino acid structure of their active site. Cathepsins range is size from 14 to 650 kDa, can have exopeptidase and endopeptidase activities, and are routed to lysosomes by a receptor that recognizes mannose 6-phosphate on the enzyme molecule (78).

Cathepsin D is an aspartate endopeptidase that exists as a proenzyme of 48-52 kDa and a two-chain active form of 34 and 14 kDa (78). Cathepsin D is found in most cells but its activity is highest in phagocytic cells such as macrophages. Activation of procathepsin D removes a 44 amino acid peptide, which is able to stimulate proliferation of breast, colon, and prostatic cancer cells (79). Secretory and basal epithelial cells of normal and BPH are generally negative or weak in cathepsin D immunoreactivity, whereas normal transitional epithelium lining ducts, basal cell hyperplasia, and normal seminal vesicle are positive for cathepsin D expression (80, 81). Areas of PIN are positive for cathepsin D and carcinomas show heterogeneity in cathepsin D expression (80), with no particularly strong expression in tumor edges or tumor outside of the prostate (81, 82). The heterogeneity of lysosomes in the prostate is further supported by observations that cathepsin D positive ductal cells stained much more positively for the lysosome membrane-associated protein LAMP-2 than LAMP-1 (83). There does not appear to be a significant relationship between cathepsin D immunoreactivity and either Gleason grade (80, 82) or disease specific progression (84). However, quantification of cathepsin D levels in prostatic carcinoma biopsies showed no difference in tissue levels of cathepsin D over BPH in one study (85), increased levels in a second (86), and a correlation with tumor grade, but not postprostatectomy pathologic stage or disease recurrence in another (87). An examination of the molecular forms of cathepsin D show that prostatic carcinoma express active cathepsin D, whereas the proenyzyme form is predominant in normal and BPH tissues (88).

Cathepsin H is a cysteine type protease that can function as an aminopeptidase as well as an endopeptidase (78). The activities of cathepsin H do not differ between normal and cancerous prostate (89), but there is increased cathepsin H immunoreactivity in PIN and in prostatic cancers (90). An enzymatically active truncated form of cathepsin H with a 12 amino acid deletion in the signal peptide region has been detected in prostate cancer.

This truncated form of cathepsin H is localized in the perinuclear cytoplasm and less associated with lysosomes, but is secreted by prostate tumor cells (90). In contrast with cathepsin F, recently described in the prostate (91, 92), and some other cysteine cathepsins (C, O, K, W, Z), cathepsin B has been systematically studied in the prostate.

Cathepsin B is a cysteine endopeptidase with broad substrate specificity that includes ECM proteins such as laminin, fibronectin and proteoglycans. Cathepsin B and other cysteine-type cathepsins are inhibited by endogenous stefin (cystatin) protein inhibitors. It is usually found in perinuclear lysosomes of normal organs and nonmalignant tumors, but is found associated with the plasma membranes of many solid organ cancers (93–97). The exocytosis of the mature form of cathepsin B from cells (98) and localization of active cathepsin B at the tumor cell periphery, including cell surface and cell processes (99) support the concept that routing of cathepsin B to the cell surface facilitates degradation of ECM proteins and progression of malignant cells from one biological compartment to another (94, 99–103).

In the prostate, cathepsin B and stefin A protein and message are localized predominantly in basal cells, and to a lesser extent in secretory cells, of normal prostate and BPH epithelia (104–108). There is heterogeneity in immunolocalization of cathepsin B and stefin A in prostatic cancers (Figures 2c–2f). Cathepsin B is localized by immunogold electron microscopy to cell processes, lysosomes, and vesicles in prostatic invasive cells (Figure 3a). The activities of cathepsins B are low in human prostate compared with other tissues (109), but its activity and that of cysteine protease inhibitors, have been found to be higher in normal vs cancer tissues (89), or that activities of cathepsin B did not differ in extracts of BPH and prostate cancer tissues, whereas, that of cyteine protease inhibitors was decreased in cancer (Figure 3b) (97). Cathepsin L activities have also been reported to be higher in normal vs cancer tissues (89), but its immunoreactivity absent in normal prostate (108). There is, however, strong localization of cathepsin B and L protein and message in neoplastic cells (105, 108, 110) in acini, isolated neoplastic cells and ragged glands in the stroma, and especially in the invasive edge of prostatic tumors (104, 105, 111). In addition, there is a shift of intracellular localization of lysosomes from the perinuclear cytoplasm to the cell periphery in prostatic carcinoma cells (97). In normal and neoplastic prostate there is co-localization of mature and pro-enzyme forms of cathepsin B in epithelial cells and a preponderance of pro-cathepsin B in stromal cells. However, mature but not pro-enzyme cathepsin B is localized in some neoplastic glands and subjacent stroma of prostatic cancers (112). Prostatic malignancy is also associated with

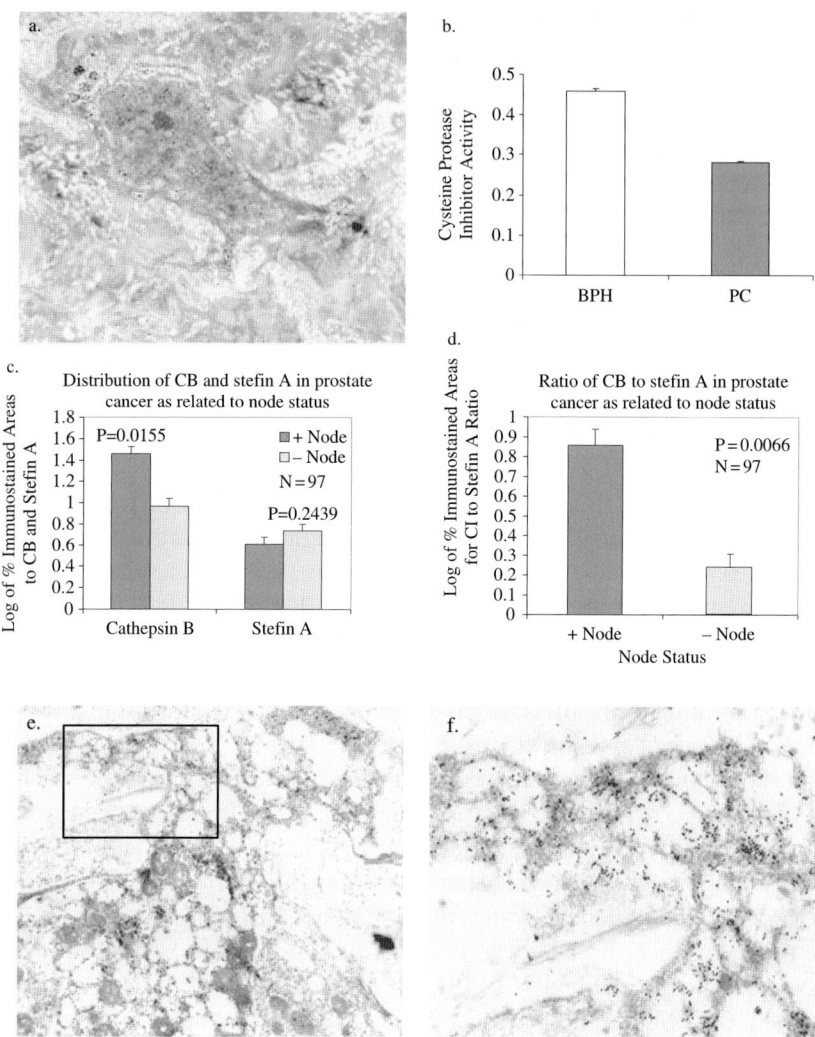

Figure 3. **A.** A micrograph illustrates an invasive prostate cancer cell localizing CB by immunogold electron microscopy. Invasive cell shows many processes, lysosome, and vesicles that have localized CB by immunogold techniques. **B.** Figure shows lower activity of cysteine protease inhibitors (CPI) in neoplastic prostate cancer (PC) when compared to benign prostatic hyperplasia (BPH). Activity is expressed in units/mg protein; columns, means; bars, SD (standard deviation) (97). An increase in CB activity in cancer may be due in part to lower levels of CPI, which may be involved in regulation of tumor aggressiveness. **C.** Figure illustrates the percent of immunostained areas for CB and stefin A in prostate tumors as related to positive and negative lymph nodes. Figure illustrates that CB was significantly higher (p = 0.0155) in tumor positive lymph nodes than in negative nodes. Differences in immunostaining for stefin A were not significant (p = 0.2439) in prostate tumors with positive and negative lymph nodes (114). Statistical analysis was conducted using Student's t-test.

increased cathepsin B and diminished cysteine protease inhibitor activites in the plasma membrane (113). Thus, there appears to be increased localization of the active form of cathepsin B at the cell surface of prostatic adenocarcinoma cells in an environment of low endogenous inhibitors, a situation that provides for localized, pericellular proteolysis of ECM proteins facilitating changes in tumor cell adhesion and mobility.

It has been recognized for some time that there is heterogeneity in clinical outcome for men with a given Gleason histologic score cancer; i.e., some men with Gleason 6 may succumb to this disease in a few years whereas others live 10 years or more. We found that within a given Gleason histologic score prostate cancer, tumors had varying levels of cathepsin B and stefin A expression, such that the ratio of the two could be $>$, $=$, or $<$ one (113). Our prediction was that tumors with a ratio of cathepsin B:stefin A $>$ one would be more biologically aggressive. Indeed, we have found a significant positive association of ratios of cathepsin B $>$ stefin A in primary prostatic cancers with the incidence of pelvic lymph node metastases (Figure 3c and 3d), and an increased rate of mortality of men whose prostatic cancers have a ratio of cathepsin B>stefin A (114). We are hopeful that the ratio of cathepsin B:stefin A will be useful in identfying the aggressive cancers within a given Gleason histologic score and that treatment regimens can subsequently be tailored accordingly.

4.3 Serine Proteases

There are two main groups of the serine class of protease that have been more highly studied in prostate pathobiology, the kallikreins, especially prostate specific antigen (PSA, hK3) and glandular kallikrein (hK2), and the

---

Figure 3. (continued) **D.** This figure shows the ratio of CB to stefin A immunostained areas in primary prostatic cancers as related to prostate cancer metastasis positive and negative lymph nodes. The figure illustrates a significantly higher ($p = 0.0066$) CB >stefin A ratio in primary prostate cancers when patients had tumor positive lymph nodes than with negative nodes. Sinha et al. (111) examined prostate cancer samples from 97 patients. Statistical analysis was conducted using Student's t-test. **E.** A portion of an invasive prostate cancer cell is present in the prostatic stroma, as evidenced by the adjacent collagen fibers, while the other portion is in the acinus. Micrograph shows secretory granules and vesicles containing PSA as evidenced by localization using anti-PSA-IgG and immunogold microscopic techniques (115). Portions of glandular epithelial cells show PSA-containing vesicles and some of them appear to be releasing PSA in prostatic stroma. PSA released in stroma may be one of the most important sources for serum PSA. Gleason score 8 tumor. **F.** Detail of an area of figure 3e illustrates distribution and leakage of PSA in prostatic stroma.

plasminogen activators. The plasminogen activator system has been most extensively investigated with respect to ECM protein modification, whereas PSA serum measurements have been utilized in detection and evaluation of prostate cancer. However, the recent identification of many new kallikreins and other serine proteases has generated new expectations for the role of these proteases in understanding prostate function and diseases.

The two plasminogen activators, tissue-type activator and urokinase are products of different genes, differ in their molecular weight, structure, and function, but cleave plasminogen through a common mechanism (38). Tissue-type activator is generally a fibrin activated, intravascular protease, but is implicated in some tissue remodeling events such as ovulation and bone remodeling. Urokinase on the other hand is a fibrin-independent protease mediating controlled extracellular proteolysis through its receptor (uPAR) localization to the cell surface where it generates cell surface bound plasmin. Plasmin hydrolyzes fibronectin, laminin, and other glycoproteins of the BM and stromal matrix, and it can activate other proteases such as proMMPs and activate and/or release growth factors bound in the ECM. Cells produce potent and specific inhibitors of plasminogen activators and plasmin, i.e., serine proteinase inhibitors (serpins), such as plasminogen activator inhibitor-type 1 (PAI-1) and – type 2 and protease nexin.

Localization of the plasminogen activator system components by immunohistochemistry in the human prostate have produced heterogeneous results. Tissue-type activator is localized in secretory cells of the central zone, but not peripheral zone in the prostate (116). Urokinase has been localized to tumor cell cytoplasm, stroma being negative, predominately in cancers with extracapsular extension (117). Similarly, uPAR is detected predominantly in cancers (118). Plasminogen activator activities are elevated in prostatic cancer compared with benign hyperplastic tissues (119, 120) and greater yet in prostatic cancer bone metastases (121). Both urokinase and tissue-type activator are present in human primary prostatic cancers (119, 121), but urokinase is the molecular form associated with prostatic tumor progression since it is proportionately greater in bone metastases over primary tumors (121) and it is the primary form of activator in established prostate tumor cell lines (reviewed in Wilson, 50). Immunologic measurements indicate that urokinase, uPAR and PAI-1 are increased in diploid prostate cancer tissues, whereas in aneuploid cancers urokinase levels remain elevated but uPAR and PAI-1 are decreased (122). There is no correlation of urokinase, tissue-type activator, uPAR, or PAI-1 tissue levels with cell cycle parameters in prostate cancer, indicating that urokinase is associated with non-cell cycle mechanisms in prostate cancer aggressive behavior (123). Increased expression of urokinase in hormone resistant prostate cancers may be due in part to amplification of this gene (124). Serum levels of urokinase and uPAR have been reported in prostate cancer patients (125, 126) and their levels calculated as densities (dividing serum level by prostate volume) are significantly associated with patients with metastatic disease and diminished survival (127).

PSA (human glandular kallikrein 3, hK3) is a member of the human glandular kallikrein gene family, which originally was thought to have 3 members and now appears to contain at least 15 (128). PSA is proteolytically processed from a prepropeptide, sequentially to an active enzyme of 237 amino acids complexed with a single carbohydrate side chain. PSA has a chymotrypsin-like proteolytic function with no kininogenase activity (129, 130), and its main known biological function is cleavage of the gel forming proteins semenogelin 1 and 2 in the ejaculate. About 60-70% of PSA in seminal plasma is in the catalytically active form, about 5% bound to protein C inhibitor, and 30% as 2 chain cleaved forms of the molecule (131). The clinical significance of PSA in the circulation of patients requires consideration of protease inhibitors, proteolytic processing, liver metabolism, and excretion in the urine (132). The majority of PSA in serum is bound to α1-antichymotrypsin or α2-macroglobulin, with the free uncomplexed PSA being enzymatically inactive. The α1-antichymotrypsin-PSA complex is immunoreactive, whereas PSA bound by α2-macroglobulin is enclosed in the structure of the inhibitor and not available for interaction with antibodies. Sera from patients with prostate cancer contain proportionately higher α1-antichymotrypsin complexed PSA and decreased free PSA, having a decreased ratio of free to total PSA as compared to men with BPH (133, 134). In patients with cancer associated elevated serum total PSA, pro-forms of PSA appear to be a considerable fraction of free PSA, whereas pro-forms of PSA were not detected in sera of those with BPH (135, 136).

PSA is able to proteolyze a number of peptides and proteins that implicate it in prostate cancer growth and invasion and metastasis. PSA may influence tumor growth since it can cleave insulin-like growth factor binding protein-3 (IGFBP-3), releasing IGF (137), activate latent tissue growth factor β (TGF-β) (138), and activate single-chain urokinase (139). A role for PSA in invasion and metastasis is indicated by its ability to degrade matrix proteins such as denatured collagen (gelatin) (140), and fibronectin and laminin (141). In contrast, PSA has antiangiogenic activity, which would impair tumor growth (142), and the levels of both PSA and α1-antichymotrypsin are considerably lower in cancer compared with normal prostate tissue (143). The demonstration of PSA localization by immunogold electron microscopy in the immediate extracellular environment (Figure 3e and 3f) is a manifestation of the PSA secreted by the invading tumor cell and supports a role for PSA in the extracellular microenvironment. In this vein, other prostatic secretory proteases such as pepsinogen II (144, 145) and trypsinogen (146) may be expected to leak from acini with malignant cells or be released from invading tumor cells into the stroma. However, the activity of extracellular PSA, or other secretory proteases, must be tightly controlled by inhibitors or proteolytic processing, for with the levels of PSA produced and that reach the circulatory system, prostate cancer should be a much more aggressive cancer than it actually is.

Another glandular kallikrein produced in a nearly prostate specific manner is hK2. hK2 has 78 % homology to PSA, but has a trypsin-like serine protease catalytic function (147, 148) and very low kininogenase activity (129, 130). The levels of hK2 protein and message increase in prostatic adenocarcinoma (149–151), which is in contrast to PSA which decreases in cancer cells (151). However, expression of pro-hK2 is greatest in primary cancers vs benign prostate or metastaic cancer (150). The increased levels of hK2 in prostate cancer cells may be due in part to amplification of the hK2 gene (151). The biologic function of hK2 may include activation of pro-PSA (152–154), and pro-hK2 (155), semen liquefaction (156), and processing of protein precursor molecules (157). hK2 may play a role in tumor cell invasion since it can directly hydrolyze ECM proteins like fibronectin (156) and may regulate the plasminogen activator system; i.e., hK2 can activate the single chain urokinase (154, 158) and inactivate PAI-1 (159). hK2 activity in turn may be regulated in part by serpins such as protease inhibitor 6 (PI6), with which hK2 complexes in prostatic tissue and which is increased in prostatic cancers (160, 161)

In addition to PSA (hK3) and hK2, hK4 (prostase), hK6 (neurosin), hK10 (NES1) and hK11 (hippostasin/PRSS20) proteins have been measured in human seminal plasma and in prostate tissue, indicating they are secretory enzymes, but there is little additional information available on their function in the prostate (162–170). hK10 immunostaining is detected in prostate secretory and neuroendocrine cells, but not in basal cells (171), and a general cytoplasmic distribution of hK6 and apical localization of hK4 are found in the prostatic acinar epithelium (162, 166). hK11 expression is found in normal and benign hyperplastic prostate (localized in prostatic secretory cells) and in prostate cancer cell lines. Interestingly, normal prostate and BPH express both prostate-type and brain-type alternatively spliced isoforms, but prostate cancer cell lines expressed only the brain-type hK11 (170). Higher levels of message but lower protein concentrations of hK4 are detected in prostatic cancers (162). The mRNA level for hK15 is upregulated in prostate cancer tissue, whereas that for hK5 is lower in prostate cancer with a negative correlation with Gleason score (172). Thus, with divergent changes in kallikrein expression in prostate adenocarcinoma, their role as markers of prostate cancer is being pursued (128). The discovery of multiple alternatively spliced mRNA for kallikreins has opened another avenue of research on possible functionally diverse proteins in this group of serine proteinases. In the prostate this includes PSA (173–176), hK2 (176, 177), hK11 (170) and hK15 (178).

Several membrane-associated serine proteases have recently been cloned and identified in the prostate. Prostasin is a glycosylphosphatidylinositol-anchored membrane associated trypsin-like serine proteinase in prostatic secretory epithelial cells that is secreted into semen (179, 180). The expression of prostasin is down regulated in prostate cancer (181). TMPRSS2 is a protease with a transmembrane domain and trypsin-like protease activity and positively regulated by androgen in LNCaP cells (182, 183). Its mRNA in human prostate tissue is selectively expressed in basal cells of the prostate epithelium, but is also localized in prostate carcinoma (184). Membrane-type serine protease 1 (MT-SP1) or matriptase is a cell surface serine extracellular protease strongly expressed in the human prostate and in human prostate tumor PC-3 cells (183, 185). This protease with trypsin-like activity can cleave gelatin, protease-activated receptor 2, and single chain urokinase, implicating it in pericellular proteolysis that would facilitate prostate tumor growth and invasion of ECM (183, 186). Hepsin is a type II cell surface trypsin-like serine proteinase that is localized in basal cells of BPH epithelium (187, 188), but its expression is found in PIN (189) and greatly over expressed in cancer (188–193). The great extent to which hespin is expressed in prostate cancers and its cell surface localization make it a prime candidate for development of new diagnostic and therapy approaches for prostate cancer.

The control of serine protease activities in normal prostate function and in tumor invasion and metastasis is influenced by protease inhibitors. Maspin, a so-called ov-serpin due to its structural homology to chicken ovalbumin, can inhibit cell surface bound urokinase (194) and is strongly expressed in basal cells of normal prostate and BPH tissues (195). Maspin protein expression is diminished in prostate cancer, the loss of which is correlated with increased Gleason score and to higher tumor stages (195). In contrast to maspin, $\alpha 1$-antichymotrypsin and PI-6 levels increase in prostatic cancers (161, 196). The role of these and other serpins such as kallistatin (197), secretory leucocyte protease inhibitor (SLPI) (198), hepatocyte growth factor activator inhibitor (HAI) (199), monocyte/neutrophil elastase inhibitor (MNEI) (200), and huWAP2 (201) expressed in prostate remain to be established for normal organ function or pathology.

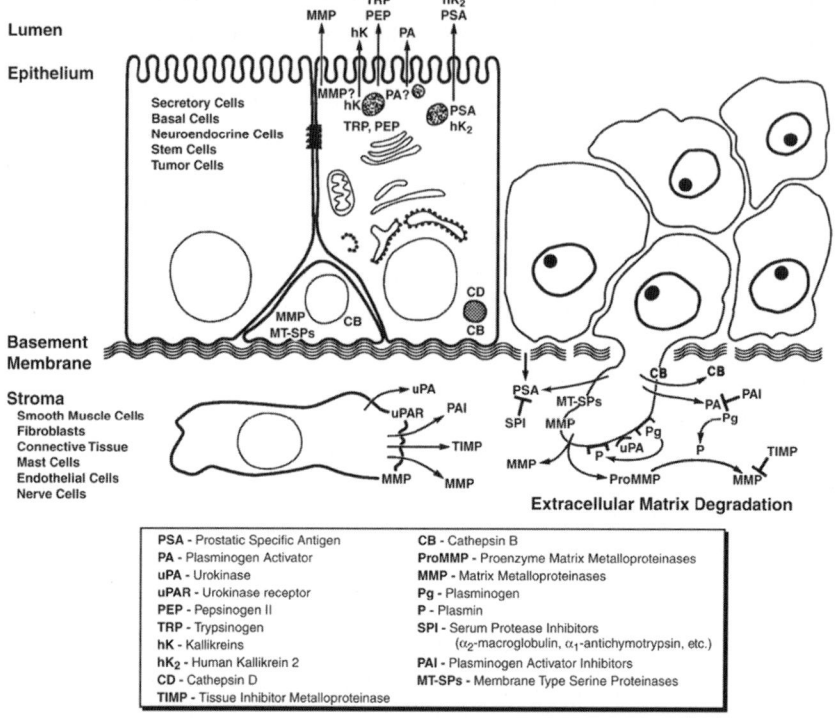

Figure 4. A diagram depicting the distribution of proteases in the normal and neoplastic prostate, and the interaction of proteases effecting degradation of ECM proteins during tumor cell invasion of the stroma. Proteases are produced in the normal prostate for secretion and are depicted in the apical cytoplasm. A number of proteases including MMP-2, cathepsin B, and membrane-type serine protease are localized predominantly in basal cells. As neoplastic changes occur in the prostate, the basement membrane becomes compromised and PSA leaks into the stroma. As the tumor becomes invasive, tumor cells penetrate the basement membrane utilizing several proteases that can function at the cells surface. Urokinase is localized to the tumor cell surface through its selective receptor, facilitating the generation of plasmin. MT-MMPs and MMP-2 associated with MT1-MMP, cell surface cathepsin B, and membrane-type serine proteases also facilitate pericellular proteolysis of ECM proteins. The activities of these proteases is controlled through their generation as pro-enzyme forms which must be activated and by specific endogenous inhibitors. These proteases and inhibitors are produced by stromal host cells, as well as tumor cells, and their cooperative function controls the generation of growth factors, cytokines, and other regulatory molecules, as well as cleavage of ECM proteins permitting physical passage of malignant cells. Reproduced from Wilson (50) with permission of Microscopy Research and Technique.

CONCLUSION

ECM components modulate cellular behavior and function by poviding information in the cellular environment essential for development, morphogenesis, tissue remodeling, and maintenance of tissue specific functions. The progression of prostate cancer is associated with the synthesis of additional ECM components like tenascin and increased turnover of others. The processing and degradation of ECM proteins by cell surface associated proteinases are an important feature of controlling tumor cell invasion and metastasis, and tumor associated angiogenesis.

MMPs, proteinases of the coagulation and firbrinolysis sytstems, and cathepsins interact in this complex process of matrix turnover in orchestrating these malignant cell processes (Figure 4). It is becoming increasingly clear that the role of these proteinases in prostate cancer is much more broad than simply permitting passage of cancer cells through matrix barriers. Early stage cancers appear to be stroma-dependent tumors since many of these proteinases are produced by stromal cells upon molecular signaling influence of cancer and inflammatory cells. As cancers progress and undergo epithelial-meshencymal transformation, cancer cells express stromal cell proteinases. Cleavage of ECM proteins releases peptides that regulate tumor cell growth and migration. Likewise, endogenous inhibitors of proteinases can influence cellular behavior directly, in addition to their function in regulating proteinase activities. Most recently a number of kallikrein and other serine proteinases have been found in the prostate, for which a role in prostate cancer remains to be examined. The more extensively studied proteinases, and perhaps many of the newly discovered ones, work in concert in proteinase cascades, and function as membrane anchored or cell surface bound proteinases, or are shed into the immediate tumor cell environment. It is hoped we can take advantage of the properties of these proteinases in prostate cancer to devise better diagnostic methods and utilize them as targets for treatment interventions.

REFERENCES

1. Sinha AA, Gleason DF, Limas C, Reddy PK, Wick MR, Hagen KA, Wilson MJ. Localization of cathepsin B in normal and hyperplastic human prostate by immunoperoxidase and protein A gold techniques. Anat Rec 1989, 223:266–75.
2. Hunt G. The role of laminin in cancer invasion and metastasis. Exp Cell Biol 1989, 57:165–76.
3. Leblond CP, Inoue S. Structure, composition, and assembly of basement membrane. Am J Anat 1989, 185:367–90.

4. Bonkoff H, Wenert N, Dhom G, Remberger K. Distribution of basement membranes in primary and metastatic carcinomas of the prostate. Hum Pathol 1992, 23: 934–9.
5. Kuhn K. Basement membrane (type IV) collagen. Matrix Biol 1995, 14:439–5.
6. Dehan P, Waltregny D, Beschin A, Noel A, Castronovo V, Tryggvason K *et al.* Loss of type IV collagen a5 and a6 chains in human invasive prostate carcinomas. Am J Pathol 1997, 151:1097–4.
7. Bonkoff H, Wernert N, Dhom G, Remberger K. Basement membranes in fetal, adult normal, hyperplastic and neoplastic human prostate. Virchows Archiv A Pathol Anat 1991, 418:375–81.
8. Nagle RB, Knox JD, Wolf C, Bowden GT, Cress AE. Adhesion molecules, extracellular matrix, and proteases in prostate carcinoma. J Cell Biochem 1994, 19:232–7.
9. Myers JC, Li D, Bageris A, Abraham V, Dion AS, Amenta PS. Biochemical and immunohistochemical characterization of human type XIX defines a novel class of basement membrane zone collagens. Am J Pathol 1997, 151:1729–40.
10. Carvalho de HF, Taboga SR, Vilamaior PSL. Collagen type VI is a component of the extracellular matrix of the prostatic stroma. Tissue Cell 1997, 29:163–70.
11. Hao J, Yang Y, McDaniel KM, Dalkin BL, Cress AN, Nagle RB. Differential expression of laminin 5 ($\alpha 3\beta 3\gamma 2$) by human malignant and normal prostate. Am J Pathol 1996, 149:1341–9.
12. Nagle RB, Hao J, Knox JD, Dalkin BL, Clark V, Cress AE. Expression of hemidesmosomal and extracellular matrix proteins by normal and malignant human prostaste tissue. Am J Pathol 1995, 146:1498–507.
13. Mizushima H, Koshikawa N, Moriyama K, Takamura H, Nagashima Y, Hirahara F, Miyazaki K. Wide distribution of laminin-5 $\gamma 2$ chain in basement membranes of various human tissues. Horm Res 1998, 50:7–14.
14. Bostwick DG, Leaske DA, Junqi Q, Sinha AA. Prostatic intraepithelial neoplasia and well differentiated adenocarcinoma maintain an intact basement membrane. Path Res Pract 1995, 191:850–5.
15. Murdoch AD, Liu B, Schwarting R, Tuan RS, Iozzo RV. Widespread expression of perlecan proteoglycan in basment membranes and extracellular matrices of human tissues as detected by a novel monoclonal antibody against domain III and by in situ hybridization. J Histochem Cytochem 1994, 42:239–49.
16. Hao J, Jackson L, Calaluce R, McDaniel K, Dalkin BL, Nagle RB. Investigation into the mechanism of the loss of laminin 5 ($\alpha 3\beta 3\gamma 2$) expression in prostate cancer. Am J Pathol 2001, 158:1129–35.
17. Martinez-Hernandez A, Ametna PS. The basement membrane in pathology. Lab Invest 1983, 48:656–77.
18. Martin GR, Rohrback DH, Terranova VP, Liotta LA. Mongr Intern Acad Pathol 1983, 24:16–30.
19. Chan L, Wong YC. Ultrastructural localization of proteoglycans by cationic dyes in the epithelial-stromal interface of the guinea pig lateral prostate. Prostate 1989, 14:147–62.
20. Kjellen L, Lindahl U. Proteoglycans: Structures and interactions. Ann Rev. Biochem 1991, 60:443–75.
21. Desjardins M, Bendayan M. Heterogeneous distribution of type IV collagen, entactin, heparan sulphate proteoglycan, and laminin among renal basement membranes as

demonstrated by quantitative immunocytochemistry. J Histochem Cytochem 1989, 37:880–97.
22. D'Ardenne AJ, Burns J, Sykes BC, Kirkpatrick P. Comparative distribution of fibronectin and type III collagen in normal human tissues. J Pathol 1983,14155–69.
23. Albrecht M, Renneberg H, Wennemuth G, Moschler O, Janssen M, Aumuller G, Konrad L. Fibronectin in human prostatic cells in vivo and in vitro: Expression, distribution, and pathological significance. Histochem Cell Biol 1999, 112:51–61.
24. Suer S, Sonmez H, Karaaslan I, Baloglu H, Kokoglu E. Tissue sialic acid and fibronectin levels in human prostatic cancer. Cancer Lett 1996, 99:135–7.
25. Burns-Cox N, Avery NC, Gingell JC, Bailey AJ. Changes in collagen metabolism in prostate cancer: A host response that MAY alter progression. J Urol 2001, 166:1698–701.
26. Van den Brule FA, Waltregny D, Castronovo V. Increased expression of galectin-1 in carcinoma-associated stroma predicts poor outcome in prostate carcinoma patients. J Pathol 2001, 193:80–7.
27. Ricciardelli C, Mayne K, Sykes PJ, Raymond WA, McCaul K, Marshall VR, Horsfall DJ. Elevated levels of versican but not decorin predict disease progression in early-stage prostate cancer. Clin Cancer Res 1998, 4:963–71.
28. Lipponen P, Aaltomaa S, Tammi R, Tammi M, Agren U, Kosma V-M. High stromal hyaluronan level is associated with poor differentiation and metastasis in prostate cancer. Eur J Cancer 2001, 37:849–56.
29. Nakada T, Kubota Y. Connective tissue proteins in the prostate gland. Int Urol Nephrol 1994, 26:183–7.
30. Luo J, Dunn T, Ewing C, Sauvageot J, Chen Y, Trent J, Isaacs W. Gene expression signature of benign prostatic hyperplasia revealed by cDNA microarray analysis. Prostate 2002, 51:189–200.
31. Djavan B, Lin V, Sietz C, Kramer G, Kaplan P, Richier J et al. Elastin gene expression in benign prostatic hyperplasia. Prostate 1999, 40:242–7.
32. Goulas A, Hatzichristou DG, Karakiulakis G, Mirtsou-Fidani V, Kalinderis A, Papakon-stantinou E. Benign hyperplasia of the human prostate is associated with tissue enrichment in chondroitin sulphate of wide size distribution. Prostate 2000, 44:104–10.
33. Tuxhorn JA, Ayala GE, Smith MJ, Dang TD, Rowley DR. Reactive stroma in human prostate cancer: Induction of myofibroblast phenotype and extracellular matrix remodelling. Clin Cancer Res 2002, 8:2912–23.
34. Ibrahim SN, Lightner VA, Ventimiglia JB, Ibrahim GK, Walther PJ, Bigner DD, Humphrey PA. Tenascin expression in prostatic hyperplasia, intraepithelial neoplasia, and carcinoma. Hum Pathol 1993, 24:982–9.
35. Xue Y, Li J, Latijnhouwers MA, Smedts F, Umbas R, Aalders TW et al. Expression of periglandular tenascin-C and basement membrane laminin in normal prostate, benign prostatic hyperplasia and prostate carcinoma. Br J Urol 1998, 81:844–51.
36. Nelson PS, Plymate SR, Wang K, True LD, Ware JL, Gan L et al. Hevin, antiadhesive matrix protein, is down-regulated in metastatic prostate adenocarcinoma. Cancer Res 1998, 58:232–6.
37. Thalman GN, Sikes RA, Devoll RE, Kiefer JA, Markwalder R, Klima I et al. Osteopontin: Possible role in prostate cancer progression. Clin Cancer Res 1999, 5:2271–77.
38. Carmeliet P, Collen D. Development and disease in protease-deficient mice: Role of the plasminogen, matrix metalloproteinase and coagulation system. Thromb Res 1998, 91:255–85.

39. Stetler-Stevenson WG. Matrix metalloproteinases in angiogenesis: A moving target for therapeutic intervention. J Clin Invest 1999, 103:1237–41.
40. Birkedal-Hansen H, Moore WGI, Bodden MK, Windsor LJ, Birkedal-Hansen B, DeCarlo A, Engler JA. Matrix metalloproteinases: A review. Crit Rev Oral Biol Med 1993, 4:197–250.
41. Nagase H, Suzuki K, Itoh Y, Kan CC, Gehring MR, Huang W, Brew K. Involvement of tissue inhibitors of metalloproteinases (TIMPS) during matrix metalloproteinase activation. Adv Exp Med Biol 1996, 389:23–31.
42. Nelson AR, Fingleton B, Rothenberg ML, Matrisian LM. Matrix metalloproteinases: Biologic activity and clinical implications. J Clin Oncol 2000, 18:1135–49.
43. Lohi JL, Wilson CL, Roby JD, Parks WC. Epilysin: A novel human matrix metalloproteinase (MMP-27) expressed in testis and keratinocytes and in response to injury. J Biol Chem 2001, 276:10134–44.
44. Egeblad M, Werb Z. New functions for the matrix metalloproteinases in cancer progression. Nat Rev Cancer 2002, 2:161–74.
45. Zucker S, Cao J, Chen WT. Critical appraisal of the use of matrix metalloproteinase inhibitors in cancer treatment. Oncogene 2000, 19:6642–5.
46. Hornebeck W, Emonard H, Monboisse J-C, Bellon G. Matrix-directed regulation of pericellular proteolysis and tumor progression. Semin Cancer Biol 2002, 12:2331–41.
47. Massova I, Kotra LP, Fridman R, Mobashery S. Matrix metalloproteinases: Structures, evolution, and diversification. FASEB J 1998, 12:1075–95.
48. Brew K, Dinakarpandian D, Nagase H. Tissue inhibitors of metalloproteinases: Structure and function. Biochim Biophys Acta 2000, 1477:267–83.
49. Welm B, Mott J, Werb Z. L biology: Vasculogenesis is a wreck without RECK. Current biol. Developmenta 2002, 12:R209–11.
50. Wilson MJ. Proteases in prostate development, function, and pathology. Micr Res Tech 1995, 30:305–18.
51. Wilson MJ, Strasser, M, Vogel, MM, Sinha AA. Calcium-dependent, independent gelatinolytic proteinase activities of the rat ventral prostate, its secretion: Characterization, effects of castration, testosterone treatment. Biol Reprod 1991, 44:776–85.
52. Wilson MJ, Garcia B, Woodson M, Sinha AA. Metalloprotease activities expressed during development and maturation of the rat prostatic complex and seminal vesicles. Biol Reprod 1992, 47:683–91.
53. Stearns ME, Wang M. Type IV collagenase (mr 72,000) expression in human prostate: Benign and malignant tissue. Cancer Res 1993, 53:878–3.
54. Boag AH, Young ID. Increased expression of the 72-kd type IV collagenase in prostatic adenocarcinoma: Demonstration by immunohistochemistry and in situ hybridization. Am J Pathol 1994, 144:585–91.
55. Montironi R, Lucarini G, Castaldini C, Galluzzi CM, Biagini G, Fabris G. Immunohistochemical evaluation of type IV collagenase (72-kd metalloproteinase) in prostatic intraepithelial neoplasia. Anticancer Res 1996, 16:2057–62.
56. Still K, Robson CN, Autzen Robinson PMC, Hamdy F. Localization and quantification of mRNA for matrix metalloproteinase-2 (MMP-2) and tissue inhibitor of matrix metalloproteinase-2 (TIMP-2) in human benign and malignant prostatic tissue. Prostate 2000, 42:18–25.
57. Bodey B, Bodey B, Jr, Siegel SE, Kaiser HE. Immunocytochemical detection of matrix metalloproteinase expression in prostate cancer. In Vivo 2001, 15:65–70.

58. Upadhyay J, Shekarriz B, Nemeth JA, Dong Z, Cummings GD, Fridman R et al. Membrane type 1-matrix metalloproteinase (MT1-MMP) and MMP-2 immunolocalization in human prostate: Change in cellular localization associated with high-grade prostatic intraepithelial neoplasia. Clin Cancer Res 1999, 5:4105–10.
59. Pajough S, Nagle RB, Breathnach R, Finch JS, Brawer MK, Bowden GT. Expression of metalloproteinase genes in human prostate cancer. J Cancer Res Clin Oncol 1991, 117:144–50.
60. Knox JD, Wolf C, McDaniel K, Clark V, Loriot M, Bowden GT, Nagle RB. Matrilysin expression in human prostate carcinoma. Mol Carcinog 1996, 15:57–63.
61. Montironi R, Fabris G, Lucarini G, Biagini G. Location of 72-kd metalloproteinase (type IV collagenase) in untreated prostatic adenocarcinoma. Pathol Res Pract 1995, 191:1140–6.
62. Wood M, Fudge K, Mohler JL, Frost AR, Garcia F, Wang M, Stearns ME. In situ hybridization studies of metalloproteinases 2 and 9 and TIMP-1 and TIMP-2 expression in human prostate cancer. Clin Exp Metastasis 1997, 15:246–58.
63. Stearns M, Stearns ME. Evidence for increased activated metalloproteinase 2 (MMP-2a) expression associated with human prostate cancer progression. Oncol Res 1996, 8:69–75.
64. Kuniyasu H, Troncoso P, Johnston D, Bucana CD, Tahara E, Fidler IJ, Pettaway CA. Relative expression of type IV collagenase, E-cadherin, and vascular endothelial growth factor/vascular permeability factor in prostatectomy specimens distinquishes organ-confined from pathologically advanced prostate cancers. Clin Cancer Res 2000, 6:2295–308.
65. Varani J, Hattori Y, Dame MK, Schmidt T, Murphy HS, Johnson KJ, Wojno KJ. Matrix metalloproteinases (MMPs) in fresh human prostate tumor tissue and organ-cultured prostate tissue: Levels of collagenolytic and gelatinolytic MMPs are low, variable and different in fresh tissue versus organ-cultured tissue. Br J Cancer 2001, 84:1076–83.
66. Hamdy FC, Fadlon EJ, Cottam D, Lawry J, Thurrell W, Silcocks PB, Anderson JB. Matrix metalloproteinse 9 expression in primary human prostatic adenocarcinoma, benign prostatic hyperplasia. Br J Cancer 1994, 69:177–82.
67. Thiery JP. Epithelial-mesenchymal transitions in tumor progression. Nat Rev Cancer 2002, 2:442–54.
68. Wilson MJ, Sellers RG, Wiehr C, Melamud O, Pei D, Peehl DM. Expression of matrix metalloproteinase-2 and –9 and their inhibitors, tissue inhibitor of metalloproteinase-1 and –2, in primary cultures of human prostatic stromal and epithelial cells. J Cell Physiol 2002, 191:208–16.
69. Sehgal I, Thompson TC. Neuropeptides induce mr 92,000 type IV collagenase (matrix metalloproteinase-9) activity in human prostate cancer cell lines. Cancer Res 1998, 58:4288–91.
70. Ishimaru H, Kageyama Y, Hayashi T, Nemoto Y, Eishi Y, Kihara K. Expression of matrix metalloproteinase-9 and bombesin/gastrin-releasing peptide in human prostate cancers and their lymph node metastases. Acta Oncol 2002, 3:289–96.
71. Wilson MJ, Norris H, Kapoor D, Woodson M, Limas C, Sinha AA. Gelatinolytic and caseinolytic proteinase activities in human prostatic secretions. J Urol 1993, 149:653–8.
72. Lokeshwar B, Selzer MG, Block NL, Gunja-Smith Z. Secretion of matrix metalloproteinases and their inhibitors (tissue inhibitor of metalloproteinases) by human

prostate in explant cultures: Reduced tissue inhibitor of metalloproteinase secretion by malignant tissues. Cancer Res 1993, 53:4493–8.
73. Festuccia C, Bologna M, Vicentia C, Tacconelli A, Miano R, Violini Mackay AR. Increased matrix metalloproteinase-9 secretion in short-term tissue cultures of prostatic tumor cells. Int J Cancer 1996, 69:386–93.
74. Hoyhtya M, Fridman R, Komarek D, Porter-Jordan K, Stetler-Stevenson WG, Liotta LA, Liang C-M. Immunohistochemical localization of matrix metalloproteinase 2 and its specific inhibitor TIMP-2 in neoplastic tissues with monoclonal antibodies. Int J Cancer 1994, 56:500–5.
75. Zhang J, Jung K, Lein M, Kristiansen G, Rudolph B, Hauptmann S et al. Differential expression of matrix metalloproteinases and their tissue inhibitors in human primary cultured prostatic cells and malignant prostate cell lines. Prostate 2002, 50:38–45.
76. McCulloch DR, Harvey M, Herrington AC. The expression of the ADAMs proteases in prostate cancer cell lines and their regulation by dihydrotestosterone. Mol Cell Endocrinol 2000, 167:11–21.
77. Marchenko GN, Ratnikov BI, Rozanov DV, Godzik A, Deryugina EI, Strongin AY. Characterization of matrix metalloproteinase-26, a novel metalloproteinase widely expressed in cancer cells of epithelial origin. Biochem J 2001, 356:705–18.
78. Schwartz MK. Tissue cathepsins as tumor markers. Clin Chim Acta 1995, 237:67–78.
79. Vetvicka V, Vetvickova J, Fusek M. Effect of procathepsin D and its activation peptide on prostate cancer cells. Cancer Lett 1998, 129:55–9.
80. Makar R, Mason A, Kittelson JM, Bowden T, Cress AE, Nagle RB. Immunohistochemical analysis of cathepsin D in prostate carcinoma. Mod Pathol 1994, 7:747–51.
81. Maygarden SJ, Novotny DB, Moul JW, Bae VL, Ware JL. Evaluation of cathepsin D and epidermal growth factor receptor in prostate carcinoma. Mod Pathol 1994, 7:930–36.
82. Moul JW, Maygarden SJ, Ware JL, Mohler JL, Maher PD, Schenkman NS, Ho CK, Cathepsin D. Epidermal growth factor receptor immunohistochemistry does not predict recurrence of prostate cancer in patients undergoing radical prostatectomy. J Urol 1996, 155:982–5.
83. Furuta K, Yang XL, Chen JS, Hamilton SR, August JT. Differential expression of the lysosome-associated membrane proteins in normal human tissues. Arch Biochem Biophys 1999, 365:75–82.
84. Theodorescu D, Broder SR, Boyd JC, Mills SE, Frierson HF. Cathepsin D and chromogranin A as predictors of long term disease specific survival after radical prostatectomy for localized carcinoma of the prostate. Cancer 1997, 80:2109–19.
85. Yang Y, Chishholm GD, Habib FK. The distribution of PSA, cathepsin -D, pS2 in BPH, cancer of the prostate. Prostate 1992, 21:201–8.
86. Chambon M, Rebillard X, Rochefort H, Brouillet JP, Baldet P, Guiter J, Maudelonde T, Cathepsin D. Cytosolic assay, immunohistochemical quantification in human prostate tumors. Prostate 1994, 24:320–5.
87. Ross JS, Nazeer T, Figge HL, Fisher HAG, Rifkin MD. Quantitative immunohistochemical determination of cathepsin D levels in prostatic carcinoma biopsies. Am J Clin Pathol 1995, 104:36–41.
88. Cherry JP, Mordente JA, Chapman JR, Choudhury MS, Tazaki H, Mallouh C, Konno S. Analysis of cathepsin D forms and their clinical implications in human prostate cancer. J Urol 1998, 160:2223–8.

89. Friedrich B, Jung K, Lein M, Turk I, Rudolph B, Hampel G *et al*. Cysteine protease inhibitors in malignant prostate cell lines, primary cultured prostatic cells, prostatic tissues. Eur J Cancer 1999, 35:138–44.
90. Waghray A, Keppler D, Sloane BF, Schuger L, Chen YQ. Analysis of a truncated form of cathepsin H in human prostate tumor cells. J Biol Chem 2002, 277:11533–8.
91. Wang B, Shi G-P, Yao PM, Li Z, Chapman HA, Bromme D. Human cathepsin F: Molecular cloning, funcitonal expression, tissue localization, and enzymatic characteristics. J Biol Chem 1998, 273:32000–8.
92. Santamaria I, Velasco G, Pendas AM, Paz A, Lopez-Ortin C. Molecular cloning and structural and functional characterization of human cathepsin F, a new cysteine proteinase of the papain family with a long propeptide domain. J Biol Chem 1999, 274:13800–9.
93. Sloane BF, Moin K, Krepela E, Rozhin Cathepsin JB. Its endogenous inhibitors: Role in tumor malignancy. Cancer Metastasis Rev 1990, 9:333–52.
94. Moin K, Cao L, Day NA, Koblinski JE, Sloane BF. Tumor cell membrane cathepsin B. Biol Chem 1998, 379:1093–9.
95. Lah TT, Kalman E, Najjar D, Gorodetsky E, Brennan P, Somers R, Kaskal I. Cell producing cathepsin D, B, L in human breast carcinoma, their association with prognosis. Human Pathol 2000, 31:149–60.
96. Hazen LGM, Bleeker FE, Lauritzen B, Bahns S, Song J, Jonker A *et al*. Comparative localization of cathepsin B protein and activity in colorectal cancer. J Histochem Cytochem 2000, 48:1421–30.
97. Sinha AA, Jamuar MP, Wilson MJ, Rozhin J, Sloane BF. Plasma membrane association of cathepsin B in human prostate cancer: Biochemical and immunogold electron microscopic analysis. Prostate 2001, 49:172–84.
98. Linebaugh BE, Sameni M, Day NA, Sloane BF, Keppler D. Exocytosis of active cathepsin B, enzyme activity at pH 7.0, inhibition and molecular mass. Eur J Biochem 1999, 264:100–9.
99. Demchik LL, Sameni M, Nelson K, Mikkelsen T, Sloane BF, Cathepsin B. Glioma invasion. Int J Dev Neurosci 1999, 17:483–94.
100. Werle B, Lotterle H, Schanzenbacher U, Lah TT, Kalman E, Kayser K *et al*. Immunochemical analysis of cathepsin B in lung tumor: An independent prognostic factor for squamous cell carcinoma patients. Br J Cancer 1999, 81:510–9.
101. Murnane MJ, Sheahan K, Ozdermirji M, Shuja S. Stage specific increase in cathepsin B messenger RNA content in human colorectal carcinoma. Cancer Res 1991, 51:1137–42.
102. Yan S, Sameni M, Sloane BF, Cathepsin B. Human tumor progression. Biol Chem 1998, 379:113–23.
103. Szpaderska AM, Fankfeter A. An intracellular form of cathepsin B contributes to invasiveness in cancer. Cancer Res 2001, 61:3493–500.
104. Sinha AA, Gleason DF, Wilson MJ, Staley NA, Furcht LT, Palm SL *et al*. Immunohistochemical localization of laminin in the basement membranes of normal, hyperplastic and neoplastic human prostate. Prostate 1989, 15:299–313.
105. Sinha AA, Gleason DF, DeLeon OF, Wilson MJ, Sloane BF. Localization of a biotinylated cathepsin B oligonucleotide probe in human prostate including invasive cells and invasive edges by in situ hybridization. Anat Rec 1993, 235:233–40.
106. Sinha AA, Quast BJ, Kordowsi JC, Wilson MJ, Reddy PK, Ewing SL *et al*. The relationship of cathepsin B and stefin A mRNA localization identifies a potentially

aggressive variant of human prostate cancer within a gleason histologic score. Anticancer Res 1999, 19:2821–30.
107. Soderstrom K-O, Laato M, Wu P, Hopsu-Havu VK, Nurmi M, Rinne A. Expression of acid cysteine proteinase inhibitor (ACPI) in the normal human prostate, benign prostatic hyperplasia and adenocarcinoma. Int J Cancer 1995, 62:1–4.
108. Fernandez PL, Farre X, Nadal A, Fernandez E, Peiro N, Sloane BF et al. Expression of cathepsins B and S in the progression of prostate carcinoma. Int J Cancer 2001, 95:51–5.
109. Shuja S, Sheahan K, Murnane MJ. Cysteine endopeptidase activity levels in normal human tissues, colorectal adenomas and carcinomas. Int J Cancer 1991, 49:341–6.
110. Chauhan SS, Goldstein LJ, Gottesman MM. Expresison of cathepsin L in human tumors. Cancer Res 1991, 51:1478–81.
111. Sinha AA, Wilson MJ, Gleason DF, Reddy PK, Sameni M, Sloane BF. Immunohistochemical localization of cathepsin B in neoplastic human prostate. Prostate 1995, 26:171–8.
112. Sinha AA, Quast BJ, Wilson MJ, Reddy PK, Gleason DF, Sloane BF. Co-distribution of pro and mature cathepsin B forms in human prostate tumors detected by confocal and immunoflluorescence microscopy. Anat Rec 1998, 252:281–9.
113. Sinha AA, Quast BJ, Wilson MJ, Fernandes ET, Reddy PK, Ewing SL et al. The ratio of cathepsin B to stefin A identifies heterogeneity within gleason histologic scores for human prostate cancer. Prostate 2001, 48:274–84.
114. Sinha AA, Quast BJ, Wilson MJ, Fernandes ET, Reddy PK, Ewing SL, Gleason DF. Prediciton of pelvic lymph node metastasis by the ratio of cathepsin B to stefin A in human prostate cancer. Cancer 2002, 94:3141–9.
115. Sinha AA, Wilson MJ, Gleason DF. Immunoelectron microscopic localization of prostate specific antigen in human prostate by the proteina-gold complex. Cancer 1987, 60:1288–93.
116. Reese JH, McNeal JE, Redwine EA, Stamey TA, Freiha FS. Tissue type plasminogen activator as a marker for functional zones, within the human prostate gland. Prostate 1988, 12:47–53.
117. Van Veldhuizen PJ, Sadasivan R, Cherian R, Wyatt A. Urokinase-type plasminogen activator expression in human prostate carcinomas. Am J Med Sci 1996, 312:8–11.
118. Mizukami IF, Barni-Wagner BA, DeAngelo LM, Liebert M, Flint A, Lawrence DA et al. Immunologic detection of the cellular receptor for urokinase plasminogen activator. Clin Immunol Immunopathol 1994, 71:96–104.
119. Camiolo SM, Markus G, Englander LS, Siuta MR, Hobika GH, Kohga S. Plasminogen activator content and secretion in explants of neoplastic and benign human prostate tissues. Cancer Res 1984, 44:311–8.
120. Koller A, Kirchheimer JC, Pfluger H, Binder BR. Tissue plasminogen activator activity in prostatic cancer. Eur Urol 1984, 10:389–94.
121. Kirchheimer JC, Pfluger H, Ritschl P, Hienert G, Binder BR. Plasminogen activator activityin bone metastases as compared to primary tumors. Invasion Met 1985, 5:344–55.
122. Plas E, Carroll VA, Jilch R, Mihaly J, Vesely M, Ulrich W et al. Analysis of fibrinolytic proteins in relation to DNA ploidy in prostate cancer. Int J Cancer 1998, 78:320–5.
123. Plas E, Carroll VA, Jilch R, Simak R, Mihaly J, Melchior S et al. Variations of components of the plasminogen activation system with the cell cycle in benign prostate tissue and prostate cancer. Cytometry (Comm Clin Cytometry) 2001, 46:184–9.

124. Helenius MA, Saramaki OR, Linja MJ, Tammela TLJ, Visakorpi T. Amplification of urokinase gene in prostate cancer. Cancer Res 2001, 61:5340–4.
125. Hienert G, Kirchheimer JC, Pfluger H, Binder BR. Urokinase-type plasminogen activator as a marker for the formation of distant metastases in prostatic carcinoma. J Urol 1988, 140:1466–9.
126. Miyake H, Hara I, Yamanaka K, Gohji K, Arakawa S, Kamidono S. Elevation of serum levels of urokinase-type plasminogen activator and its receptor is associated with disease progression and prognosis in patients with prostate cancer. Prostate 1999, 39:123–9.
127. Miyake H, Hara I, Yamanaka K, Arakawa S, Kamidono S. Elevation of urokinase-type plasminogen activator and its receptor densities as new predictors of disease progression and prognosis in men with prostate cancer. Int J Oncol 1999, 14:535–41.
128. Diamandis E.P., Yousef G.M., Human tissue Kallikreins: a family of new cancer biomarkers. Clin Chem 2002, 48:1198–205.
129. Deperthes D, Marceau F, Frenette G, Lazure C, Tremblay RR, Dube JY. Human kallikrein hK2 has low kininongenase activity while prostate-specific antigen has none. Biochim Biophys Acta 1997, 1343:102–6.
130. Charlesworth MC, Young CYF, Miller VM, Tindall DJ. Kininogenase activity of prostate-derived human glandular kallikrein (hK2) purified from seminal fluid. J Androl 1999, 20:220–9.
131. Stenman U-H. Prostate-specific antigen, clinical use and staging: An overview. Br J Urol 1997, 79(Suppl 1):53–60.
132. Rittenhouse HG, Finlay JA, Mikolajczyk SD, Partin AW. Human kallikrein 2 (hK2) and prostate-specific antigen (PSA): Two closely related, but distinct kallikreins in the prostate. Crit Rev Clin Lab Sci 1998, 35:275–368.
133. Garnick MB, Fair WR. Prostate cancer: Emerging concepts. Part II. Ann Intern Med 1996, 125:205–12.
134. Becker C, Lilja H. Individual prostate-specific antigen (PSA) forms as prostate tumor markers. Clin Chem 1997, 257:117–32.
135. Peter J, Unverzagt C, Krogh TN, Vorm O, Hoesel W. Identification of precursor forms of free prostate-specific antigen in serum of prostate cancer patients by immunosorption and mass spectrometry. Cancer Res 2001, 61:957–62.
136. Niemela P, Lovgren J, Karp M, Lilja H, Pettersson K. Sensitive and specific enzymatic assay for the determination of precursor forms of prostate-specific antigen after an activation step. Clin Chem 2002, 48:1257–64.
137. Cohen P, Graves HC, Peehl DM, Kamarei M, Giudice LC, Rosenfeld RG. Prostate-specific antigen (PSA) is an insulin-like growth factor binding protein-3 protease found in seminal plasma. J Clin Endocrinol Metab 1992, 75:1046–53.
138. Killian CS, Corral DA, Kawinski E, Constantine RI. Mitogenic response of osteblast cells to prostate-specific antigen suggests an activation of latent TGF-beta and a proteolytic modulation of cell adhesion receptors. Biochem Biophys Res Commun 1993, 192:940–7.
139. Yoshida E, Ohmura S, Sugiki M, Maruyama M, Mihara H. Prostate-specific antigen activates single-chain urokinase-type plasminogen activator. Int J Cancer 1995, 63:863–5.
140. Tauber PF, Zaneveld LJD. Coagulation and liquefaction of human semen, pp. 153–66. In: *Human Semen and Fertility Regulation in Men*. Hafez ESE, ed., St. Louis: Mosby, 1976.

141. Webber MM, Waghray A, Bello D. Prostate-specific antigen, a serine protease, facilitates human prostate cancer cell invasion. Clin Cancer Res 1995, 1089–94.
142. Fortier AH, Nelson BJ, Grella DK, Holaday JW. Antiangiogenic activity of prostate-specific antigen. J Natl Cancer Inst 1999, 91:1635–40.
143. Meehan KL, Holland JW, Dawkins HJS. Proteomic analysis of normal and malignant prostate tissue to identify novel proteins lost in cancer. Prostate 2002, 50:54–63.
144. Samloff IM, Liebman WM. Purification and immunohistochemical characterization of group II pepsinogens in human seminal fluid. Clin Exp Immunol 1972, 11:405–14.
145. Reese JH, McNeal JE, Redwine EA, Samloff LM, Stamey TA. Differential distribution of pepsinogen II between the zones of the human prostate and the seminal vesicle. J Urol 1986, 136:1148–51.
146. Paju A, Bjartell A, Zhang W-M, Nordling S, Borgstrom A, Hansson J, Stenman U-H. Expression and characterization of trypsinogen produced in the human male genital tract. Am J Pathol 2000, 157:2011–21.
147. Frenette G, Deperthes D, Tremblay RR, Lazure Dube CJY. Purification of enzymatically active kallikrein hK2 from human seminal plasma. Biochim Biophys Acta (Gen Subj) 1997, 1334:109–5.
148. Mikolajczyk SD, Millar LS, Kumar A, Saedi MS. Human glandular kallikrein, hK2< shows arginine-restricted specificity and forms complexes with plasma protease inhibitors. Prostate 1998, 34:44–50.
149. Darson MF, Pacelli A, Roche P, Rittenhouse HG, Wolfert RL, Young CY et al. Human glandular kallikrein 2 (hK2) expression in prostatic intraepithelial neoplasia and adenocarcinoma: A novel prostate cancer marker. Urology 1997, 49:857–62.
150. Darson MF, Pacelli A, Roche P, Rittenhouse HG, Wolfert RL, Saeid MS et al. Human glandular kallikrein 2 expression in prostate adenocarcinoma and lymph node metastases. Urology 1999, 53:939–44.
151. Herrala AM, Prvari KS, Kyllonen AP, Vihko PT. Comparison of human prostate specific glandular kallikrein 2 and prostate specific antigen gene expression in prostate with gene amplification and overexpression of prostate specific glandular kallikrein 2 in tumor tissue. Cancer 2001, 92:2975–84.
152. Kumar A, Mirolajczk SD, Goel AS, Millar LS, Saedi MS. Expression of pro form of prostate-specific antigen by mammalian cells and its conversion to mature, active form by human kallikrein 2. Cancer Res 1997, 57:3111–4.
153. Lovgren J, Rajakoski K, Karp M, Lundwall A, Lilja H. Activation of the zymogen form of prostate-specific antigen by human glandular kallikrein 2. Biochem Biophys Res Commun 1997, 238:549–5.
154. Takayama TK, Fujikawa K, Davie EW. Characterization of the precursor of prostate-specific antigen activation by trypsin and by human glandular kallikrein. J Biol Chem 1997, 272:21582–8.
155. Mikolajczyk SD, Millar LS, Marker KM, Grauer LS, Goel AS, Cass MMJ et al. ALA217 is important for the catalytic function and autoactivation of prostate-specific human kallikrein 2. Eur J Biochem 1997, 246:440–6.
156. Deperthes D, Frenette G, Brilliard-Bourdet M, Bourgeous L, Gauthrier F, Tremblay RR, Dube JY. Potential involvement of kallikrein hK2 in the hydrolysis of the human seminal vesicle proteins after ejaculation. J Androl 1996, 17:659–65.
157. Lovgren J, Airas K, Lilja H. Enzymatic action of human glandular kallikrein 2 (hK2). Substrate specificity and regulation by ZN2+ and e xtracelluar protease inhibitors. Eur J Biochem 1999, 262:781–9.

158. Frenette G, Tremblay RR, Lazure C, Dube JY. Prostatic kallikrein (hK2), but not prostate-specific antigen (hK3), activates single-chain urokinase-type plasminogen activator. Int J Cancer 1997, 71:897–9.
159. Mikolajczyk SD, Millar LS, Kumar A, Saedi MS. Prostatic human kallekrein 2 inactivates and complexes with plasminogen activator inhibitor-1. Int J Cancer 1999, 81:438–42.
160. Mikolajczyk SD, Millar LS, Marker KM et al. Identification of a novel complex between human kallikrein 2 and protease inhibitor-6 in prostate cancer tissue. Cancer Res 1999, 59:3927–30.
161. Saedi MS, Zhu Z, Marker K, Liu R-S, Carpenter PM, Rittenhouse H, Mirolajczyk SD. Human kallikrein 2 (hK2), but not prostate-specific antigen (PSA), rapidly complexes with protease inhibitor 6 (PI6) released from prostate carcinoma cells. Int J Cancer 2001, 94:558–63.
162. Obiezu C, Soosaipillai A, Jung K, Stephan C, Scorilas A, Howarth DHC, Diamandis EP. Detection of human kallikrein 4 in healthy and cancerouos prostatic tissues by immunofluorometry and immunohistochemistry. Clin Chem 2002, 48:1232–40.
163. Diamandis EP, Yousef GM, Soosaipillai AR, Grass L, Porter A, Little S, Sotiropoulou G. Immunofluorometric assay of human kallikrein 6 (zyme/protease M/neurosin) and preliminary clinical applications. Clin Biochem 2000, 33:369–75.
164. Goyal J, Smith KM, Cowan JM, Wazer DE, Lee SW, Band V. The role for NES1 serine protease as a novel tumor suppressor. Cancer Res 1998, 58:4782–6.
165. Nelson P, Gan L, Ferguson C, Moss P, Gelinas R, Hood L, Wang K. Molecular cloning and characterization of prostase, an androgen-regulated serine protease with prostate-restricted expression. Proc Natl Acad Sci USA 1999, 96:3114–9.
166. Petraki CD, Karavana VN, Skoufogiannis PT, Little SP, Howarth DJC, Yousef GM, Diamandis EP. The spectrum of human kallikrein 6 (zyme/protease M/neurosin) expression in human tissues as assessed by immunohistochemistry. J Histochem Cytochem 2001, 49:1431–41.
167. Luo L-Y, Grass L, Howarth JC, Thibault P, Ong H, Diamandis EP. Immunofluoremetric assay of human kallikrein 10 and its identification in biological fluids and tissues. Clin Chem 2001, 47:237–46.
168. Diamandis EP, Okkui A, Mitsui S, Luo L-Y, Soosaipillai A, Grass L et al. Human kallikrein 11: A new biomarker of prostate and ovarian carcinoma. Cancer Res 2002, 62:295–300.
169. Mitsui S, Yamada T, Okui A, Kominami K, Uemura H, Yamaguchi N. A novel isoform of a kallikrein-like protease, TLSP/hippostasin, (PRSS20), is expressed in the human brain and prostate. Biochem Biophys Res Commun 2000, 272:205–11.
170. Nakamura T, Mitsui S, Okui A, Kominami K, Nomoto T, Ukimura O et al. Alternative splicing isoforms of hippostasin (PRSS20/KLK11) in prostate cancer cell lines. Prostate 2001, 49:72–8.
171. Petraki CD, Karavana VN, Luo L-Y, Diamandis EP. Human kallikrein 10 expression in normal tissues by immunohistochemistry. J Histochem Cytochem 2002, 50:1247–61.
172. Yousef GM, Scorilas A, Chang A, Rendl L, Diamandis M, Jung K, Diamandis EP. Down-regulation of the human kallikrein gene 5 (KLK5) in prostate cancer tissues. Prostate 2002, 51:126–32.
173. Riegman PHJ, Vlietstra RJ, Van der Korput JAGM, Romijn JC, Trapman J. Characterization of the prostate-specific antigen gene: A novel human kallikrein-like gene. Biochem Biophys Res Commun 1989, 159:95–102.

174. Heuze N, Olayat S, Gutman N, Zani M-L, Courty Y. Molecular cloning and expression of an alternative hKLK3 transcript coding for a variant protein of prostate-specific antigen. Cancer Res 1999, 59:2820–4.
175. Heuze-Vouc'h N, Leblond V, Olayat S, Gauthier F, Courty Y. Characterization of PSA-RP2, a protein related to prostate-specific antigen and encoded by alternative hKLK3 transcripts. Eur J Biochem 2001, 268:4408–13.
176. David A, Mabjeesh N, Azar I, Biton S, Engel S, Bernstein J et al. Unusual alternative splicing within the human kallikrein ggenes KLK2 and KLK3 gives rise to novel prostate-specific proteins. J Biol Chem 2002, 277:18084–90.
177. Liu XF, Essand M, Vasmatzis G, Lee B, Pastan I. Identification of three new alternate human kallikrein 2 transcripts: Evidence of long transcript and alternative splicing. Biochem Biophys Res Commun 1999, 264:833–9.
178. Yousef GM, Scorilas A, Jung K, Ashworth LK, Diamandis EP. Molecular cloning of the human kallikrein 15 gene (KLK15): Upregulation in prostate cancer. J Biol Chem 2001, 276:53–61.
179. Yu JX, Chao L, Chao J. Prostasin is a novel human serine proteinase from seminal fluid. Purification, tissue dustribution, and localization in prostate gland. J Biol Chem 1994, 269:18843–8.
180. Chen L-M, Skinner ML, Kauffman SW, Chao J, Chao L, Thaler CC, Chai KX. Prostasin is a glycosylphosphatidylinositol-anchored active serine protease. J Biol Chem 2001, 276:21434–42.
181. Chen L-M, Hodge GB, Guarda LA, Welch JL, Greenberg NM, Chai KX. Down-regulation of prostasin serine protease: A potential invasion suppressor in prostate cancer. Prostate 2001, 48:93–103.
182. Paoloni-Giacobino A, Chen H, Peitsch MC, Rossier C, Antonarakis SE. Cloning of the TMPRSS2 gene, which encodes a novel serine protease with transmembrane, LDLRA, and SRCR domains and maps to 21Q22.3. Genomics 1997, 44:309–20.
183. Lin B, Ferguson C, White JT, Wang S, Vessella R, True LD et al. Prostate-localized and androgen-regulated expression of the membrane-bound serine protease TMPRSS2. Cancer Res 1999, 59:4180–84.
184. Lin C-Y, Anders J, Johnson M, Sang QA, Dickson RB. Molecular cloning of cDNA for matriptase, a matrix-degrading serine protease with trypsin-like activity. J Biol Chem 1999, 274:18231–6.
185. Takeuchi T, Shuman MA, Craik CS. Reverse biochemistry: Use of macromolecular protease inhibitors to dissect complex biological processes and identify a membrane-type serine protease in epithelial cancer and normal tissue. Proc Natl Acad Sci USA 1999, 96:11054–61.
186. Takeuchi T, Harris JL, Huang W, Yan KW, Coughlin SR, Craik CS. Cellular localization of membrane-type serine protease 1 and identification of protease-activated receptor-2 and single-chain urokinase-type plasminogen activator as substrates. J Biol Chem 2000, 275:26333–42.
187. Kim DR, Sharmin S, Inoue M, Kido H. Cloning and expression of novel mosaic serine proteases with and without a transmembrane domain from human lung. Biochim Biophys Acta 2001, 1518:204–9.
188. Dhanasekaran SM, Barrette TR, Ghosh D, Shah R, Varambally S, Kurachi K et al. Delineation of prognostic biomarkers in prostate cancer. Nature 2001, 412:822–6.
189. Magee JA, Araki T, Patil S, Ehrig T, True L, Humphrey PA et al. Expression profiling reveals hepsin overexpression in prostate cancer. Cancer Res 2001, 61:5692–6.

190. Luo J, Duggan DJ, Chen Y, Sauvageot J, Ewing CM, Bittner ML *et al*. Human prostate cancer and benign prostatic hyperplasia: Molecular dissection by gene expression profiling. Cancer Res 2001, 61:4683–8.
191. Welsh JB, Sapinoso LM, Su aI, Kern SG. Analysis of gene expression identifies candidate markers and pharmacological targets in prostate cancer. Cancer Res 2001, 61:5974–8.
192. Stamey TA, Warrington JA, Caldwell MC, Chen Z, Fan Z, Mahadevappa M *et al*. Molecular genetic profiling of gleason grade 4/5 prostate cancers compared to benign prostatic hyperplasia. J Urol 2001, 166:2171–7.
193. Ernst T, Hergenhahn M, Kenzelmann M, Cohen CD, Bonrouhi M, Weninger A *et al*. Decrease and gain of gene expression are equally discriminatory markers for prostate carcinoma: A gene expression analysis of total and microdissected prostate tissue. Am J Pathol 2002, 160:2169–80.
194. McGowen R, Biliran J, Jr, Sager R, Sheng S. The surface of prostate carcinoma DU145 cells mediates the inhibition of urokinase-type plasminogen acitvtor by maspin. Cancer Res 2000, 60:4771–8.
195. Machtens S, Serth J, Bokemeyer C, Bathke W, Minssen A, Kollmannsberger C *et al*. Expression of the P53 and maspin protein in primary prostate cancer: Correlation with clinical features. Int J Cancer 2001, 95:337–42.
196. Bjork T, Hulkko S, Bjartell A, Di Sant'Agnese A, Abrahamsson P-A, Lilja H. ALPHA1-antichymotrypsin production in PSA-producing cells is common in prostate cancer but rare in benign prostatic hyperplasia. Urology 1994, 43:427–34.
197. Chai KX, Chen LM, Chao J, Chao L. Kallistatin: A novel human serine proteinase inhibitor. Molecular cloning, tissue distribution, and expression in escherichia coli. J Biol Chem 1993, 268:24498–505.
198. Ohlsson K, Bjartell A, Lilja H. Secretory leucocyte protease inhibitor in the male genital tract: PSA-induced proteolytic processing in human semen and tissue localization. J Androl 1995, 16:64–74.
199. Shimomura T, Denda K, Kitamura A, Kawaguchi T, Kito M, Kondo J *et al*. Hepatocyte growth factor activator inhibitor, a novel kunitz-type serine protease inhibitor. J Biol Chem 1997, 272:6370–6.
200. Cooley J, Takayam TK, Shapiro SD, Schecter NM, Remold-O'Donell E. The serpin MNEI inhibits elastase-like and chymotrypsin-like serine proteases through efficient reactions at two active sites. Biochemistry 2001, 40:15762–70.
201. Lundwall A, Clauss A. Identification of a novel protease inhibitor gene that is highly expressed in the prostate. Biochem Biophys Res Commun 2002, 290:452–6.

Chapter 12

THE BIOLOGY OF BONE METASTASES FROM PROSTATE CANCER AND THE ROLE OF BISPHOSPHONATES

Noel W. Clarke[1] and Herbert A. Fleisch[2]
[1]*Christie Hospital, Withington, Manchester, UK;*
[2]*Department of Pathophysiology, University of Berne, Berne, Switzerland*

Abstract: Bone metastases from prostate cancer are a associated with morbidity and death from the disease. Prostate cancer cells are found in the circulation from an early stage but their number increases significantly as the extent of the disease increases. Once in the circulation they are cleared rapidly, binding to endothelial surfaces by an integrin mediated mechanism, before migrating through basement membranes to the interstitium. Cells need to be motile and present in significant numbers for metastases to form within the bone marrow and close to the bone, the cytokine milieu is altered, disturbing the balanced bone physiology. The osteoblast overactivity produced is accompanied by gross osteoclast mediated bone destruction and marrow suppression. The osteoblast / osteoclast dysfunction is linked through actions of receptor activator of the nuclear factor Kappa B ligand (RANK ligand), endothelin-1, osteoprotogerin and parathyroid hormone-related protein (PTHrP). Clinically, metastatic infiltration induces marrow failure, bone fractures and spinal cord compression. The latter is a grave complication which needs rapid intervention in selected cases to achieve the best outcome. Bisphosphonates can reduce the skeletal complication rate. They work mainly by an osteoclast inhibitory effect although some have anti-tumor activity *in vitro*. Those containing an Imidazole ring are the most potent. The treatment of prostate cancer by androgen ablation also has an adverse effect on skeletal function. Bone loss is significant in men whose testosterone is reduced: this effect can be prevented by use of bisphosphonates such as Pamidronate and Zoledronic acid. Palliation of bone pain is important in end-stage disease. Localised radiotherapy and bone seeking radioisotopes may be effective in many cases. Ultimately however, the outlook is poor and most men will die from their disease within 6 months of the onset of progression of androgen insensitive disease in bone.

Key words: prostate cancer, bone, metastasis, radiotherapy, spinal cord compression, bisphosphonates, pathological fracture, integrins, RANK ligand

1. BIOLOGY OF BONE METASTASES

1.1 Introduction

Bone metastases from prostate cancer are a major unresolved clinical problem.

90% of men with skeletal deposits from the disease will die within five years of first presentation with skeletal metastases (1) and 84% of men dying from prostate cancer will have post-mortem evidence of metastatic disease in the skeleton (2). Morbidity and death is usually the direct result of the invasion of the red bone marrow by malignant metastatic prostatic epithelial cells, which proliferate in the bone marrow and in relation to the bone surface. Once established, they grow in large numbers, disturbing the integrated structure and function of the bone marrow and the bony skeleton itself, producing the classical clinical picture of marrow failure, bone pain, pathological fracture and spinal cord compression.

1.2 Prevalence

The bony skeleton is the third commonest site of malignant invasion overall and in prostate cancer, the reported incidence of bone metastases varies between 35–85% (3, 4). Scintigraphic studies have shown that the areas most commonly affected are the axial skeleton (especially the lumbar spine) (60%) followed by the ribs (50%), appendicular skeleton (38%) and skull (14%) (5). The mode of dissemination to the skeleton is haematogenous and their distribution correlates closely with the distribution of the red marrow in bone (6, 7). The affinity for the red marrow is the most likely factor determining the distribution of the metastatic spread. Great emphasis has been placed on the Batsons' theory of "valveless" venous spread (8). However, the high incidence of metastases in the lumbar spine and pelvis is likely to be a consequence of the anatomical proximity and the pattern of venous drainage which dictates that this area of the skeleton has a higher exposure to cells released from the prostate and therefore has a higher number of epithelial cellular "hits" on the bone marrow endothelium itself. It is known that prostate epithelial cell/bone marrow endothelial binding is a rapid process (9) and that a critical number of cellular "hits" are needed to form a metastatic colony (10). The environment for metastatic implantation and growth is therefore at its height in the red bone marrow of the pelvis and lumbar spine. It is this combination of factors, which is likely to account for the observed pattern of metastatic distribution.

1.3   Pathophysiology

Metastatic epithelial cells in the circulation first impinge on the bone marrow endothelium where they are arrested by an initial "docking" step mediated by cell surface carbohydrate/lectin moieties. This is followed by a "locking" step mediated by integrins. This is a selective process, with tumor cells binding to specific endothelial cells at the preferred metastatic site (11, 12). This binding occurs rapidly and is mediated by the Beta 1 integrin component (9) although other integrins may also be involved (13). The tumor cells bind to endothelial junctional regions, following which they actively migrate through the gap junctions in a process which is, at least in part, mediated by degradative enzymes such as matrix metalloproteinases (14).

Once through the endothelial barrier the cells require several key elements to be present to develop into an overt metastasis. There are a number of uncertainties in this area and it has been shown by RT-PCR based and whole cell extraction studies that malignant epithelial cells can remain dormant in the bone marrow for considerable periods of time. However, there are certain key elements which are required for propagation to enable development in to a metastasis: these include a critical cell number and cell-cell cross talk via specific integrins (15), cellular motility (16) and the presence of active degradative enzymes (14).

Once established the micrometastasis develops in the bone marrow space, often in close association with the bone surface (Figure 1) where the microenvironment is disturbed locally. It has been postulated that the first event in this process is osteoclast mediated resorption leading to release of stimulatory cytokines from the bone surface and a cycle of resorption/tumor stimulation. However, in personal observation of serial micrometastases from human skeleton biopsies taken from men with prostate cancer (Clarke, Personal Communication), this phenomenon has not been observed. The first event in the process is always a stimulation of fibroblastic elements in the bone marrow and local stimulation of osteoblasts (Figures 1, 2). As the metastases develops it induces an imbalance of the carefully regulated skeletal cycle wherein bone resorption is linked closely to formation in a "coupled" manner, with the result that there is accelerated bone formation and resorption occurring synchronously. This is caused by changes in local cytokine production and interaction.

A number of stimulating factors have been identified in relation to "osteoblastic" metastases in prostate cancer. The factors selectively stimulate the mesodermal cell lineages thereby increasing osteoblast and fibroblast activity. They include fibroblast growth factors, transforming growth factor-beta (TGF-β), bone morphorgenetic protein (BMP) and endothelin-1 (17).

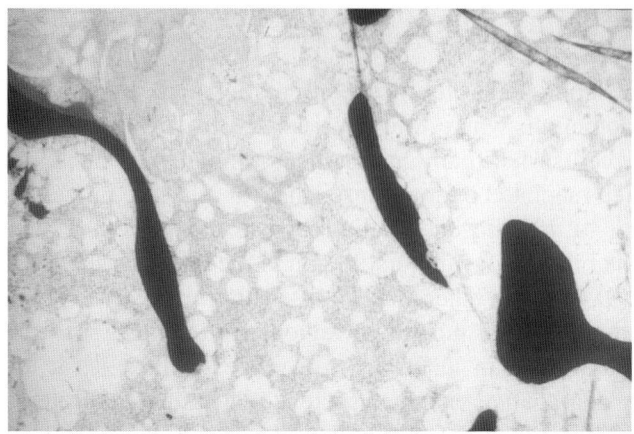

Figure 1. Section of an iliac crest bone biopsy from a patient with metastatic prostate cancer. An early metastatic deposit can be seen in the bone marrow space. This is disturbing the bone metabolism in a localised way as illustrated by the increase in collagen deposition on the surface of the bone trabeculum occurring as a consequence of osteoblast stimulation in the immediate vicinity of the tumor itself. This appearance is characteristic of the appearance observed in early metastatic deposits.

This over activity is responsible for the measurable increase in bone volume (18, 19) and for the accelerated bone mineralisation rate as measured by double tetracycline labelling (20). The tumor-generated bone deposited is abnormal "woven" bone (Figure 3). This is characteristic of bone produced in high turn over states and it is responsible for the well described sclerotic appearance measured histomorphometrically (19) and biochemically (21) and seen radiologically in over 90% of patients with this disease (22).

The traditional view of prostate cancer as an "osteoblastic" disease has obscured the fact that the disease is responsible for major bone destruction. This was suggested initially on the basis of preliminary histological studies (23) and was subsequently proven on equivocally on the basis of histomorphometric measurement of human metastatic bone biopsies (18, 19) and biochemical measurement of bone resorption products in humans (21, 24). The paradox of increasing bone volume in the presence of bone resorption is explained by histomorphometric studies (19) showing that the resorption of the existing skeleton is accompanied by synchronous replacement of abnormal woven bone, which, itself, undergoes further resorption (Figures 4 a, b and c). This produces a measurable increase in bone volume in the presence of wholesale destruction of the normal skeleton.

The lytic process, like the formative "blastic" process arises as a consequence of abnormal levels of soluble growth factors produced by the

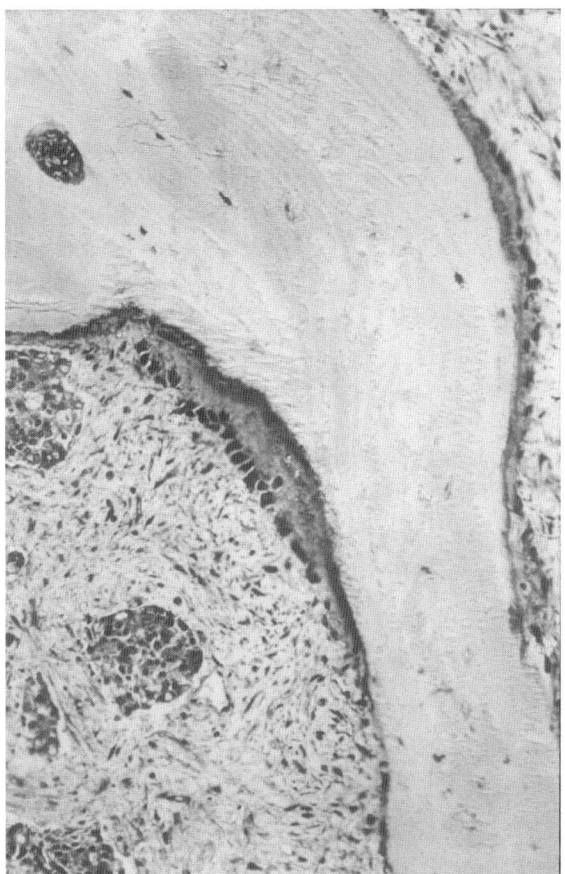

Figure 2. An established metastasis from a man with metastatic bone disease from prostate cancer. The bone marrow is replaced by neoplastic cells which have induced marked osteoblast activity on the bone surface where the osteblasts are rapidly laying down collagen which will subsequently be calcified to form abnormal "woven" bone.

invading tumor. This in turn stimulates abnormal osteoclast activity, which is responsible for the bone resorption. Osteoclast recruitment, differentiation and activation by tumors is incompletely understood. One hypothesis is that there is stimulation by macrophage colony stimulating factor (M-CSF), the receptor activator of the nuclear factor Kappa B (NFkB) ligand (RANK ligand) and osteoprotegerin (25, 26). Osteoblasts secrete the RANK-ligand which then induces osteoclast differentiation by binding the RANK surface receptor on the osteoclast precursor. This in turn stimulates osteoclastogenesis (26). The protein, osteoprotegerin plays a key regulatory role in this process by competing for the RANK binding site on

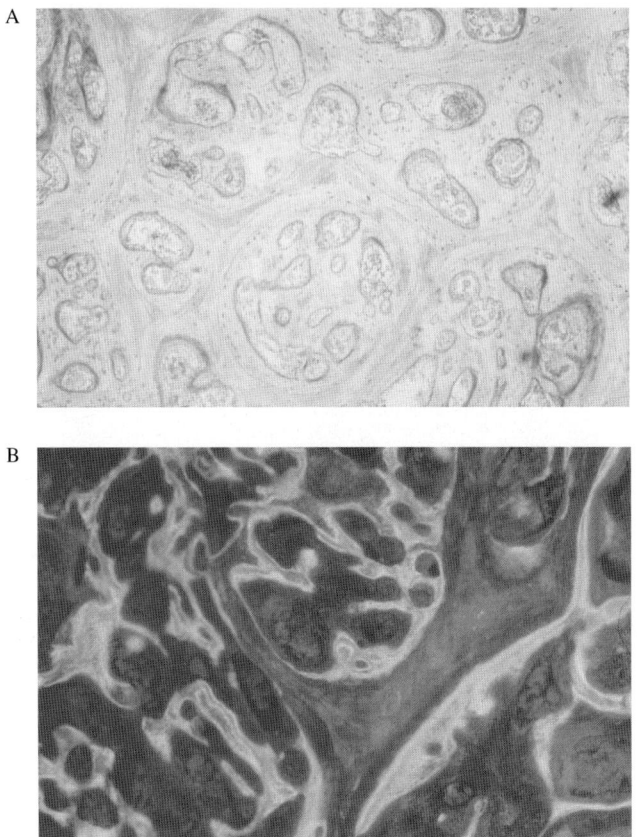

Figure 3. **A.** Typical appearance of osteosclerosis in a metastatic deposit from prostate cancer. The woven bone has been laid down on the surface of the bone in an "uncoupled" manner ie without prior resorption. Uncoupled resorption can also be observed elsewhere in the specimen. **B.** A similar metastatic specimen to that observed in Figure 3b. This patient has received pulsed doses of tetracycline which is taken up in new bone and shows up as yellow when observed using fluorescent microscopy. The specimen shows widespread and rapid bone formation as a consequence of hyperstimulation of osteoblasts. These in turn lay down bone in a very rapid manner as "woven" bone. This type of bone lacks the ordered structure and integrity of lamellar bone (see Figures 4 b to d).

osteoclast precursors. A co-factor in this process may be parathyroid hormone-related protein (PTH-rP). Cancer cells are unable to express RANK ligand and cannot therefore stimulate osteoclastogenesis by this route. However, when PTH-rP is added to murine osteoblasts and haemopoietic progenitors in culture, osteoclasts differentiate in the absence of other stimulatory agents (27), suggesting that PTH-rP has a facilitatory role. PTH-rP is a

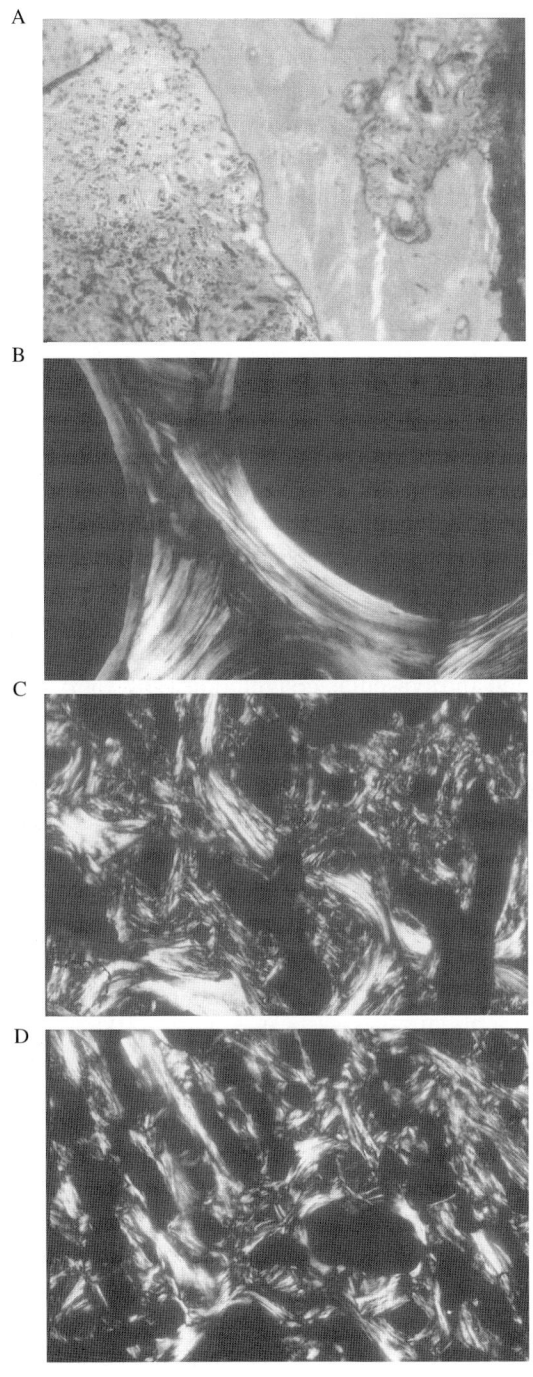

Figure 4. (Caption on page 260)

major factor in bone resorption in breast cancer (17) and is expressed in both primary and bone metastases in prostate cancer (28, 29).

1.4 Clinical and Metabolic Effects

Morbidity and death from prostate cancer is most commonly linked to metastatic spread to the bony skeleton. The disturbance in balanced skeletal and bone marrow function manifests as bone marrow failure, altered calcium metabolism, pathological fracture and spinal cord compression. The treatment of the disease using androgen ablation or blockade also has implications for skeletal integrity in the longer term.

1.5 Bone Marrow Failure

This arises as a direct consequence of red marrow infiltration by the metastatic prostate cancer cells (Figure 5). These displace the erythroid and blast cell precursors, thereby inducing dysfunction and depletion in leukoid and erythroid lineages. The most common clinical manifestation of this is anaemia although immunological dysfunction, platelet malfunction and overt disseminated intravascular coagulation (DIC) are also sequelae. The anaemia is often responsible for lethargy and shortness of breath (particularly when the hemoglobin falls below 8 g/dl). At this level it is usual to consider transfusion to enable symptomatic improvement (30). This is used to good effect as a palliative measure (31).

A further approach is the use of erythropoetin (EPO) (32). Combined androgen blockade is known to have a suppressive effect on erythroid function and this has been shown to be responsive to EPO. A limited number of studies have examined the use of this agent in the hormone refractory setting. In a small study (33) 4 of 9 patients receiving treatment over a 12 week period had a 2 g/dl increase in their haemoglobin levels. In a further, larger study, patients receiving EPO at a dose of 5000 units 3 times per week

◄―――――――――――――――――――――――――――――――――――

Figure 4. **A.** Tunnelling bone resorption secondary to osteoclast hyper-stimulation by metastatic prostate cancer in the skeleton. Osteoclasts can be seen at the apex of the tunnelled resorption cavity. These are being stimulated by paracrine factors from the adjacent prostate cancer cells. **B-D.** The paradox of accelerated resorption in the presence of increasing bone volume is explained in this series of bone sections viewed under crossed polarised light. The ordered bone lamellar structure can be seen clearly in 4b. In c and d the lamellar skeleton has been progressively resorbed (fragments of the original lamellar bone structure can be seen through out) and replaced by woven bone. This, in turn, is undergoing resorption at the same time.

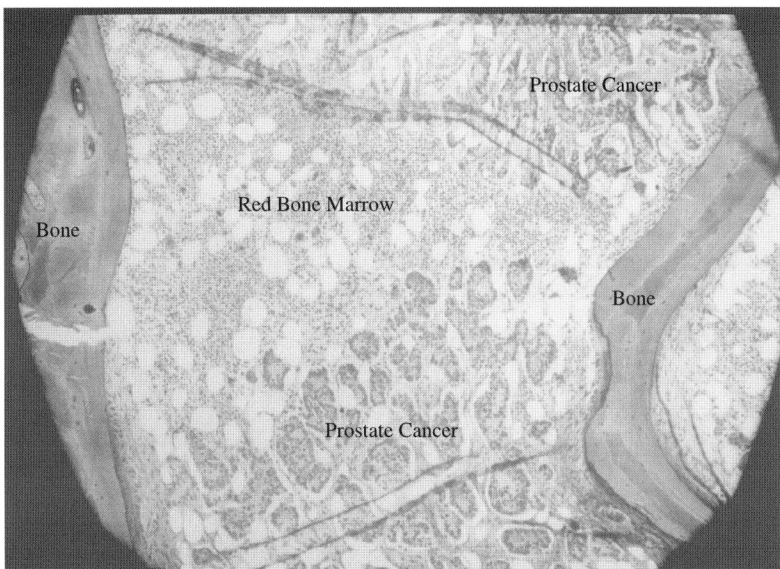

Figure 5. Bone biopsy from a bone metastasis in hormone refractory prostate cancer. The trabeculae of the cancellous bone frame the marrow space containing normal red bone marrow (centre to upper left) and encroaching prostate cancer cells (lower central and upper right). The prostate cancer cells are displacing the red bone marrow progressively. The advancing front of malignant cells replaces the normal red marrow until the marrow space ultimately becomes populated completely by prostate cancer cells which in turn, induce osteoblast and osteoclast hyper-activity (as seen on the contiguous bone surfaces). It should be noted that the marrow replacement is not a compression phenomenon, as shown by the preservation of the architecture of the normal red marrow at the cancer/bone marrow interface. The marrow displacement is responsible for the anaemia and general haematological dysfunction seen commonly in HRPC.

were found to benefit significantly without major side effects. Quality of life in the 43% of patients experiencing an increase of >2 g/dl was improved (34). However, given the life expectancy of the patients and the cost of therapy, the treatment cost/benefit ratio must be considered. It is because of this that EPO therapy has not yet gained wide acceptance in the treatment of anaemia arising from hormone refractory prostate cancer (HRPC).

1.6 Skeletal Dysfunction

The derangement of skeletal function described above has an effect on calcium metabolism. By contrast with other cancers such as breast, which often induce hypercalcaemia, prostate cancer patients often have a measurably low serum calcium. This is because the excessive bone formation in metastases actually induces a 'calcium sink' effect (35), which utilises the excess calcium released by the ongoing lytic process. For this reason, hypercalcaemia is uncommon in prostate cancer, occurring in only 1–5% of patients (36). The increased calcium mobilisation does however lead to mild hyperparathyroidism and a chronic increase in bone resorption in areas of the skeleton not involved by cancer which, in turn, potentiates the decrease in bone the volume of patients affected by the disease (19).

1.7 Pahological Fracture

Pathological fracture has formerly been perceived as a relatively uncommon event in prostate cancer with a proposed incident figure of 3% (37), contrasting with a rate of 9% in malignancies overall and 16% in breast cancer (38, 39). However, more recent analysis has shown that pathological fracture is a much more common problem than was previously thought. In HRPC the fracture rate has been reported to be as high as 33% with approximately 2/3 occurring in the vertebral column and 1/3 in the long bones (40). This risk is exacerbated by the long-term use of androgen suppression (41) and when fracture occurs, it is associated with a significant reduction in patient survival (42). An emerging body of evidence now suggests that the incidence of fracture can be reduced by the use of bisphosphonates (see below). Other treatments include prophylactic local irradiation of lytic metastases in the shafts of long bones and in the neck of the femur. However, when a pathological fracture occurs in a long bone, it is important to treat this by rapid orthopaedic fixation or joint replacement (Figure 6). This is highly effective in reducing pain and restoring mobility. Fixation is usually supplemented by treatment with local radiotherapy 2–4 weeks after the surgery.

1.8 Spinal Cord Compression

This is a devastating complication of metastatic bone disease (Figure 7). Prostate cancer is the commonest cause of cord compression arising from cancer and the clinical manifestations can occur in up to 10–17% of patients (37, 43). It is possible to identify patients at risk by simple clinical parameters. In a retrospective review of 68 patients (44) it was shown that heavy skeletal tumor load, long-standing duration of continuous androgen suppression and low hemoglobin concentration effectively identified an 'at risk' population and that subsequent Magnetic Resonance Imaging scanning

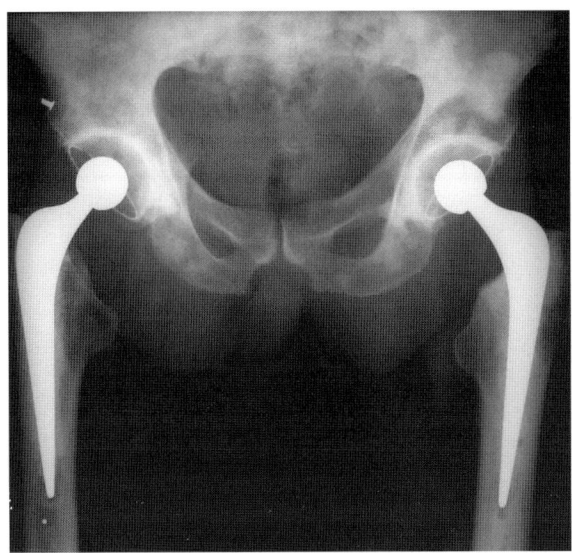

Figure 6. Radiograph of a 63 year old man with hormone refractory prostate cancer illustrating the problem of long bone fracture. Multiple sclerotic bone metastases are seen throughout the pelvis. Pathological fractures secondary to tumor mediated bone destruction have occurred separately in the necks of both femora over a 12 month period. These have been treated by prosthetic joint replacement and subsequent local radiotherapy.

of such patients facilitated identification of men whose disease might be treated locally (e.g., with radiotherapy) before development of irreversible neurological deterioration. There is also some evidence to suggest that addition of a bisphosphonate to this group of patients will decrease the risk of cord compression still further (37, 45).

Unfortunately, many patients present with acute problems, the underlying pathophysiological cause being a collapse of an affected vertebral body or encroachment of the tumor in the spinal canal itself. This tends to cause maximal trouble in the thoracic spine where the spinal canal is at its most narrow (46). The prodromal symptoms tend to manifest as an excruciating 'band-like' pain around the lower abdomen (90% of cases) although more subtle manifestations include isolated peripheral neuropathy/lower limb weakness or spontaneous loss of normal bladder and/or bowel function (46). Management of the acute situation is by Dexamethasone and focal radiotherapy. In suitable cases this may be supplemented by consideration of surgical decompression. Once more, a reasoned balance must be struck in relation to outcome and survival, as the durability of response to surgery

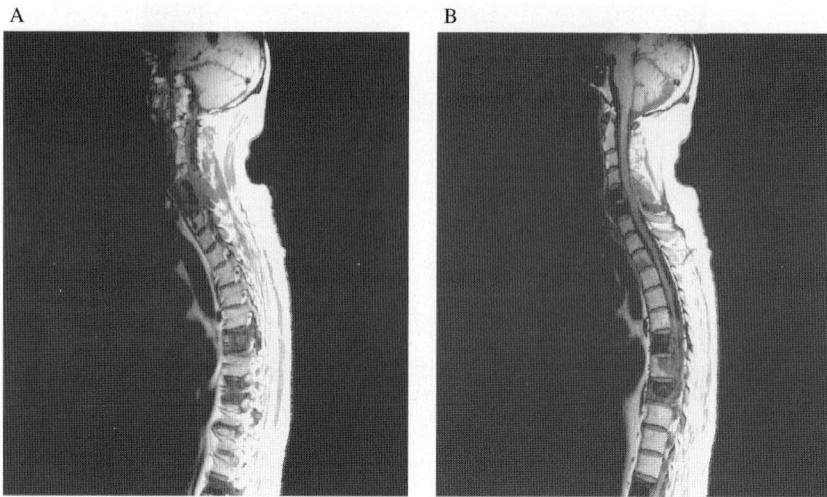

Figure 7. Spinal cord compression in HRPC. The serial scans from the same patient show destructive lesions in multiple vertebrae and illustrate that compression often occurs at multiple levels simultaneously. Early treatment is required for the best clinical outcome but paraplegia at presentation is usually an indicator of poor outcome.

is often limited. In a study of 69 patients (52 with HRPC) (47) presenting with spinal cord compression, only 52% had a functional improvement in motor power after treatment, the majority seeing this within the first week of therapy. Many of the patients had multiple levels of compression (Figure 7) and MRI was the most effective means of diagnosing this accurately. Patients of younger age (less then 65) with single compression levels fared better and when these factors were excluded, there was no additional benefit arising from high irradiation dose (>30 gray) or surgical decompression (47). In a further study of 37 patients undergoing surgical decompression of the spinal cord, only 8 of 19 men with HRPC had a recovery of mobility post-operatively. The peri-operative mortality was 8% and a high proportion of the men with hormone refractory disease died within the first year after surgery notwithstanding the outcome of the decompression. Predictors of good outcome were the ability to walk pre-operatively and rapid intervention after the onset of symptoms. Immobility with an onset of less than 24 hours and established paraplegia were particularly bad signs, the latter being a 'consistently accurate indication of poor prognosis' in the long-term (48). This raises the question of whether or not laminectomy is justified in HRPC patients with this problem. The answer must be 'yes' but only in certain circumstances. The younger, more ambulant male, preferably with a single compression site is the one most likely to benefit provided that the decompression is undertaken as soon as possible after the onset of symptoms.

1.9 Bone Pain

Many patients with prostatic bone metastases will experience bone pain at some point in the course of their disease (5, 49). Its aetiology is incompletely understood. The extent of disease in the skeleton does not necessarily correlate with the pain experienced (50) but whether the pain is associated with a single isolated metastasis or with a heavy skeletal load, it is often a source of considerable morbidity requiring multi-disciplinary treatments by Urologists, Oncologists and Palliative Care teams in order to bring symptoms under control. The therapies available are manifold but the main treatment modalities are the use of external beam or systemically administered radiotherapy, analgesics, bisphonates and other second-line therapies including chemotherapy. These are discussed in more detail in Chapter 15.

2. ROLE OF BISPHOSPHONATES

2.1 Introduction

Bisphosphonates have been used extensively in cancer treatment in recent years, particularly in the field of breast cancer and myeloma. Their use in prostate cancer has been uncertain but in recent years, the utility of this class of compounds has begun to emerge.

2.2 Preclinical Aspects Relevant for Their Use in Tumor Bone Disease

The geminal bisphosphonates are a new class of drugs which has been developed in the past three decades for diagnostic and therapeutic use in various diseases of bone and calcium metabolism, among others tumor bone disease. Their main effect is to inhibit bone resorption. This action is made use of in tumor bone disease, in order to inhibit tumoral osteolysis and its consequences.

2.2.1 Chemistry

The bisphosphonates, previously misnamed diphosphonates, are compounds characterized by a P-C-P bond (Figure 8).

The basic P-C-P structure allows many possible variations, especially by changing the two lateral chains R1 and R2 on the carbon atom. Small changes in the structure of the bisphosphonates can lead to extensive alterations in their physicochemical, biological, therapeutic, and toxicological characteristics. Ten bisphosphonates are commercially available for therapy in humans, and six namely etidronate, clodronate, ibandronate, incadronate, pamidronate and zoledronate are available for tumor-induced bone disease.

The bisphosphonates display a strong affinity to solid calcium phosphates. This explains their physicochemical effects. Indeed, after binding, many of the bisphosphonates act as crystal poisons and inhibit the precipitation and aggregation as well as the dissolution of calcium phosphate solid phase, this even at very low concentration (51, 52, 53, 54).

The P-C-P bond of the bisphosphonates is relatively stable towards heat and most chemical reagents, and completely resistant to enzymatic hydrolysis.

The fact that bisphosphonates affect bone *in vivo* was reported for the first time in 1968 and 1969 (51, 53).

2.2.2 Effects on Calcification *in vitro* and *in vivo*

Bisphosphonates prevent experimentally induced calcification of many soft tissues, amongst others arteries, kidneys, and skin, both when given parenterally and orally (51, 52). If administered at a sufficient dose, certain bisphosphonates, such as etidronate, can also impair the mineralization of normal calcified tissues (55). This inhibition of mineralization is present for most active compounds and occurs at a concentration of around 5–20 mg of compound phosphorus per kg administered parenterally. The inhibition of mineralization appears to be due chiefly to the physicochemical inhibition of crystal growth.

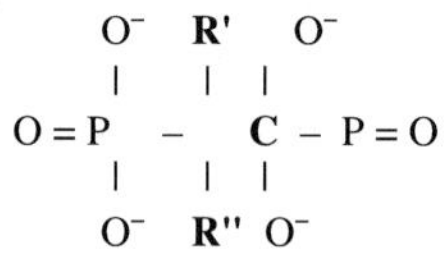

$$O=P\begin{pmatrix}O^-\\|\\|\\O^-\end{pmatrix}-\overset{\overset{\displaystyle R'}{|}}{\underset{\underset{\displaystyle R''}{|}}{C}}-P=O\begin{pmatrix}O^-\\|\\|\\O^-\end{pmatrix}$$

Figure 8. Structure of bisphosphonates.

2.3 Inhibition of Bone Resorption

2.3.1 Normal and Experimentally Induced Bone Resorption

The fact that bisphosphonates inhibit calcium phosphate crystal dissolution in vitro had led us to hypothesize that these compounds might also act on bone resorption *in vivo*. The hypothesis of an effect on bone destruction proved correct, but the mechanism of action is different from that originally conceived, since it is not based on the physicochemical inhibtion of crystal dissolution but to a cellular effect.

Bisphosphonates block bone resorption induced by various means in organ culture (53, 54). An inhibition can also be found when the effect of isolated osteoclasts is investigated on various mineralized matrices *in vitro*.

Bisphosphonates also strongly inhibit bone resorption *in vivo*, both in normal animals and in experimental models of increased bone resorption. In growing rats they block the degradation of both bone and cartilage and thus arrest the remodeling of the metaphysis, which becomes club-shaped and radiologically more dense than normal (56). This effect is used as a model to study the potency of new compounds (57).The inhibition of endogenous bone resorption has also been documented, initially by Ca^{45} kinetic studies and hydroxyproline excretion (58), later by many other means. The effect occurs within 24–48 hours (59) and is therefore slower than that of calcitonin. The decrease in resorption is accompanied by an increase in both calcium balance (58) and mineral content of bone. This is possible because of an increase in intestinal absorption of calcium. Unless given in excess, bisphosphonates improve biomechanical properties both in normal animals and in experimental models of osteoporosis. The first model was in rats immobilized by sciatic nerve section (60) and was followed by many others such as ovariectomy, orchidectomy, corticosteroid administration and others. Bisphosphonates inhibit bone loss in all of them. They also impair bone resorption experimentally induced by various other means, such as parathyroid hormone, the first one used (53, 54).

2.3.2 Tumor-Induced Bone Resorption

It was already known in the early 1980s that bisphosphonates very effectively inhibit tumoral bone resorption both *in vitro* and *in vivo*. All bisphosphonates which had previously been found to inhibit bone resorption in other systems were active, among others among others alendronate, clodronate, etidronate, ibandronate, incadronate, olpadronate, pamidronate, risedronate and zoledronate.

When added to culture medium, bisphosphonates inhibit the bone resorbing effect of supernatants of various cancers in mice calvaria *in vitro* (61). Numerous studies demonstrate that bisphosphonates also inhibit tumoral bone resorption *in vivo*. The most common models used involve the administration of various tumor cells either subcutaneously, intra-arterially or in the vicinity of bone. The former induces hypercalcemia, the second bone metastases and the latter local bone resorption and invasion. The first such studies performed showed that the humoral hypercalcemia induced by subcutaneously implanted Walker 256 carcinoma cells or by implanted Leydig tumor cells (62) could be partially prevented. The effect is generally more pronounced on calciuria than on calcaemia due to the effect that the bisphosphonates influence only the elevated bone resorption, but not the increase in renal reabsorption of calcium. Bisphosphonates also prevent or slow down bone resorption due to actual tumor invasion, as shown in numerous models. The first one used was the injection of Walker carcinosarcoma cells into the rat iliac artery, a procedure whereby the cells are implanted into the bone (63). Effectiveness is also obtained when the tumor cells are implanted directly into bone (64, 65) or into into the vicinity of bone (66). Many kinds of tumor cells have been used, among others bladder tumor (66), various mammary tumors (55), myeloma (67), melanoma (68) and prostate carcinoma (69, 70, 71). More recently the models have been improved by using nude mice (70, 71, 72). In all these models bone resorption is decreased by the various bisphosphonates used.

One of the questions pertains to the effect on the skeletal tumor burden. While earlier results showed no effect or even some increase, the newer ones display a decrease (72, 73).

2.3.3 Activity and Structure

The activity of individual bisphosphonates varies greatly from compound to compound. For etidronate, the first bisphosphonate to be used in clinical practice, the dose inhibiting bone resorption is low and very close to that inducing a block of normal mineralization. Therefore, one of the aims of bisphosphonate research has been to find compounds with a higher antiresorptive activity, without a higher inhibition of mineralization. This has proved to be possible. Thus, today there are compounds which have a 5–10,000 times higher antiresorptive activity than etidronate as assessed in the rat. This is the case for zoledronate (74) and minodronate. Today all very active compounds contain a nitrogen. The potency of various bisphosphonates in the rat are the following starting with the least potent: etidronate, tiludronate, clodronate, pamidronate, neridronate, incadronate, olpadronate, alendronate, ibandronate, risedronate, minodronate, zoledronate. The ranking is very similar in humans, at least with respect to their relative place in the scale of potency. However the difference in potency between the least effective (etidronate) and the most potent (zoledronate) is less in humans and depends on the disease for which the compounds are used. This difference is much smaller for osteoporosis, than for Paget's disease and tumor induced hypercalcemia.

2.3.4 Mechanisms of Action in the Inhibition of Bone Resorption

It appears now that the inhibition of bone resorption is not due to the inhibition of crystal dissolution as initially postulated, but is cellular. The bisphosphonates affect the osteoclast whereby four mechanisms appear to be involved: 1) Inhibition of osteoclast recruitment; 2) Inhibition of osteoclast adhesion; 3) Shortening of the life span of osteoclasts by inducing programmed cell death (apoptosis [75]); 4) Inhibition of osteoclast activity. All four effects could be due either to a direct action on the osteoclast or its precursors, or possibly indirectly through action on cells which modulate the osteoclast recruitment and/or activity such as the osteoblast (76).

Great progress in our understanding of the intracellular mechanisms of the bisphosphonates has been made by the discovery that nitrogen-containing bisphosphonates inhibit the mevalonate pathway (77) due to an inhibition of farnesyl pyrophosphate synthase (78, 79). This leads to a decrease of the formation of isoprenoid lipids such as farnesyl- and geranylgeranylpyrophosphates. These are required for the post-translational prenylation (transfer of fatty acid chains) of proteins, including the GTP-binding proteins Ras, Rho, Rac and Rab, which are important for many cell functions, including cytoskeletal assembly and intracellular signaling. Therefore, N-containing bisphosphonates will induce a series of changes leading to decreased activity, probably the main effect, and to earlier apoptosis in several cell types, including osteoclasts. In osteoclasts the lack of geranylgeranylpyrophosphate appears to be responsible for the effects (80).

In contrast, some non-nitrogen-containing bisphosphonates, such as clodronate, etidronate, and tiludronate, can be incorporated into the phosphate chain of ATP-containing compounds so that they become nonhydrolyzable. The new P-C-P containing ATP analogs impair cell function and may lead to apoptosis and cell death (81). Thus, the bisphosphonates can be classified into two major groups with different modes of action.

2.3.5 Mechanisms of Action in Tumoral Bone Resorption

As described above, bisphosphonates inhibit the bone destruction induced by various tumors both *in vitro* and in animals. This is accompanied by a decrease in the development of metastases and of tumor burden. This could be due to various causes. One is that, since less bone is destroyed, the place for tumoral expansion is limited. Another explanation involves the self-supporting cycle called "seed and soil mechanism" by which growth factors present in bone, such as TGF-β and insulin-like growth factors (IGFs), are liberated during bone resorption and stimulate thereafter the multiplication of tumor cells. As a consequence to a decrease in bone resorption, this cycle would be interrupted (82, 83). Another cause could be the fact that bisphosphonates can inhibit the adhesion of some cells, among them tumor cells, *in vitro* (84, 85). The effect is specific for mineralized matrices, and the potency of various bisphosphonates on adhesion is well correlated with the potency to inhibit bone resorption *in vivo*. Furthermore, various bisphosphonates have recently been found to inhibit the multiplication *in vitro* of a number of tumor cells (86), among other prostate cells (87). In addition the bisphosphonates also induce apoptosis and death of tumor cells *in vitro* (88, 89), the effect showing a synergy with paclitaxel (90). These effects occur also *in vivo* (91) and appear to be mediated, at least in part, by the effect on the mevalonate pathway (101). Even more recently a new mode of action has been proposed based on the finding that bisphosphonates can inhibit angiogenesis induced in various ways *in vitro* (92, 93). Possibly the known inhibitory effect of bisphosphonates on matrix metalloproteinases is involved in this process. Since angiogenesis is important in the development of metastases, it could be that bisphosphonates are acting also in this manner.

Thus the possibility exits that bisphosphonates may have a direct effect on tumor cells. However, since the effect is often seen only at relatively high concentrations of bisphosphonates, it has yet to be shown that these effects are functioning and relevant *in vivo*. An important question is also whether any of these mechanisms could affect tumor cells not present in bone.

2.3.6 Specificity of Action in Bone

An interesting fact is that despite this large spectrum of cellular effects *in vitro*, bisphosphonates act almost exclusively on calcified tissues. This selectivity stems from the strong affinity of these compounds for calcium phosphate, which allows them to be cleared very rapidly from blood and to be incorporated specifically into calcified tissues, especially bone.

They concentrate both under the osteoblasts and osteoclasts (94). When bisphosphonate-loaded bone is resorbed, the compounds will be released into the surrounding solution (Figure 9). They can thus reach high local concentration and be taken up by the osteoclasts and the osteoblasts. This mechanism would explain not only their specificity for skeletal tissues, but also why their effect starts only within one to two days and can last for a very long time even after only one administration.

On the other hand the bisphosphonates deposit only in very small amounts in other tissues in view of their short presence in blood. This can add to the explanation for the relatively low toxicity of these compounds.

2.4 Bisphosphonates in Prostate Cancer

The utility and use of this class of drugs in prostate cancer has increased in recent years. The main indications are in treatment of advanced metastatic disease (reduction of pain, pathological fracture and cord compression) whilst latterly, it has also become apparent that this class of drugs also has an important role in reducing the skeletal morbidity associated with long-term androgen withdrawal.

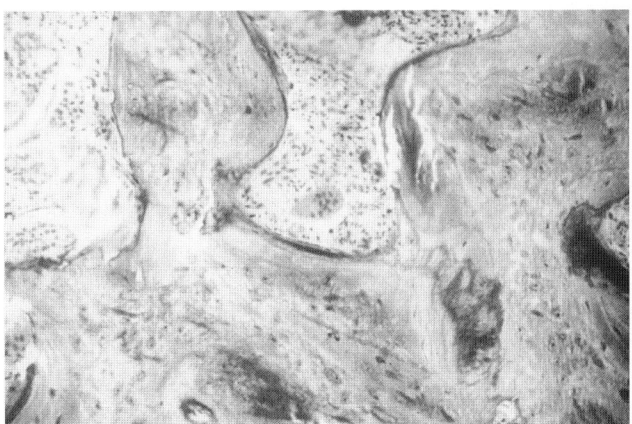

Figure 9. Bone biopsy specimen through a bone metastasis in a patient who has undergone 6 months therapy with the bisphosphonate, Pamidronate. A bisphosphonate affected osteoclast can be seen clearly. The cell is rounded, has multiple central nuclei and is unable to bind to the bone surface and resorb it.

2.4.1 Control of Bone Pain

The use of bisphosphonates in alleviating bone pain has been surrounded by uncertainty. A number of open-label studies using the earlier and less potent agents, Clodronate (95, 96) and Pamidronate (97) have reported a beneficial effect and these results have been supported by positive findings using more powerful later generation drugs. In an open label study of 25 patients using the intravenous bisphosphonate 'Ibandronate', reductions in bone pain were seen in 92% of patients with concomitant diminution in analgesic requirements and improvement in performance (98). However, such findings have not been replicated in larger controlled studies with Clodronate (99, 100) or Pamidronate (101). This may however, be a consequence of the lower potency of these agents by comparison with stronger drugs such as Zoledronate and Ibandronate. In a large scale randomised trial using Zoledronate, currently the most potent bisphosphonate available, there was a significant decrease in pain requirement for those receiving the drug, although quality of life and performance were not affected significantly (45). The reason for the variability of the results is not completely clear. Notwithstanding this, bisphosphonates do have a place in the management of pain in HRPC. It seems that the patient most likely to benefit from this class of drugs used as a pain relieving therapy is the one with painful bone metastases which are difficult to control by other means.

2.4.2 Reduction of Pathological Fracture and Cord Compression

It has been known for some time that this class of drugs reduces bone resorption in HRPC (21), but their clinical utility in terms of benefit to the patient by reducing skeletal related morbid events has been open to question. Early controlled studies using less potent agents in small number studies (e.g., 102) showed no effect from treatment by comparison with controls. Latterly, larger studies have shown some differences even with less potent agents. A randomised UK MRC study assigned 311 patients with HRPC to receive the bisphosphonate Clodronate or placebo with results showing a small reduction in time to symptomatic bone progression (103). In a second study using the same agent with chemotherapy (Mitoxantrone and Prednisone), subset analysis showed that moderate to severe bone pain was improved although the palliative effects were not different (99). In a large randomised placebo controlled study using the newer, more potent bisphosphonate, Zoledronic Acid, results have shown that serial use of the drug as monotherapy (in addition to standard palliative care) produced an 11% reduction in the incidence of skeletal related events by comparison with controls (45). This leads to the question of whether or not all patients with HRPC should receive bisphosphonates with a similar potency to the newer agents Zoledronate and Ibandronate. The view of some experts is that the cost/benefit from such a policy would be insufficiently great (104). However, the same authors accept that there are patients who are likely to benefit from such a regimen. These patients would include those with heavy skeletal tumor load, particularly in the thoraco-lumbar spine and femoral bones and those who have been on long-term Luteinizing hormone-releasing hormone (LHRH) therapy or maximal androgen blockade. One future way of focusing this therapy may be to utilise serum and urinary markers to predict the "at risk" population. Patients with high markers of bone turnover are known to represent a population with an increased risk of developing pathological fracture (105) and it may be that targeting this group will result in the most effective outcome.

2.4.3 Bisphosphonates in Androgen Ablation

The knowledge that long term androgen deficiency has an osteoporotic effect on the male skeleton has been known for many years following reports of early ostoporotic fractures in castrate young men. It is therefore surprising that this phenomenon has only been studied relatively recently in men undergoing androgen deprivation for prostate cancer.

The loss of bone mineral density following acute androgen deprivation was reported in females being treated for endometriosis with LHRH agonist therapy (106) and in males undergoing androgen deprivation for benign prostatic hyperplasia (107). The effect in men with prostate cancer was shown subsequently in a controlled study involving the use of serial bone biopsies, biochemical analysis of bone breakdown markers and administration of the Bisphosphonate, Pamidronate (108). The reported results showed that there was a marked increase in bone breakdown in the months following orchidectomy and that this was accompanied by a fall in the bone volume in the non-metastatic skeleton. This effect was osteoclast mediated and the osteoclast mediated osteolysis responsible for the measured phenomenon could be inhibited to a degree by the administration of a bisphosphonate.

Bisphosphonate usage did not become widespread after this because of the view that life expectancy in men with bone metastases was relatively limited. They were therefore unlikely to run in to problems with osteoporosis. However, the concept of androgen administration at an earlier time point in the treatment of prostate cancer, allied to an increasing realisation that bone volume loss in this disease is a problem (109) and that it leads to an increase in the rate of osteoporotic fracture (110), has changed the thinking in urological cancer management. It is now accepted that bone density loss is of the order of 3 to 5% annually following androgen deprivation (111). This is associated with a doubling of the risk of osteoporotic fracture (112) and an increase in the overall fracture rate with time (111). The presence of a skeletal fracture, whether pathological or osteoporotic, has an adverse effect on survival of men with prostate cancer (113).

Bisphosphonates are effective in decreasing the bone loss associated with androgen deprivation therapy. In the previously mentioned study of 28 men with bone metastases undergoing androgen withdrawal therapy with or without Pamidronate (108), it was shown that patients receiving Pamidronate 30 mg weekly for 4 weeks then monthly for a further 5 months following androgen withdrawal had lower indices of bone breakdown and a preservation of bone volume measured (histomorphometrically). Two other studies published subsequently have shown similar effects. In a randomized controlled study of 47 men receiving Pamidronate 60 mg iv 12 weekly, there was a decrease in the bone loss in the hip and lumbar spine regions of men receiving bisphosphonate (114). In the second study, a single infusion of Pamidronate at the point of hormone manipulation was also effective in reducing bone turnover and minimising the loss of bone volume (115). There is therefore, clear evidence of efficacy in this clinical situation and further studies using the more potent Bisphosphonates are under way. The results of these studies are awaited. On the basis of the published evidence, an increasing number of patients are receiving this class of drugs in an adjuvant manner. There are, however, a number of questions which remain to be answered. Which is the most effective agent, how often does the treatment need to be administered and for what duration? Is there a population of patients whose risk is particularly high and what is the effect of synchronous, emerging therapies such as long term steroid usage and cytotoxic chemotherapy? Such questions are important and will hopefully be answered in the future by well conducted, randomised controlled trials in men with the disease.

3. CONCLUSION

Bone metastases from prostate cancer are common and are a source of considerable morbidity. The understanding of their pathogenesis and natural history is improving but the overall knowledge and comprehension of the mechanisms of skeletal spread and subsequent marrow and skeletal dysfunction thereby induced is incomplete. The bisphosphonate class of drugs have many interesting and novel properties. There is evidence that these properties may be of significant benefit in prostate cancer, both in the palliation of the end stage effects of the disease in the skeleton and in the prevention of the adverse effects of bone loss associated with treatment of the disease by androgen deprivation and other therapies.

REFERENCES

1. Blackard CE, Byar DP, Jordan WP Jr. VACURG. Orchiectomy for advanced prostatic carcinoma. A reevaluation. Urology 1973, 1:553–60.
2. Abrams HL, Spiro R, Goldstein N. Metastases in carcinoma. Analysis of 1000 autopsied cases. Cancer 1950, 3:74–85.
3. Galasko CSB, ed. Development of skeletal metastases, pp. 22–51. *Skeletal Metastases*. London: Butterworth, 1986.
4. Carlin B, Andriole GL. The national history of skeletal complications and management of bone metastases in patients with prostate cancer. Cancer 2000, 88:2989–94.
5. Tofe J. Correlation of neoplasms with incidence and localisation of skeletal metastases: An analysis of 1355 bisphosphonate scans. J Nucl Med 1975, 16:986–9.
6. Willis RA. Secondary tumours in bone, pp. 229–50. In: *The Spread of Tumours in the Human Body, 3rd Edition*. Willis RA, ed., London: Butterworth, 1973.
7. Dodds PR, Coride VJ, Lytton B. The role of the vertebral veins in the dissemination of prostate cancer. J Urol 1981, 126:753–5.
8. Batson OV. The function of the vertebral veins and their role in the spread of metastases. Ann Surg 1940, 112:138–49.
9. Scott LJ, Clarke NW, Shanks JH, Testa NG, Lang SH. Interaction of human prostatic epithelial cells with bone marrow endothelium: Banding and invasion. Br J Cancer 2001, 84:1417–23.
10. Lang SH, Clarke NW, George NJR, Allen TD, Testa NG. Interaction of prostatic epithelial cells from benign and malignant tumor tissue with bone- marrow stroma. Prostate 1998, 34:203–13.
11. Nicholson GL, Winkelhoake JL. Organ specification of blood borne tumor metastasis determined by cell adhesions. Nature 1975, 255:230–2.
12. Auerbach R, Lu WC. Specification of adhesions between murine tumor cells and capillary endothelium: An in vitro correlate of preferential metastasis in vivo. Cancer Res 1987, 47:1492–6.
13. Trikha M *et al*. Role of alpha II (b) beta-3 integrin in bone metastasis. Prostate 1998, 35:1982–5.
14. Hart CA, Scott LJ, Bagley S, Brydon AAG, Clarke NW, Lang SH. Role of proteolytic enzymes in human prostate bone metastasis formation: In vivo and in vitro studies. Br J Cancer 2002, 86:11361–40.
15. Lang SH, Clarke NW, George NJR, Testa NG. Primary prostatic epithelial cell binding of human bone marrow stroma and the role of the X2B1 integrin. Clin Exp Metastasis 1997, 15:218–27.

16. Lang SH, Clarke NW, George NJR, Testa NG. Scatter factor influences the formation of prostate epithelial cell colonies of bone marrow stroma in vitro. Clin Exp Metastasis 1999, 17:333–40.
17. Guise TA, Mundy GR. Cancer and bone. Endocr Rev 1998, 19:18–54.
18. Charhon SA, Chapoy MC, Devlin EE *et al*. Histomorphometric analysis of sclerotic bone metastasis from prostatic carcinoma from prostate cancer with special reference to osteomalacia. Cancer 1983, 51:918–24.
19. Clarke NW, McClure J, George NJR. Morphometric evidence from bone resorption and replacement in prostate cancer. Br J Urol 1991, 68:74–80.
20. Clarke NW, McClure J, George NJR. Osteoblast function and osteomalacia in prostate cancer. Eur Urol 1993, 24:286–90.
21. Clarke NW, McClure J, George NJR. Disodium pamidronate identifies differential osteoclastic bone resorption in metastatic prostate cancer. Br J Urol 1992, 69:64–70.
22. Cook GB, Watson FR. Events in the natural history of prostate cancer: Rising salvage, mean age distribution and contingency co-efficient. J Urol 1968, 99:87–96.
23. Galasko CSB. Mechanisms of one destruction in the development of skeletal metastases. Nature 1976, 263:507–10.
24. Urwin GH, Percival RC, Harris S *et al*. Generalised increase in bone resorption in carcinoma of the prostate. Br J Urol 1985, 57:721–3.
25. Tietelbaum SL. Bone resorption by osteoclasts. Science 2000, 289:1504–8.
26. Suda T *et al*. Modulation of osteoclast differentiation and function modulation by new members of the tumor factor receptor by new members of the tumor necrosis factor receptor and ligand families. Endocr Rev 1999, 20:345–57.
27. Thomas RJ *et al*. Breast cancer cells interact with osteoblasts to support osteoclast formation. Endocrinol 1999, 140:4451–8.
28. Bryden AAG, Islam SH, Shanks JH, George N, Clarke NW. Expression of pthrp. In bone metastases from prostate cancer. Prostate Cancer Prostate Dis 2002, 40:673–6.
29. Bryden AAG, Hoyland J, Freemant AJ, George N, Clarke NW. Role of pthrp in primary and metastatic prostate cancer. Br J Cancer 2002, 86:1136–42.
30. Globel BH. Bleeding disorders, pp. 575–607. In: *Cancer Nursing – Principles and Practice (Ed 3)*. Groenwald S, Frogge M, Goodman M, Yarbru C, eds, Boston: Jones Bartlett, 1993.
31. Esper P, Pienta KJ. Supportive core in the patient with hormone refractory prostate cancer. Semin Urol Oncol 1997, 15:56–64.
32. Alpoers P, Chappell R, Schaibold H. Erythropoietin in urology oncology. Eur Urol 2001, 39:1–8.
33. Beshara S, Letochka H, Linde T. Anaemia associated with advanced prostatic adenocarcinoma effects of recombinant human erythropoietin. Prostate 1997, 31:153–60.
34. Johannsson JE, Wersall P, Brandberg Y. Efficiency of erythropoietin beta on haemoglobin, Q o L and transfusion needs inpatients with anaemia Due To HRPC – a randomised study. Scand J Urol Nephrol 2001, 35:288–94.
35. Spencer H, Lewin I. Derangements of calcium metabolism in patients with neoplastic bone involvement. J Chronic Dis 1963, 16:713–26.
36. Mahadevia P, Ramaswamy A, Greenwald E, Wollner D, Markham D. Hypercalcaemia in prostate cancer. Arch Intern Med 1983, 143:1339–42.
37. Soerdjbalie-Maikeov V, Pelger RE, Lycklama A, Nijeholt GA *et al*. Strontium 89 (medastron) and the bisphosphonate olpandronate reduce the incidence of spinal cord

compression in patients with hormone-refractory prostate cancer metastatic to the skeleton. Eur J Nucl Med Mol Imaging 2002, 29:494–8.
38. Coleman RE, Rubens RD. The clinical course of bone metastases from breast cancer. Br J Cancer 1987, 55:61–6.
39. Neville-Webb HC, Holden I, Coleman RE. The anti-tumour activity of bisphosphonates. Cancer Treat Rev 2002, 28:305–19.
40. Berrutt A, Dogliotti L, Tucci M et al. Metabolic bone disease induced by prostate cancer: Rational for use of bisphosphonates. J Urol 2001, 166:2023–31.
41. Townsend MF, Saunders WH, Northway RU et al. Fractures associated with LHRH agonists used in prostate cancer. Bone 1997, 79:545–50.
42. Oefefein MG, Ricchiuttiv, Conrand WV et al. Skeletal fractures negatively correlate uwith overall survival in men with prostate cancer. J Urol 2002, 168:1005–7.
43. Osbourn J, Getzenberg RH, Trump DL et al. Spinal and compression in prostate cancer. J Neurol Oncol 1995, 23:135–47.
44. Bayley A, Milosevic M, Bland R, Logue JPL et al. A prospective study of factors predicting clinically occult spinal and compression in patients with metastatic prostate carcinoma. Cancer 2001, 92:303–10.
45. Saad F, Gleason DM, Murray R et al. Of randomised placebo controlled trial of zoledronic acid in patients with hormone refractory metastatic prostate cancer. J Natl Cancer Inst 2002, 94:1458–68.
46. Kuban Da AM, Siegried SV. Characteristics of spinal cord compression in adenocarcinoma of the prostate. Urology 1986, 28:364–9.
47. Huddart RA, Rajan B, Lau M et al. Spinal cord decompression and carcinoma of the prostate: Treatment outcome and prognostic factors. Radiothe Oncol 1997, 44:292–36.
48. Iacovou J, Marks JC, Abrams PH et al. Cord compression and carcinoma of prostate: Is laminectomy justified. Br J Urol 1985, 57:733–6.
49. Pollen JJ, Schmidt JD. Bone pain in metastatic cancer of the prostate. Urology 1979, 13:129–34.
50. Shuttleworth ED, Blandy JP. Carcinoma of the prostate, pp. 57:773–736. In:.Blandy JP, ed., London: Urology Blackwell Scientific Publ, 1976.
51. Francis MD, Russell RGG, Fleisch H. Diphosphonates inhibit formation of calcium phosphate crystals in vitro and pathological calcification in vivo. Science 1969, 165:1264–6.
52. Fleisch H, Russell RGG, Bisaz S, Mühlbauer RC, Williams DA. The inhibitory effect of phosphonates on the formation of calcium phosphate crystals in vitro and on aortic and kidney calcification in vivo. Eur J Clin Invest 1970, 1:12–18.
53. Fleisch H, Russell RGG, Francis MD. Diphosphonates inhibit hydroxyapatite dissolution in vitro and bone resorption in tissue culture and in vivo. Science 1969, 165:1262–4.
54. Russell RGG, Mühlbauer RC, Bisaz S, Williams DA, Fleisch H. The influence of pyrophosphate, condensed phosphates, phosphonates and other phosphate compounds on the dissolution of hydroxyapatite in vitro and on bone resorption induced by parathyroid hormone in tissue culture and in thyroparathyroidectomised rats. Calcif Tissue Res 1970, 6:183–96.
55. Garanttini S, Guaitani A, Mantovani A. Effect of etidronate disodium on the interactions between malignancy and bone. Am J Med 1987, 82:29–33.
56. Schenk R, Merz WA, Mühlbauer R, Russell RGG, Fleisch H. Effect of ethane-1-hydroxy-1,1-diphosphonate (EHDP) and dichloromethylene diphosphonate

(CL2MDP) on the calcification and resorption of cartilage and bone in the tibial epiphysis and metaphysis of rats. Calcif Tissue Res 1973, 11:196–214.
57. Schenk R, Eggli P, Fleisch H, Rosini S. Quantitative morphometric evaluation of the inhibitory activity of new aminobisphosphonates on bone resorption in the rat. Calcif Tissue Int 1986, 38:342–9.
58. Gasser AB, Morgan DB, Fleisch HA.Richelle LJ. The influence of two diphosphonates on calcium metabolism in the rat. Clin Sci 1972, 43:31–45.
59. Mühlbauer RC, Fleisch H. A method for continual monitoring of bone resorption in rats: Evidence for a diurnal rhythm. Am J Physiol 1990, 259:R679–89.
60. Mühlbauer RC, Russell RGG, Williams DA, Fleisch H. The effects of diphosphonates, polyphosphates and calcitonin on „immobilisation osteoporosis" in rats. Eur J Clin Invest 1971, 1:336–44.
61. Jung A, Mermillod B, Barras C, Baud M, Courvoisier B. Inhibition by two diphosphonates of bone lysis in tumor conditioned media. Cancer Res 1981, 41:3233–7.
62. Martodam RR, Thornton KS, Sica DA, D'Souza SM, Flora L, Mundy GR. The effects of dichloromethylene diphosphonate on hypercalcemia and other parameters of the humoral hypercalcemia of malignancy in the rat leydig cell tumor. Calcif Tissue Int 1983, 35:512–19.
63. Jung A, Bornand J, Mermillod B, Edouard C, Meunier PJ. Inhibition by diphosphonates of bone resorption induced by the walker tumor of the rat. Cancer Res 1984, 44:3007–11.
64. Guaitani A, Polentarutti N, Filippeschi S, Marmonti L, Corti F, Italia C et al. Effects of disodium etidronate in murine tumor models. Eur J Cancer Clin Oncol 1984, 20:685–93.
65. Krempien B, Wingen F, Eichmann T, Müller M, Schmähl D. Protective effects of a prophylactic treatment with the bisphosphonate 3-amino-1-hydroxypropane-1,1-bisphosphonic acid on the development of tumor osteopathies in the rat: Experimental studies with the walker carcinosarcoma. Oncology 1988, 256:41–6.
66. Nemoto R, Uchida K, Tsutsumi M, Koiso K, Satou S, Satou T. A model of localized osteolysis induced by the MBT-2 tumor in mice and its responsiveness to etidronate disodium. J Cancer Res Clin Oncol 1987, 113:539–43.
67. Radl J, Croese JW, Zurcher C.Van den Enden-Vieveen MHM, Brondijk RJ, Kazil M, Haaijman JJ, Reitsma PH, Bijvoet OLM. Influence of treatment with APD-bisphosphonate on the bone lesions in the mouse 5T2 multiple myeloma. Cancer 1985, 55:1030–40.
68. Hiraga T, Tanaka S, Yamamoto M, Nakajima T, Ozawa H. Inhibitory effects of bisphosponate (YM175) on bone resorption induced by a metastatic bone tumor. Bone 1996, 18:1–7.
69. Pollard M, Luckert PH. Effects of dichloromethylene diphosphonate on the osteolytic and osteoplastic effects of rat prostate adenocarcinoma cells. J Natl Cancer Inst 1985, 5:949–54.
70. Nemoto R, Sato S, Nishijima Y, Miyakawa I, Koiso K, Harada M. Effects of a new bisphosphonate (ahbubp) on osteolysis induced by human prostate cancer cells in nude mice. J Urol 1990, 144:770–4.
71. Lee YP, Schwarz EM, Davies M, Jo M, Gates J, Zhang X et al. Use of zoledronate to treat osteoblastic versus osteolytic lesions in a severe-combined-immunodeficient mouse model. Cancer Res 2002, 62:5564–70.

72. Sasaki A, Boyce BF, Story B, Wright KR, Chapman M, Boyce R et al. Bisphosphonate risedronate reduces metastatic human breast cancer burden in bone in nude mice. Cancer Res 1995, 55:3551–7.
73. Sasaki A, Kitamura K, Alcalde RE, Tanaka T, Suzuki A, Etoh Y, Matsumura T. Effect of a newly developed bisphosphonate, YH 529, on osteolytic bone metastases in nude mice. Int J Cancer 1998, 77:279–85.
74. Green JR, Müller K, Jaeggi KA. Preclinical pharmacology of CGP 42'446, a new, potent, heterocyclic bisphosphonate compound. J Bone Miner Res 1994, 9:745–51.
75. Hughes DE, Wright Uy KRHL, Sasaki A, Yoneda Roodman Mundy Boyce TGDGRBF. Bisphosphonates promote apoptosis in murine osteoclasts in vitro and in vivo. J Bone Miner Res 1995, 10:1478–87.
76. Sahni M, Guenther HL, Fleisch H, Collin P, Martin TJ. Bisphosphonates act on rat bone resorption through the mediation of osteoblasts. J Clin Invest 1993, 91:2004–11.
77. Luckman SP, Coxon FP, Ebetino FH, Russell RGG, Rogers MJ. Heterocycle-containing bisphosphonates cause apoptosis and inhibit bone resorption by preventing protein prenylation: Evidence from structure-activity relationships in J774 macrophages. J Bone Miner Res 1998, 13:1668–78.
78. Van Beek E, Pieterman E, Cohen L, Löwik C, Papapoulos S. Farnesyl pyrophosphate synthase is the molecular target of nitrogen-containing bisphosphonates. Biochem Biophys Res Commun 1999, 264:108–1.
79. Bergstrom JD, Bostedor RG, Masarachia PJ, Reszka AA, Rodan G. Alendronate is a specific, nanomolar inhibitor of farnesyl diphosphate synthase. Arch Biochem Biophys 2000, 373:231–41.
80. Fisher JE, Rogers MJ, Halasy JM, Luckman SP, Hughes DE, Masarachia PJ et al. Alendronate mechanism of action: Gernylgeraniol, an intermediate in the mevalonate pathway, prevents inhibition of osteoclast formation, bone resorption, and kinase activation in vitro. Proc Natl Acad Sci 1999, 96:133–8.
81. Frith JC, Mönkkönen J, Blackburn GM, Russell RGG, Rogers MJ. Clodronate and liposome-encapsulated clodronate are metabolised to a toxic ATP analog, ADENOSINE5' (-dichloromethylene) triphosphate, by mammalian cells in vitro. J Bone Miner Res 1997, 12:1358–67.
82. Mundy GR, Yoneda T. Facilitation and suppression of bone metastasis. Clin Orthop Relat Res 1995, 312:34–44.
83. Guise TA, Mundy GR. Cancer and bone. Endocr Rev 1998, 19:18–54.
84. Van der Pluijm G, Vloedgraven H, van Beek E, van der Wee-Pals L, Löwik C, Papapoulos S. Bisphosphonates inhibit the adhesion of breast cancer cells to bone matrices in vitro. J Clin Invest 1996, 98:698–705.
85. Boissier S, Magnetto S, Frappart L, Cuzin B, Ebetino FH, Delmas PD. Bisphosphonates inhibit prostate and breast carcinoma cell adhesion to unmineralized and mineralized bone extracellular matrices. Cancer Res 1997, 57:3890–4.
86. Derenne S, Amiot M, Barille S, Collette M, Robillard N, Berthaud P et al. Zoledronate is a potent inhibitor of myeloma cell growth and secretion of IL-6 and MMP-1 by the tumoral envronment. J Bone Miner Res 1999, 14:2048–65.
87. Lee MV, Fong EM, Singer FR, Guenette RS. Bisphosphonate treatment inhibits the growth of prostate cancer cells. Cancer Res 2001, 2602–8.
88. Shipman CM, Rogers MJ, Apperley JF, Russell RGG, Croucher PI. Bisphosphonates induce apoptosis in human myeloma cell lines: A novel anti-tumour activity. Br J Haematol 1997, 98:665–72.

89. Fromigue O, Lagneaux L, Body J-J. Bisphosphonates induce breast cancer cell death in vitro. J Bone Miner Res 2000, 15:2211–21.
90. Jagdev SP, Coleman RE, Shipman CM, Rostami-H A, Croucher PI. The bisphosphonate, zoledronic acid, induces apoptosis of breast cancer cells: Evidence for synergy with paclitaxel. Br J Cancer 2001, 84:1126–34.
91. Hiraga T, Williams Mundy GRP, Yoneda T. The bisphosphonate ibandronate promotes apoptosis in MDA-MB-231 human breast cancer cells in bone metastases. Cancer Res 2001, 61:4418–24.
92. Wood J, Bonjean K, Ruetz S, Bellahcène A, Devy L, Foidart JM et al. Novel antiangiogenic effects of the bisphosphonate compound zoledronic acid. J Pharmacol Exp Ther 2002, 302:1055–61.
93. Okamoto T, Yamagishi Y, Inagaki Y, Amano S, Takeuchi M, Kikuchi S et al. Incadronate disodium inhibits advanced glycation end products-induced angiognesis in vitro. Biochem Biophys Res Commun 2002, 297:419–24.
94. Masarachia P, Weinreb M, Balena R, Rodan GA. Comparison of the distribution of 3h-alendronate and 3h-etidronate in rat and mouse bones. Bone 1996, 19:281–90.
95. Lycklama T, Tammela TL, Lincholm TS, Seppanen J. The effect of combined intravenous and oral clodronate treatment on bone pain in patients with metastatic prostate cancer. Ann Chir Gynaecol 1994, 83:316–19.
96. Cesswell SM, English PJ, Hall RR et al. Relief and quality of life assessment following intravenous and oral clodronate in hormone escape metastatic prostate cancer. Pain 1995, 76:360–5.
97. Purhoit OP, Anthony C, Radstone CR et al. High dose intravenous pamidronate for metastatic bone pain. Br J Cancer 1994, 70:554–8.
98. Heidenreich A, Elert A, Hoffmann R. Ibandronate in the treatment of prostate cancer associated with painful osseous metastases. Prostate Cancer Prostate Dis 2002, 2:231–5.
99. Ernst DS, Brasher P, Hagan N et al. A randomised controlled trail of intravenous clodronate in patients with metastatic bone disease and pain. J Pain Symptom Manage 1997, 13:319–26.
100. Kylmala T, Taube T, Tammela T, et al. Concomitant intravenous and oral clodronate in the relief of bone pain – a double-blinded placebo controlled cross-over study in patients with prostate cancer. Br J Cancer 1997, 76:939–42.
101. Lipton A, Glover D, Garvey H et al. Pamidronate in the treatment of bone metastases: Results of 2 dose ranging trials in patients with breast or prostate cancer. Ann Oncol 1994, 5(Suppl. 7):35–53.
102. Smith JA. Palliation of painful bone metastases from prostate cancer using sodium etidronate: Results of a randomised, prospective placebo controlled study. J Urol 1989, 141:85–7.
103. Dearnaley DP, Sydes MR. Preliminary evidence that oral clodronate delays symptomatic progression of bone metastases from prostate cancer. First results of the MRC PRO5 trail. Am Soc Clin Oncol 2001, 1693.
104. Canil CM, Tannock IF. Should bisphosphonates be used routinely in patients with prostate cancer metastatic to bone. J Natl Cancer Inst 2002, 94:1422–3.
105. Coleman RE. Metastatic bone disease and the role of biochemical markers of bone metabolism in benign and malignant diseases. Cancer Treat. Revs 2001, 27:133–5.
106. Johannsen JS, Riis BJ, Hassager C et al. The effect of a gonadotropin-releasing hormone agonist analog (nafarelin) on bone metabolism. J Clin Endocrinol Metab 1988, 67:701–6.

107. Goldray D, Weisman Y, Jacard N *et al*. Decreased bone marrow chemistry in elderly men treated with the gnrh agonist decapeptyl (d-trp-6-gnrh). J Clin Endocrinol Metab 1993, 76:288–92.
108. Clarke NW, McClure J, George NJ. The effects of orchidectomy on skeletal metabolism in metastatic prostate cancer. Scand. J Urol. Nephrology 1993, 27:475–83.
109. Daniell HW. Osteoporosis after orchidectomy for prostate cancer. J Urol 1997, 157:439–41.
110. Townsend MF, Saunders WH, Northway RO *et al*. Fractures associated with LHRH agonist used in the treatment of prostate cancer. Bone 1997, 79:545–8.
111. Ross RW, Small EJ. Osteoporosis in men treated with androgen deprivation therapy for prostate cancer. J Urol 2002, 167:1952–6.
112. Ricchiuti VS, Conrad PW, Oefelein M. Skeletal fractures associated with androgen suppression induced osteoporosis – the chemical incidence and risk factors for prostate cancer patients. J Urol 2001, 165:290–4.
113. Oefelein M, Ricchiuti V, Conrad W, Resnick MI. Skeletal fractures negatively correlate with overall survival in men with prostate cancer. J Urol 2002, 168:1005–7.
114. Smith MR, McGovern FJ, Zeetman MD *et al*. Pamidronate to prevent bone loss during androgen deprivation therapy for prostate cancer. N Engl J Med 2001, 948–54.
115. Diamond TH, Winters J, Smith A *et al*. The anti-osteoporotic efficacy of intravenous pamidronate in men with prostate carcinoma receiving combined androgen blockade: A double-blind, randomised, placebo controlled cross-over study. Cancer 2001, 92:1444–50.

Chapter 13

HORMONE THERAPY FOR PROSTATE CANCER

Mike Shelley[1], Charles L. Bennett[2], Derek Nathan[3], Oliver Sartor[4]

[1] *Cochrane Prostatic Diseases and Urological Cancers Group, Cochrane Unit, Research Department, Velindre NHS Trust, Cardiff, Wales, UK*
[2] *The Chicago VA Healthcare System/Lakeside Division, the Robert H Lurie Comprehensive Cancer Center, the Division of Hematology/Oncology of the Department of Medicine, Chicago, IL, USA*
[3] *The Institute for Health Services Research and Policy Studies of Northwestern University, Chicago, IL, USA*
[4] *The Louisiana State University Stanley Scott Cancer Center, New Orleans, Louisiana, USA*

Abstract: For the last six decades the standard palliative option for patients with advanced prostate cancer has centered on androgen deprivation strategies. The different approaches for achieving androgen deprivation, which include surgical castration or medical castration (oestrogen agonists, antiandrogens, LHRH analogues and agonists), appear to be therapeutically equivalent, inducing symptomatic relief in up to 80% of patients. However, androgen deprivation is associated with significant side-effects such as cardiotoxicity, gynaecomastia and impotence. For patients with localised disease, androgen deprivation has been explored in the neo-adjuvant and adjuvant setting. There is no convincing evidence that neo-adjuvant hormone therapy combined with radical prostatectomy provides long-term efficacy. Adjuvant hormone therapy with bicalutamide has shown a 42% reduction in the risk of disease progression compared to placebo, but long-term follow up is required to establish an improvement in overall survival. Results from randomised controlled trials of neo-adjuvant and adjuvant hormone therapy with radiotherapy suggest benefits in terms of freedom from disease and perhaps survival, particularly in patients with locally advanced or lymph node positive disease. Data from randomised trials and meta-analyses do not provide strong evidence that immediate hormone therapy clearly improves overall survival, although progression-free survival may be prolonged in patients with lymph node positive disease. There is no consensus on the use of combined androgen blockage (CAB), despite the wealth of data in the literature, and the small survival advantage reported in some meta-analyses needs to be balanced against the side-effects of CAB and the consequent reduction in quality of life. Intermittent androgen deprivation (IAD) has been used to delay the onset of androgen-independent tumor growth and reduce the side-effects associated with continuous therapy. Although repeat clinical responses have been documented and quality of life may be improved with this treatment, IAD must be considered experimental.

Key words: prostate cancer, hormone therapy, neo-adjuvant, adjuvant, combined androgen blockade, intermittent androgen deprivation

It has been known for over 60 years that prostate carcinoma is sensitive to circulating androgens (1) and that reducing the level of plasma androgens retards the growth of prostatic carcinoma. This has led to the routine clinical practice of androgen deprivation as an important treatment approach for patients with carcinoma of the prostate.

The major plasma androgen is testosterone, approximately 95% of which is secreted by the testes and the remainder by the adrenal glands. Circulating testosterone diffuses passively into prostate cancer cells and is rapidly converted to 5α-dihydrotestosterone (DHT), by the enzyme 5α-reductase localized on the nuclear membrane DHT selectively binds to the nuclear androgen receptor (AR) with an affinity five times that of testosterone. This binding induces a conformational change and dimerization of the AR, revealing a DNA binding domain, allowing the complex to functionally interact with specific nucleotides sequences known as hormone response elements or HRE. The HRE are genetically located on the promoter region and the interaction results in the up-regulation of growth factors, such as fibroblast growth factor-7 and possibly epidermal growth factor and insulin growth factor-1, influencing prostatic cell proliferation (2). Depriving androgen sensitive prostate carcinoma cells of androgens leads to prostatic atrophy and cell death by apoptosis.

1. ANDROGEN DEPRIVATION THERAPIES

Androgen deprivation is achieved either surgically or clinically, with drugs that interfere with the production or function of androgens. Surgical castration (bilateral orchidectomy) offers an effective treatment for advanced carcinoma of the prostate with approximately 70% of patients showing beneficial responses (1). In an early Veterans Administration Co-operative Urological Research Group (VAGURG) study, orchidectomy was associated with a 73% response rate and a 35% 5-year overall survival compared with 66% and 20%, respectively, for patients receiving placebo (3). Additional follow-up of this study, however, indicated similar response rates but improved pain relief and performance status with orchidectomy (4). Orchidectomy is now considered the gold standard by which all other treatments are compared, and in a recent EORTC study of 328 patients, orchidectomy was found to have a similar time to metastatic progression and overall survival rate compared to cyproterone acetate and stiboestrol (5). Orchidectomy can be accomplished as an outpatient procedure and reduces circulating testosterone by 95% within 3 to 12 hours. Additional advantages, apart from the speed and ease of this method, include low cost and favourable patient compliance. However, orchidectomy is associated with feminization, gynaecomastia, hot flushes, impotence and loss of libido (6). Psychologically, 50% of men regret the decision to undergo orchidectomy compared with other treatment options (7), although these effects may be ameliorated, to some extent, by the implantation of testicular protheses (8).

Estrogens were shown to affect the progression of prostate cancer in the 1940s, and provided an alternative to orchidectomy in patients unable to accept this procedure. The synthesis of diethylstilbestrol (DES) in 1938, provided the first oral estrogen for the treatment of prostate cancer. The main action of DES is suppression of luteinizing hormone (LH) from the pituitary gland leading to the subsequent reduction in testosterone synthesis and secretion by the testes. DES also increases the level of circulating sex-hormone binding globulin (SHBG) which reduces the concentration of free plasma testosterone. There is also evidence for a direct cytotoxic action of DES on prostate carcinoma cells *in vitro* probably through promotion of cell cycle arrest and apoptosis (9). This agent was shown to be active clinically at a daily dose of 3 mg, with 70–80% of patients with metastatic disease experiencing symptomatic relief (10). The early VACURG trials provided significant information on the activity of DES but also highlighted the severe side-effects of this therapy particularly the thromboembolic cardiovascular complications, limiting its' usefulness. The cardiotoxicity of DES toxicity is not amelioratied by the co-administration of low dose warfarin (11), however, there has been renewed interest with DES in those patients who have failed combined androgen blockade with reported response rates of 66% by prostate-specific antigen (PSA) criteria (12).

The severity of side-effects associated with DES has led to its general replacement with luteinizing hormone-releasing hormone (LHRH) analogues such as leuprolide and gorserelin. These agents provide medical castration by stimulating LHRH receptors in the pituitary gland, which initially induce a testosterone surge, but on continued use, downregulate LHRH receptors, paradoxically leading to a reduction in the testicular formation of testosterone. The initial testosterone surge may last for up to

2 weeks and gives rise to the 'flare phenomenon' in some patients, which may lead to increased tumor growth, worsening of bone pain and local symptoms (13). LHRH analogues alone, are therefore not recommended as first line therapy for patients at risk of spinal cord compression, urinary obstruction or with painful bone metastases. Anti-androgens may be given prior to LHRH analogues to reduce the severity of the testosterone flare. A systematic review and meta-anlaysis of ten randomised controlled trials, reported no significant difference in overall survival between orchidectomy and LHRH agonists (14). All currently available LHRH analogues appear to be clinically equivalent and there are fewer cardiovascular complications and gynecomastia with LHRH analogues compared to estrogen therapy, but they are associated with hot flushes, loss of libido and impotence. Since LHRH analogues need to be administered daily, significant efforts have been made to produce slow release preparations and clinical trials indicate that depot forms reduce and maintain testosterone at castrate levels for several months (15).

There are a number of antiandrogenic agents available with clinical activity in patients with prostate cancer and generally fall into two categories; steroidal antiandrogens and non-steroidal antiandrogens (NSAA). Progestational steroidal antiandrogens include cyproterone acetate, medroxyprogesterone acetate, hydroxprogesterone acetate and chlormadione acetate, and have been used as primary therapy for prostate cancer at some point in the past (16). They inhibit the secretion of LH from the pituitary gland in addition to competitively inhibiting the binding of DHT to the prostate androgen receptor resulting in reduced synthesis of testosterone. Only cyproterone acetate has been critically evaluated clinically and reduces the flare associated with LHRH agonists and can maintain potency in about 40% of patients (17). Cyproterone acetate it is not available in all countries due to the cardiovascular complications seen with this agent. The NSAA flutamide, nilutamide and bicalutamide, sometimes referred to as 'pure antiandrogen', also compete with testosterone and DHT binding to the intracellular prostatic androgen receptor. In addition, they interfere with the testosterone negative feedback mechanism of the hypothalamic- pituitary axis which results in an increase in LHRH, LH and a self-limiting increase in testosterone. As a monotherapy, flutamide has been reported to be equivalent to DES in two studies (18, 19), however, a third randomized study reported inferior results for flutamide with response rates of 50% and 62% (DES) (20). In a randomized study with a follow-up period of 8.5 years, nilutamide combined with orchidectomy improved patient survival compared to orchidectomy plus placebo (21) but appears to have more serious side-effects than the other NSAAs (22). Bicalutamide is the most recently available pure antiandrogen and is well tolerated with a halflife (7 days) that allows daily dosing. As a monotherapy, bicalutamide is comparable to castration (orchidectomy or 3.6mg goserelin) in terms of time to progression (hazard ratio 1.20) and overall survival (hazard ratio 1.31), but has significantly less inhibition of libido and physical capacity (23). The main side-effects of the pure antiandrogens are breast pain and gynecomastia, fatigue, back and pelvic pain and gastrointestinal disturbances. Bicalutamide may have a palliative role in reducing pain in patients in who have failed first-line hormonal therapy (24).

The ultimate aim of hormone therapy is to improve survival in potentially curable patients and improve the quality of life of patients receiving palliative treatment. As a result hormonal therapy for prostate cancer is continually evolving due to the advent of PSA monitoring and early detection, new agents for androgen deprivation and investigational schedules for hormone manipulation. In this dynamic arena there are a number of controversies relating to androgen deprivation such as neo-adjuvant/adjuvant therapy, the timing of hormone therapy, combined androgen blockade, and intermittent therapy and the sections that follow will review these topics.

2. NEO-ADJUVANT AND ADJUVANT HORMONE THERAPY

Radical prostatectomy is a primary treatment modality for localized disease with the aim of complete tumor resection. Neo-adjuvant hormone therapy has been used to reduce tumor volume and improve the outcome following radical prostatectomy. Although neo-adjuvant therapy with prostatectomy has been widely used, the data from randomized trials, at present, do not provide conclusive evidence for its' long term efficacy. From 1994 to 1997, at least seven centres have reported randomized trials of neoadjuvant therapy prior to radical prostatectomy (25–31). Four trials used an LHRH agonist plus an antiandrogen whereas the other three trials used a single agent of either a LHRH agonist, an antiandrogen or estramustine (Table 1). Neo-adjuvant hormone therapy decreased the rate of positive margins in 6 out 7 trials, all of which were statistically significant. The average decrease was from 41% (range 14 to 65%) to 21% (range 8 to 28%), however, the benefit appears to be restricted to patients with

Table 1. Randomised trials of neo-adjuvant hormone therapy (NeoA.) prior to prostatectomy (RP)

Trial	Pt. No		Regime	Positive Margins %		Seminal Vesicle Invasion		Lymph Node metastases	
	NeoA.	RP		NeoA.	RP	NeoA.	RP	NeoA.	RP
Labrie (25)	90	71	Leuprolide Flutamide	8	34*	0	6	7	3
Hugosson (26)	56	55	Triptorelin Cyproterone	23	41*	–	–	15	5
Soloway (27)	138	144	Leuprolide Flutamide	18	48*	15	22	6	6
Van Poppel (28)	65	62	estramustine	28	37	–	–	–	–
Dalkin (29)	28	28	Goserelin	18	14*	18	14	–	–
Goldenberg (30)	101	91	Cyproterone	28	65*	28	14*	3	–
Witjes (31)	164	190	Goserelin Flutamide	27	46*	–	–	23*	7

* Significantly different

clinical stage T2b lesions, since no significant improvements were seen with T3 disease (28, 31).

No improvement in the rate of seminal vesicle invasion was seen with neo-adjuvant therapy, nor any significant reduction in the rate of lymph node metastases compared to controls. Longer follow-up of these studies, ranging from 3 to 7 years, indicated that neo-adjuvant therapy did not significantly improve the biochemical recurrence rate and suggests that the routine induction of androgen deprivation before prostatectomy may not be clinically useful (32–34)

The majority of randomized trials administered neo-adjuvant therapy for 3 months, although there does not appear to any rational basis for this. However, significant pathological changes in prostate cancer tissue induced after 3 months of neo-adjuvant therapy have been reported and include reduced cell vacuolization, intra-luminal crystalloids and a lower prevalence of capsular penetration (35). Two studies have investigated extending the period of neo-adjuvant androgen deprivation. The first randomized 547 men to either 3 months or 8 months neo-adjuvant therapy with monthly leuprolide and daily flutamide (36). Twenty three percent of patients in the 3 month group were reported to have positive surgical margins compared to 12% in the 8 month group ($p = 0.01$). A higher incidence of positive lymph nodes was identified in the 3 month group (3%) compared to the 8 month group (0.4%, $p = 0.038$). The results of this trial were too immature to comment on biochemical recurrence rates. The second trial was a prospective cohort study of 756 men, 240 of whom received neo-adjuvant androgen deprivation therapy for either 3 months or 5 months, and 516 treated with radical prostatectomy alone (37). The neo-adjuvant group had a reduced rate of pathological indicators of prognosis compared to the surgery alone group, the 5 month group having significantly lower rates than the 3 month group. At a median follow-up of 4 years, the risk of PSA failure was significantly in favour of 5 months neo-adjuvant therapy compared to surgery alone (hazard ratio 0.6, 95% confidence interval 0.30 to 0.94), whereas there was no significant different for the 3 month group and surgery. This suggests a clinical benefit of prolonged androgen deprivation but needs to be tested in a randomized trial.

The reduction in tumor volume by neo-adjuvant therapy and the associated change in pathology do not appear to influence the ease of prostatectomy. The time required for surgery, the total blood loss and the percentage of patients achieving nerve-sparing surgery are not affected by neo-adjuvant therapy (27, 31).

Men who are at high risk of cancer recurrence following radical prostatectomy are appropriate candidates for adjuvant hormone therapy. The role of adjuvant hormone therapy in this setting has been recently reviewed in a retrospective analysis of 707 cases attending the Mayo Clinic (38). The data suggest that adjuvant therapy has a significant impact on PSA progression and cause-specific survival in pT3b patients with seminal vesicle invasion and lymph node disease. After adjusting for patient age, preoperative PSA, margins, grade and ploidy, the risk ratio for stage pT3b patients undergoing radical prostatectomy was 0.3 (95% confidence interval 0.2 to 0.7) for prostate cancer death, in favour of hormone therapy. However, these results should be viewed with caution, since they are derived from a retrospective nonrandomized study.

A recent randomized trial reported on the efficacy of immediate adjuvant hormone therapy with goserelin or bilateral orchidectomy compared with observation, after radical prostatectomy and pelvic lymphadenectomy in 98 patients with positive lymph nodes (39). After a median follow-up of 7.1 years, overall survival was significantly improved in patients receiving the adjuvant hormone therapy compared to the observation group (85% versus 64.7%, $p = 0.02$). Adjuvant therapy also significantly reduced the cancer-specific survival (6.3% versus 34%, $p = 0.01$) and decreased the rate of disease recurrence (14.9% versus 89.4%, $p = < 0.001$). However, this trial has been criticized for the small number of patients randomized, the Gleason score imbalance between groups, the relatively short follow-up time and the low overall survival (40).

There has been considerable interest in the use of NSAA as adjuvant therapy for patients with localized disease. A large international program consisting of 3 randomised trials, has evaluated the efficacy of 150mg bicalutamide given as immediate therapy, either alone or as adjuvant therapy to prostatectomy, radiotherapy or watchful waiting in 8,113 men with localized or locally advanced prostate cancer (41). Patients were randomized to receive daily bicalutamide or placebo in addition to standard care. Across the entire program, 922 patients (11.4%) showed evidence of objective disease progression, as determined by bone scan, including 363 in the bicalutamide arm and 559 in the placebo group (hazard ratio 0.58, 95% confidence interval 0.51 – 0.66, $p < 0.0001$). This translates into a significant reduction of 42% in the risk of disease progression with bicalutamide compared with those receiving standard care alone. The main side-effects associated with bicalutamide were gynecomastia plus breast pain (53%), breast pain alone (20%), and gynecomastia alone (13%), and were reported to be mild to moderate in 90% of cases. The incidence of hot flushes was 9% with bicalutamide and 5% in the standard care alone group, with corresponding levels for decreased libido and impotence of 4% versus 1% and

9% versus 6%. As yet, there is no difference in survival between the two groups since relatively few deaths have occurred (6%) and the majority of these were unrelated to prostate cancer. Longer follow-up will determine whether the reduction in risk of disease progression seen with bicalutamide translates into an overall survival benefit. Androgen deprivation therapy has been combined with radiotherapy in a number of trials (Table 2). The rationale for using neo-adjuvant therapy is to debulk the tumor and increase the efficacy of radiotherapy, whereas with adjuvant therapy a synergistic interaction results in increased apoptosis.

It is quite difficult to separate the role of these two mechanisms in many clinical trials because of overlap. In some neo-adjuvant therapy trials, androgen deprivation may be continued during radiotherapy. In others trials, early adjuvant therapy is started concomitantly with later fractions of radiotherapy. Further, androgen deprivation may commence prior to radiotherapy and may continue during and after radiotherapy. It is uncertain whether one sequence is superior.

The RTOG 86-10 randomised study was designed to evaluate androgen deprivation, with goserelin plus flutamide, in the neo-adjuvant setting and during radiotherapy (42). In patients with Gleason score 2–6, androgen deprivation was associated with a highly significant improvement in local control, disease progression and overall survival compared to patients receiving radiotherapy alone.

Four randomized studies evaluated neo-adjuvant therapy plus continued hormone therapy during and after radiotherapy. A Medical Research Council (MRC) study (43) randomized 277 men with locally advanced prostate cancer (T2 – T4 NXMO) to orchidedctomy (90), radiotherapy alone (88) or combined therapy (99). Androgen ablation with orchidectomy, either alone or in combination with radiotherapy, significantly reduced the incidence of metastases compared to radiotherapy alone. The 7–year overall survival rates were not significantly different between the three groups and ranged approximately from 30–40%, suggesting that androgen deprivation with radiotherapy is no better than androgen deprivation alone. A French 3-armed, randomized study also examined the benefits of neo-adjuvant and adjuvant hormone therapy with radiotherapy (44). Patients were randomly allocated radiotherapy alone, 3 months of neo-adjuvant total androgen blockage prior to radiotherapy or a combination therapy 3 months before, during, and 6 months after radiotherapy. Those patients receiving total androgen blockage had significantly lower rate of positive biopsies at 12 and 24 months ($p < 0.0001$). A small Swedish trial randomized 91 patients with non-metastatic prostate cancer to neo-adjuvant androgen deprivation

Table 2. Randomised trials of neo-adjuvant and adjuvant androgen deprivation (AD) combined with radiotherapy

Trial	Patients	Interventions Compared	Outcome
Pilepich (42)	471, T2-T4 +/− lymph node disease	RT + Goreselin + Flutamide vs RT alone	Local control, DP and OS significantly better with AD.
Fellows (43)	277 locally advanced (T2-T4 NXM0)	Orichectomy vs RT* vs Combined therapy	No significant difference in 7-year overall survival
Granfors (45)	91, T1 – T4, pN0 -3 M0	Orichectomy + RT vs RT alone	Combined therapy significantly improved DP and OS in lymph node positive patients
Laverdiere (44)	120, stage B1-T2a, B2/T2c and C-T3/T4	RT alone vs neoadjuvant LHRH agonist + flutamide vs combination (before, during and after RT)	Significantly higher positive biopsy rate with RT alone.
Hanks (46)	1554, T2C – T4	2 months zoladex + flutamide prior to RT – randomized to 2 years Zoladex or no therapy	AA significantly improved D-FS, DP, distant metastases and biochemical failure rate.
Zagars (47)	78, stage C	RT alone vs RT + DES	D-FS significantly better with AA. No significant difference in OS
Bolla (48)	415, T1-T4N0	RT alone vs RT + goserelin	AA significantly improved local control, D-FS and OS
Lawton (49)	977, T3	RT alone vs RT + goserelin	Significant improvement in local control and D-FS but not OS

RT Radiotherapy, DP Disease Progression, OS Overall Survival, D-FS Disease-Free survival.

(orchidectomy) plus radiotherapy or radiotherapy alone (45). After a median follow-up of 9.3 years, clinical progression was seen in 61% of patients receiving radiotherapy alone and 31% receiving the combined treatment. There was a significant difference in overall survival in favour of the combined therapy ($p = 0.007$) but this was confined to lymph node positive patients.

The fourth trial was a recent RTOG prospective study (protocol 92–02) in which all patients received Zoladex (goserelin acetate) and flutamide before and during radiotherapy, and were then randomized to 2 years additional Zoladex or no therapy (46). Those patients receiving the long-term androgen deprivation had a significant improvement in disease-free survival (54% vs 34%, $p = 0.001$), local progression (6% vs 13%, $p = 0.0001$), distant metastases (11% vs 17%, $p = 0.001$) and biochemical failure (21% vs 46%, $p = 0.0001$). These studies support the use of neo-adjuvant and continued use of androgen deprivation with radiotherapy in patients with locally advanced prostate cancer.

Three randomized trials, representing 1468 patients, have examined adjuvant androgen deprivation following radiotherapy. One study used DES 2–5 mg daily for 9 to 93 months (47) and 2 used medical castration with goserelin for 3 years post-radiotherapy (48) or until disease progression (49). All three trials reported a significant improvement in local control and disease-free survival associated with androgen deprivation, but only one showed a significant overall survival advantage (48). A recent study compared 418 patients with locally advanced, but nonmetastatic, prostate cancer who received short-term androgen deprivation with radiotherapy in the RTOG 86–10 trial with 575 patients receiving long-term androgen deprivation plus radiotherapy from the RTOG 85–31 trial (50). The authors report that long-term therapy significantly improved biochemical disease free survival (bNED control), distant metastatic failure, and cause-specific failure rates in locally advanced nonmetastatic disease.

The results from randomized trials demonstrate that neo-adjuvant/ adjuvant hormone therapy with radiotherapy significantly improves freedom from disease and, in some trials, overall survival, although the benefits may be restricted to high grade, locally advanced or lymph node positive disease. The problem in interpreting these results is the lack of a control arm with androgen ablation alone since this therapy could have produced results similar to the combined therapy. Only one trial included an androgen deprivation arm and this showed no improvement in overall survival although the trial was small with low statistical power (43). Further studies are needed to address this issue.

3. THE TIMING OF HORMONE THERAPY

The question of whether to start hormone therapy in prostate cancer patients immediately following diagnosis or to wait until disease progression is still being debated. Because hormone therapy is associated with substantial side-effects, it needs to be established that initiating treatment early in the management of these patients prolongs survival without compromising quality of life.

The first trial to address this question was the VAGURG I study in which patients were randomized to DES 5 mg, DES plus orchidectomy, placebo plus orchidectomy, or placebo (51). The placebo group received delayed DES when clinical signs of progression were observed. This study showed no difference in survival between those receiving DES or placebo and gave rise to the concept that 'watchful waiting' was a valid therapeutic option. In the second VACURG study patients were randomized to different doses of DES (0.2 mg, 1 mg or 5 mg) or placebo, the latter receiving treatment on disease progression (52). The DES 5 mg arm was stopped early due to excess cardiovascular toxicity, but the immediate androgen suppression with 1mg DES was associated with an increase in overall survival compared to the deferred group (placebo). However, these studies have been extensively criticized for either delaying hormone therapy too long in the placebo group, which would favour immediate therapy.

There are a number of more recent randomized trials that provide further data on the efficacy of immediate therapy compared to watchful waiting. A MRC trial randomized 934 men with histologically confirmed adenocarcinoma of the prostate, to receive either immediate androgen deprivation with orichectomy or an LHRH analogue plus and antiandrogen for tumor flare, or deferred therapy when the disease had progressed sufficiently to warrant clinical intervention (53). There was no information on the frequency of patient follow-up or how disease progression was detected. There was a significant benefit in terms of a reduction in tumor progression from M0 to M1 disease for patients receiving immediate androgen ablation therapy. In patients with no evidence of metastatic disease an initial survival benefit for immediate hormone therapy was also reported. Those with metastatic disease had fewer adverse disease complications with immediate therapy. However in a later update with longer follow-up, the significant overall survival advantage for M0 patients had disappeared (54). A number of reservations have been expressed concerning this trial, including the number of patients (6%) in the deferred arm that died without receiving hormone therapy, and that some of the complications, such as pathological fracture, could have been reduced in the deferred arm if hormone therapy had been given at an earlier time.

Several randomized trials previously discussed, comparing neo-adjuvant/adjuvant hormone therapy with observation, may, in fact, be considered as comparing immediate with delayed hormone therapy since in the observation group of each study, androgen deprivation was initiated at first sign of disease progression (45, 47–49). Three of these trials reported a significant improvement in overall survival with immediate androgen deprivation, although in one this was restricted to Gleason 8–10 patients (49).

Two meta-analyses have evaluated immediate versus delayed androgen deprivation. The first one used data from three randomized trials and performed an analysis on 5-year hazard rates, using a random effect model that reduces to a fixed effect model when the studies were homogenous (55). The combined hazard ratio was 0.91 (95% confidence interval 0.815 – 1.026) where a ratio of less than 1.0 indicates that immediate therapy is superior, although statistical significance was not reached. The second meta-analysis included four randomized trials and was published on the Cochrane Library (56). The percent overall survival at 5 and 10 years for the immediate androgen deprivation group were 44% and 18% compared to 37% and 12% for the deferred group. The pooled estimate for the difference in overall survival was only significant at 10 years (odds ratio 1.50, 95% confidence interval 1.04–2.16). It is important to note that this review did not include the most recent updated data available for the MRC study (54).

The data from all relevant randomized trials and meta-analyses do not provide convincing evidence that immediate hormone therapy clearly improves overall survival. The evidence dose suggests that immediate therapy prolongs progression-free survival in patients with lymph node positive disease and may therefore improve quality of life. In addition, in patients with metastatic disease, particularly to the bone, there may be a role for immediate therapy in reducing complications, such as spinal compression and pain.

4. COMBINED ANDROGEN BLOCKADE

There is good *in vitro* and *in vivo* evidence to suggest that C_{19}-steriods produced in the adrenal glands are metabolised in the human prostate gland to DHT (57). Using radiolabelled androstenedione and dehydroepiandrosterone in patients, it has been suggested that up to 30–40% of the prostatic DHT is derived from adrenal androgens (58). It has also been shown that prostate biopsies from castrate patients contain significant amounts of

DHT which could only have been derived from adrenal origin. Theses data indicate that the secretion of adrenal androgens could provide a potential proliferative action on prostatic carcinoma cells via DHT interaction with intracellular androgen receptors. This alternative source of DHT could explain, in part, the progression seen in some patients despite castration. Adrenal ablation, in addition to castration, should theoretically reduce prostate growth stimulation to a minimum, and this concept forms the basis for the Combined Androgen Blockage (CAB) approach to treating advanced prostate cancer. Clinical interest in CAB was initiated by Labrie *et al.* (59) and consisted of concomitant administration of an LHRF agonist to inhibit pituitary secretion of LH and an antiandrogen to block the action of intraprostatic DHT. The introduction of CAB as a possible alternative approach to castration alone, has invoked much interest and controversy amongst urological oncologists.

In the report by Labrie *et al.* (59), 37 previously untreated patients with advanced (Stages C or D) prostatic cancer, received CAB with nilutamide or flutamide plus burserelin and produced a remission rate of 97%. These results stimulated a more detailed clinical evaluation of CAB and, to date, there have been 27 randomised trials comparing CAB with monotherapy in 7,987 patients with advanced prostate cancer. Despite this plethora of data, the controversy surrounding the clinical value of CAB still exists.

The information, from so many randomized trials, has provided ample data to perform several overviews (60–62) and detailed meta-analyses (55, 63–68) in order to provide a pooled summary of the available evidence (Table 3).

The Prostate Cancer Trialist Collaborative Group (PCTCG) (66) performed a meta-analysis using individual patient data from 27 randomised trials. Orchidectomy or an LHRH agonist was combined with nilutamide in 8 trials, with flutamide in 12 trials and cyproterone acetate in 7 trials. The 5-year overall survival was 25.4% for CAB and 23.6% for androgen deprivation monotherapy, giving a non-significant absolute difference of 1.8%. The results from the cyproterone actetate studies were slightly in favour of monotherapy with 5-year survival rates of 15.4% for CAB and 18.1% for androgen deprivation alone. Trials of either nilutamide or flutamide tended to support CAB with 5-year survival rates of 27.6% and 24.7% giving an absolute difference of 2.9%. The authors comment that due to the range of uncertainty, the results for overall survival, although real, could range from anywhere between 0% and 5% in support of CAB. Advocates of CAB have criticised this study for combining steroidal antiandrogens and NSAAs, and for including all studies in the meta-analysis because control groups varied in the duration of antiandrogen therapy for tumor flare.

Table 3. Meta-analyses comparing Combined Androgen Blockade (CAB) with Monotheraphy (M)

Study	RCTs	Patients	Method	Survival
Bertagna (63)	7	1056	OR: published data.	CAB reduced overall mortality by 11%.
Caubet (64)	13	3427	RR:Published data.:	Significantly favours CAB. RR 0.78–0.84
Bennett (65)	9	4128	RR: published data.	10% improvement in OS with CAB
PCTCG {Prostate Cancer Trialist Collaborative Group (66)	27	8275	IPD used on ITT basis	5-year OS 25.4% CAB, 23.6% monotherapy
Samson (68)	21	6871	HR: published data	Significant improvement at 5 years with CAB (HR 0.871)

IPD Individual Patients Data, ITT Intention to Treat, RR relative Risk, HR Hazard Ratio, OR Odds Ratio

A meta-analysis of the survival benefit of CAB using NSAA was reported by Caubet *et al.* (64) using published data from 13 randomised studies, 9 of which provided sufficient data for survival meta-analysis. Using two statistical methods, this study estimated the relative risk (RR) when comparing treatment with NSAA plus either an LHRH agonist or ochidectomy versus treatment with an LHRH agonist or orchidectomy alone. For overall survival, the first method (proportional hazard model) used data from seven trials and gave a RR of 0.78 (95% confidence interval 0.67–0.90, $p < 0.001$) and the second method (log hazard ratio estimate) gave and RR 0.84 (95% confidence interval 0.76–0.93, $p < 0.001$). Both methods were significantly in favour of CAB. This study also showed a significant improvement in tumor response ($p < 0.0002$) and progression-free survival ($p < 0.001$) with CAB. A smaller meta-analysis of seven double-blind, randomized trials published in 1994, compared the combination of orchidectomy plus nilutamide versus orchidectomy plus placebo as first-line hormonal therapy for metastatic prostate cancer (63). The combination therapy significantly improved pain of metastatic origin and disease progression. There was an 11% reduction in the annual odds of overall mortality in the group receiving combined therapy, although this was not statistically significant (odds ratio 0.89; 95% confidence interval 0.75–1.07).

One meta-analysis assessed the benefit of CAB with flutamide versus castration alone with data from 9 published trials, representing 4,128 patients with advanced prostate cancer (65). Castration was achieved in six studies with goserelin, in one study with leuprolide, and in four studies by orchidectomy. The pooled estimate for overall survival gave a relative risk of 0.90 (95% confidence interval, 0.79–1.00) significantly in support of CAB. This translates into a 10% improvement in overall survival with CAB using flutamide. A more recent systematic review and meta-analysis (68) that updates two previous frequently cited reports (55, 67), compared the effect of monotherapy with CAB on time to progression, cause-specific survival and overall survival using data from 27 randomised trials. Three of six trial reporting cause-specific survival, and used orchidectomy in the control arm and a NSAA in the combination arm, showed a significant difference in favour of CAB. Two of six trials reporting progression-free survival, and one out of sixteen trials reporting time to progression, indicated a significant improvement with CAB. Data for overall survival were derived from 20 trials and showed no significant difference at 2 years (hazard ratio 0.970; 95% confidence interval 0.866–1.087). However, there was a modest, but significant improvement at 5 years in 10 trials in favour of CAB (hazard ratio 0.871, 95% confidence interval 0.805–0.942) Sensitivity analyses indicated that the type of therapy, stage of disease and study quality, did not appear to influence the results. The adverse events leading to patient's withdrawal ranged from 0 to 14% and were considerably less with monotherapy. At the present time there is no method to predict which patients may benefit from CAB and the small increase in survival advantage observed with CAB has to be weighed against the side-effects and the consequent reduction in quality of life. Despite the large amount of data available, there is no consensus on the use of CAB and ultimately will depend on the consenting patient and the individual clinician.

5. INTERMITTENT ANDROGEN DEPRIVATION THERAPY

Continuous androgen deprivation produces excellent short-term results for advanced prostate cancer but the long-term outcome is limited by the development of disease unresponsive to androgen manipulation. Preclinical studies have suggested that continuous androgen deprivation may lead to stimulation of signaling pathways that give rise to androgen-independent tumors and that using intermittent androgen deprivation (IAD) may inhibit these pathways delaying the onset of androgen-independent disease (69). This has been translated into the clinical setting where patients are treated with androgen deprivation for a period of time until clinical or biochemical evidence indicates a maximum response, at which point the treatment is stopped. Active monitoring is continued until there is evidence of disease progression, when androgen deprivation therapy is started again. This cycle is repeated until, inevitably, androgen-independent disease develops. The major aims of IAD are to maintain androgen-responsiveness, to reduce the toxicity associated with continuous hormone therapy, in particular restoration of sexual function between treatment cycles, as well as to decrease treatment costs.

The first trial investigating the efficacy of intermittent androgen deprivation was reported in 1986 by Klotz and colleagues (70). Twenty patients with advanced prostate cancer received intermittent therapy with either DES or flutamide which was continued for 2 to 70 months until metastatic bone pain abated, local obstructive symptoms resolved and pulmonary metastases completely disappeared. Hormonal therapy was resumed for recurrent symptoms associated with metastatic disease, local progression or reappearance of pulmonary metastases. The time off therapy until first evidence of progression ranged from 1 to 24 months (median 8 months). All relapsed patients responded to the re-introduction of therapy. Ten men became impotent on treatment, 9 of whom resumed sexual activity within

3 months of stopping treatment. A number of additional prospective trials have now reported on the use of intermittent androgen deprivation (71–76) although none have been performed in a randomised design (Table 4). A range of reversible hormone therapies have been used to induce androgen suppression, with a first cycle duration of approximately 8 months and up to six IAD cycles achievable (76). The treatment interval varies and the time off treatment tends to decrease with consecutive cycles. The majority of trials report consistent responses during IAD, and a significant improvement in libido whilst off treatment in men who had normal libido before therapy. There was also an improvement in overall well-being during the periods between androgen suppression.

The early development of androgen-independent disease appears to be associated with invasive high-grade tumors and metastases. Prognostic factors that may influence outcome, remain to be determined, although there is a suggestion from the limited data available that a poor PSA response to initial androgen deprivation, may correlate with a worse prognosis. Whether IAD prolongs the onset of androgen-independent disease and affects survival remains unclear and needs to be assessed in randomized studies. The SWOG 9346 randomised trial comparing intermittent androgen

Table 4. Clinical trials of Intermittent Androgen Deprivation (IAD)

Trial	Patients, Stage	IAD regime	First treatment		Time of treatment (mths)	Response to retreatment
			Length (mths)	Response (pts)		
Klotz (70)	20, B1–D2	DES or flutamide	10	20	7.8	12
Higano (71)	22, B–D2	Leuprolide flutamide	9–12	15	6	12
Crook (72)	54 locally recurrent	Leuprolide nilutamide	8	41	8.8	20 of 35
Kurek (73)	44, prostatectomy relapse or pT1b	Leuprorelin cyproterone	9	NR	11.8	NR
Goldenberg (74)	47, A2- D2	MAB	>6	30	7.5	NR
Horwich (75)	16, metastatic	Leuprorelin cyproterone	5.5	11	8	10
Grossfeld (76)	61, T1–T3	MAB or leuprolide	8	NR	9	45

therapy with continuous therapy is ongoing, but it will be some time before mature results are available. Although repeat clinical responses have been documented with IAD, and a suggestion that quality of life may be improved with this treatment, IAD must be considered experimental until data are available to prove its equivalence with continuous androgen deprivation.

6. SUMMARY AND CONCLUSIONS

Androgen deprivation is an effective treatment for patients with advanced prostate cancer but is also being frequently used at earlier stages of disease. Castration still appears to be the principal approach to androgen suppression. Orchidectomy is simple to perform but is irreversible and is associated with a reduced quality of life. DES was the first real alternative to castration but its use is severely limited by cardiovascular complications. The advent of LHRH agonists provided an additional means of castration without the cardiovascular side-effects of DES, but these agents induce an initial tumor flare which requires the simultaneous administration of an anti-androgen. The NSAA are effective in reducing testosterone to castrate levels, and are widely used either alone or in combination with LHRH agonists. Bicalutamide, in particular, appears to be well tolerated, and maintains sexual potency in many men. Orchidectomy, estrogen agonists, NSAA and LHRH agonists are reported to have therapeutic equivalence but the mechanism by which they ablate testosterone function differs.

The routine practice of screening and monitoring prostate cancer patients with PSA has led to earlier diagnosis and detection of disease progression. This has fueled debate on the appropriate time for initiation of hormone therapy. There are several situations when a clinician is faced with the decision whether to initiate androgen deprivation therapy or not. These could be before, during or after primary therapy, at the first indication of an elevated PSA or PSA doubling time, or when disease progression becomes clinically evident. There is a tendency for early treatment to be beneficial, but there is no definitive answer as to when to initiate hormone therapy for PSA progression or in patients with asymptomatic metastases. However, patients with a rising PSA after definitive therapy and a high risk of recurrence may be candidates for early hormone therapy. For patients with locally advanced disease or positive lymph nodes, hormone therapy adjuvant to definitive treatment appears to be beneficial. There is no doubt that patients with symptomatic metastatic disease should be treated with hormone therapy immediately.

Choosing the appropriate class and schedule of androgen deprivation therapy is important as this may affect clinical outcome and quality of life, and should be a joint decision between the informed patients and the clinician. Combined androgen blockade appears to be only marginally better in terms of survival than continuous therapy with LHRH agonists but is more toxic. Therefore, the decision to use CAB therapy must weigh the balance between the slight survival benefit and the reduced quality of life.

It is important to note that hormone therapy for advanced prostate cancer is not curative and is associated with serious side-effects that include osteoporosis, sexual dysfunction and reduced physical health (77). Consequently, the long tern use of androgen deprivation therapy leads to a significant reduction in quality of life. Intermittent androgen deprivation, although at an early stage of evaluation, is associated with repeated responses and may improve overall quality of life, by reducing toxicities during periods off treatment as well as improving a feeling of well being. Whether intermittent androgen deprivation impacts on survival remains unknown and needs to be tested in randomized studies.

REFERENCES

1. Huggins CCVH. Studies on prostatic cancer: (1) The effect of estrogen and androgen injection on the serum phosphates in metastatic carcinoma of the prostate. Cancer Res 1941, 1:293–297.
2. Griffiths K, Coffey DS, Cockett. ATK. The regulation of prostatic growth, pp. 73–115. In: *Third International Consultation on Benign Prostatic Hyperplasia (BPH)*. Cockett ATK, Khoury SYA, eds, Paris: SCI, 1996.
3. Veterans Administration Cooperative Urological research Group. Treatment and survival of patients with cancer of the prostate. Surg Gynecol Obstet 1967, 124: 1011–1017.
4. Blackard CE, Byar DPWPJ. Orchidectomy for advanced prostatic carcinoma: A re-evaluation. Urology 1973, 1:553–560.
5. Robinson MR, Smith PH, Richards B, Newling DW, de Pauw M, Sylvester R. The final analysis of the EORTC genito-urinary tract cancer co-operative group phase III clinical trial (protocol 30805) comparing orchidectomy, orchidectomy plus cyproterone acetate and low dose stilboestrol in the management of metastatic carcinoma of the prostate. Eur Urol 1995, 28:273–83.
6. Smith JA Jr. Hormonal therapy of prostate cancer: Current concepts and future prospects. Clin Ther 1988, 10:281–6.
7. Clark JA, Wray NP, Ashton CM. Living with treatment decisions: Regrets and quality of life among men treated for metastatic prostate cancer. J Clin Oncol 2001, 19:72–80.
8. Kunkel EJ, Bakker JR, Myers RE, Oyesanmi O, Gomella LG. Biopsychosocial aspects of prostate cancer. Psychosomatics 2000, 41:85–94.

9. Robertson CN, Roberson KM, Padilla GM, O'Brien ET, Cook JM, Kim CS, Fine RL. Induction of apoptosis by diethylstilbestrol in hormone-insensitive prostate cancer cells. J Natl Cancer Inst 1996, 88:908–17.
10. Resnick MI, Grayhack JT. Treatment of stage IV carcinoma of the prostate. Urol Clin North Am 1975, 2:141–61.
11. Klotz L, McNeill I, Fleshner N. A phase 1-2 trial of diethylstilbestrol plus low dose warfarin in advanced prostate carcinoma. J Urol 1999, 161:169–72.
12. Rosenbaum E, Wygoda M, Gips M, Hurbert A, Tochner Z, Gabizon A. Diethylstibestrol is an active agent in prostate cancer patients after failure to complete androgen blockage. In. Am Soc Clin Oncol 2000, abstract 1372.
13. Bubley GJ. Is the flare phenomenon clinically significant. Urology 2001, 58 (Suppl 1):5–9.
14. Seidenfeld J, Samson DJ, Hasselblad V, Aronson N, Albertsen PC, Bennett CL, Wilt TJ. Single-therapy androgen suppression in men with advanced prostate cancer: A systematic review and meta-analysis. Ann Intern Med 2000, 132:566–77.
15. Tunn UW, Bargelloni U, Cosciani S, Fiaccavento G, Guazzieri S, Pagano F. Comparison of LH-RH analogue 1-month depot and 3-month depot by their hormone levels and pharmacokinetic profile in patients with advanced prostate cancer. Urol Int 1998, 60(Suppl 1):9–16.
16. Geller J, Albert JD. Endocrine therapy: Predictors of response to prostatic cancer. Semin Urol 1983, 1:291–7.
17. Jacobi GH, Altwein JE, Kurth KH, Basting R, Hohenfellner R. Treatment of advanced prostatic cancer with parenteral cyproterone acetate: A phase III randomised trial. Br J Urol 1980, 52:208–15.
18. Jacobo E, Schmidt JD, Weinstein SH, Flocks RH. Comparison of flutamide (SCH-13521) and diethylstilbestrol in untreated advanced prostatic cancer. Urology 1976, 8:231–3.
19. Lund F, Rasmussen F. Flutamide versus stilboestrol in the management of advanced prostatic cancer. A controlled prospective study. Br J Urol 1988, 61:140–2.
20. Chang A, Yeap B, Davis T, Blum R, Hahn R, Khanna O et al. Double-blind, randomized study of primary hormonal treatment of stage D2 prostate carcinoma: Flutamide versus diethylstilbestrol. J Clin Oncol 1996, 14:2250–7.
21. Dijkman GA, Janknegt RA, De Reijke TM, Debruyne FM. Long-term efficacy and safety of nilutamide plus castration in advanced prostate cancer, and the significance of early prostate specific antigen normalization. International anandron study group. J Urol 1997, 158:160–3.
22. Dole EJ, Holdsworth MT. Nilutamide: An antiandrogen for the treatment of prostate cancer. Ann Pharmacother 1997, 31:65–75.
23. Iversen P, Tyrrell CJ, Kaisary AV, Anderson JB, Van Poppel H, Tammela TL et al. Bicalutamide monotherapy compared with castration in patients with nonmetastatic locally advanced prostate cancer: 6.3 Years of followup. J Urol 2000, 164:1579–82.
24. Kucuk O, Fisher E, Moinpour CM, Coleman D, Hussain MH, Sartor AO et al. Phase II trial of bicalutamide in patients with advanced prostate cancer in whom conventional hormonal therapy failed: A southwest oncology group study (SWOG 9235). Urology 2001, 58:53–8.
25. Labrie F, Cusan L, Gomez JL, Diamond P, Suburu R, Lemay M et al. Neoadjuvant hormonal therapy: The canadian experience. Urology 1997, 49(3A Suppl):56–64.

26. Hugosson J, Abrahamsson PA, Ahlgren G, Aus G, Lundberg S, Schelin S*et al*. The risk of malignancy in the surgical margin at radical prostatectomy reduced almost three-fold in patients given neo-adjuvant hormone treatment. Eur Urol 1996, 29:413–9.
27. Soloway MS, Sharifi R, Wajsman Z, McLeod D, Wood DP Jr, Puras-Baez A. Randomized prospective study comparing radical prostatectomy alone versus radical prostatectomy preceded by androgen blockade in clinical stage B2 (T2BNXM0) prostate cancer. The lupron depot neoadjuvant prostate cancer study group. J Urol 1995, 154 (Pt 1):424–8.
28. Van Poppel H, De Ridder D, Elgamal AA, Van de Voorde W, Werbrouck P, Ackaert K *et al*. Neoadjuvant hormonal therapy before radical prostatectomy decreases the number of positive surgical margins in stage T2 prostate cancer: Interim results of a prospective randomized trial. The belgian uro-oncological study group. J Urol 1995, 154(Pt 1):429–34.
29. Dalkin BL, Ahmann FR, Nagle R, Johnson CS. Randomized study of neoadjuvant testicular androgen ablation therapy before radical prostatectomy in men with clinically localized prostate cancer. J Urol 1996, 155:1357–60.
30. Goldenberg SL, Klotz LH, Srigley J, Jewett MA, Mador D, Fradet Y *et al*. Randomized, prospective, controlled study comparing radical prostatectomy alone and neoadjuvant androgen withdrawal in the treatment of localized prostate cancer. Canadian urologic oncology group. J Urol 1996, 156:873–7.
31. Witjes WP, Schulman CC, Debruyne FM. Preliminary results of a prospective randomized study comparing radical prostatectomy versus radical prostatectomy associated with neoadjuvant hormonal combination therapy in T2-3 N0 M0 prostatic carcinoma. The european study group on neoadjuvant treatment of prostate cancer. Urology 1997, 49(3A Suppl):65–9.
32. Soloway MS, Pareek K, Sharifi R, Wajsman Z, McLeod D, Wood DP Jr, Puras-Baez A. Neoadjuvant androgen ablation before radical prostatectomy in cT2bNxMo prostate cancer: 5-Year results. J Urol 2002, 167:112–6.
33. Aus G, Abrahamsson PA, Ahlgren G, Hugosson J, Lundberg S, Schain M *et al*. Three-month neoadjuvant hormonal therapy before radical prostatectomy: A 7-year follow-up of a randomized controlled trial. BJU Int 2002, 90:561–6.
34. Klotz LH, Goldenberg SL, Jewett M, Barkin J, Chetner M, Fradet Y *et al*. CUOG randomized trial of neoadjuvant androgen ablation before radical prostatectomy: 36-Month post-treatment PSA results. Canadian urologic oncology group. Urology 1999, 53:757–63.
35. Vailancourt L, Ttu B, Fradet Y, Dupont A, Gomez J, Cusan L *et al*. Effect of neoadjuvant endocrine therapy (combined androgen blockade) on normal prostate and prostatic carcinoma. A randomized study. Am J Surg Pathol 1996, 20:86–93.
36. Gleave ME, Goldenberg SL, Chin JL, Warner J, Saad F, Klotz LH *et al*. Randomized comparative study of 3 versus 8-month neoadjuvant hormonal therapy before radical prostatectomy: Biochemical and pathological effects. J Urol 2001, 166:500–6.
37. Meyer F, Bairati I, Bedard C, Lacombe L, Tetu B, Fradet Y. Duration of neoadjuvant androgen deprivation therapy before radical prostatectomy and disease-free survival in men with prostate cancer. Urology 2001, 58(Suppl 1):71–7.
38. Zincke H, Lau W, Bergstralh E, Blute ML. Role of early adjuvant hormonal therapy after radical prostatectomy for prostate cancer. J Urol 2001, 166:2208–15.
39. Messing EM, Manola J, Sarosdy M, Wilding G, Crawford ED, Trump D. Immediate hormonal therapy compared with observation after radical prostatectomy and pelvic

lymphadenectomy in men with node-positive prostate cancer. N Engl J Med 1999, 341:1781–8.
40. Walsh PC, DeWeese TL, Eisenberger MA. A structured debate: Immediate versus deferred androgen suppression in prostate cancer-evidence for deferred treatment.[comment]. J Urol 2001, 166:508–15; discussion 515–6.
41. See WA, Wirth MP, McLeod DG, Iversen P, Klimberg I, Gleason D *et al.* Bicalutamide as immediate therapy either alone or as adjuvant to standard care of patients with localized or locally advanced prostate cancer: First analysis of the early prostate cancer program. J Urol 2002, 168:429–35.
42. Pilepich MV, Winter K, John MJ, Mesic JB, Sause W, Rubin P *et al.* Phase III radiation therapy oncology group (RTOG) trial 86-10 of androgen deprivation adjuvant to definitive radiotherapy in locally advanced carcinoma of the prostate. Int J Radiat Oncol Biol Phys 2001, 50:1243–52.
43. Fellows GJ, Clark PB, Beynon LL, Boreham J, Keen C, Parkinson MC *et al.* Treatment of advanced localised prostatic cancer by orchiectomy, radiotherapy, or combined treatment. A medical research council study. Urological cancer working party–subgroup on prostatic cancer. Br J Urol 1992, 70:304–9.
44. Laverdiere J, Gomez JL, Cusan L, Suburu ER, Diamond P, Lemay M *et al.* Beneficial effect of combination hormonal therapy administered prior and following external beam radiation therapy in localized prostate cancer. Int J Radiat Oncol Biol Phys 1997, 37:247–52.
45. Granfors T, Modig H, Damber JE, Tomic R. Combined orchiectomy and external radiotherapy versus radiotherapy alone for nonmetastatic prostate cancer with or without pelvic lymph node involvement: A prospective randomized study. J Urol 1998, 159:2030–4.
46. Hanks, Lu J, Matchtay M, Venkatesan V, Pinover W, Byhardt R *et al*, eds, RTOG protocol 92-02: A phase III trial of the use of long-term androgen supression following neoadjuvant hormonal cytoreduction and radiotherapy in locally advanced carcinoma of the prostate, p. Abstract 1284. *American Society of Clinical Oncology.* New Orleans: 2000.
47. Zagars GK, Johnson DE, von Eschenbach AC, Hussey DH. Adjuvant estrogen following radiation therapy for stage C adenocarcinoma of the prostate: Long-term results of a prospective randomized study. Int J Radiat Oncol Biol Phys 1988, 14:1085–91.
48. Bolla M, Collette L, Blank L, Warde P, Dubois JB, Mirimanoff RO *et al.* Long-term results with immediate androgen suppression and external irradiation in patients with locally advanced prostate cancer (an EORTC study): A phase III randomised trial. Lancet 2002, 360:103–6.
49. Lawton CA, Winter K, Murray K, Machtay M, Mesic JB, Hanks GE *et al.* Updated results of the phase III radiation therapy oncology group (RTOG) trial 85-31 evaluating the potential benefit of androgen suppression following standard radiation therapy for unfavorable prognosis carcinoma of the prostate. Int J Radiat Oncol Biol Phys 2001, 49:937–46.
50. Horwitz EM, Winter K, Hanks GE, Lawton CA, Russell AH, Machtay M. Subset analysis of RTOG 85-31 and 86-10 indicates an advantage for long-term vs. Short-Term adjuvant hormones for patients with locally advanced nonmetastatic prostate cancer treated with radiation therapy. Int J Radiat Oncol Biol Phys 2001, 49:947–56.
51. Byar DP. Proceedings: The veterans administration cooperative urological research group's studies of cancer of the prostate. Cancer 1973, 32:1126–30.

52. Byar DP, Corle DK. Hormone therapy for prostate cancer: Results of the veterans administration cooperative urological research group studies. NCI Monogr 1988, (7):165–70.
53. Medical Research Council Prostate Cancer Working Party Investigators Group. Immediate versus deferred treatment for advanced prostatic cancer; initial results of the medical research council trial. Br J Urol 1997, 79:235–246.
54. Kirk D, on behalf of the Medical Research Council Prostate Cancer Working Party Investigators Group. Immediate vs deferred hormone treatment for prostate cancer: How safe is androgen deprivation. BJU Int 2000, 86(Suppl 3):220.
55. Agency for Health Care Research Quality (AHRQ). *Relative Effectiveness and Cost-Effectiveness of Methods of Androgen Suppression in the Treatment of Advanced Prostate Cancer.* Rockville, Maryland: Agency for Health Care Research and Quality (AHRQ), 1999. Report No.: 4.
56. Nair B, Wilt T, MacDonald R, Rutks I, eds, Early versus deferred androgen suppression in the treatment of advanced prostate cancer, *Cochrane Library.* Oxford Update Software Ltd, 2002.
57. Harper ME, Pike A, Peeling WB, Griffiths K. Steroids of adrenal origin metabolized by human prostatic tissue both in vivo and in vitro. J Endocrinol 1974, 60:117–25.
58. Geller J, Albert J, Vik A. Advantages of total androgen blockade in the treatment of advanced prostate cancer. Semin Oncol 1988, 15(Suppl 1):53–61.
59. Labrie F, Dupont A, Belanger A, Lacoursiere Y, Raynaud JP, Husson JM*et al.* New approach in the treatment of prostate cancer: Complete instead of partial withdrawal of androgens. Prostate 1983, 4:579–94.
60. Hucher M, de Gery A, Bertagna C. Anandron (nilutamide) combined with orchiectomy in stage D prostate cancer patients. Overview of seven randomized placebo controlled studies. Cancer 1993, 72(Suppl):3886–7.
61. Iversen P. Combined androgen blockade in the treatment of advanced prostate cancer - an overview. Scand J Urol Nephrol 1997, 31:249–54.
62. Laufer M, Denmeade SR, Sinibaldi VJ, Carducci MA, Eisenberger MA. Complete androgen blockade for prostate cancer: What went wrong. J Urol 2000, 164:3–9.
63. Bertagna C, Degery A, Hucher M, Francois JP, Zanirato J. Efficacy of the combination of nilutamide plus orchidectomy in patients with metastatic prostatic cancer: A meta-analysis of seven randomized double-blind trials. Br J Urol 1994, 73:396–402.
64. Caubet JF, Tosteson TD, Dong EW, Naylon EM, Whiting GW, Ernstoff MS, Ross SD. Maximum androgen blockade in advanced prostate cancer: A meta-analysis of published randomized controlled trials using nonsteroidal antiandrogens. Urology 1997, 49:71–8.
65. Bennett CL, Tosteson TD, Schmitt B, Weinberg PD, Ernstoff MS, Ross SD. Maximum androgen-blockade with medical or surgical castration in advanced prostate cancer: A meta-analysis of nine published randomized controlled trials and 4128 patients using flutamide. Prostate Cancer Prostatic Dis 1999, 2:4–8.
66. Prostate Cancer Trialist Collaborative Group. Maximum androgen blockade in advanced prostate cancer: An overview of the randomised trials. Lancet 2000, 355:1491–8.
67. Schmitt B, Wilt TJ, Schellhammer PF, DeMasi V, Sartor O, Crawford ED, Bennett CL. Combined androgen blockade with nonsteroidal antiandrogens for advanced prostate cancer: A systematic review. Urology 2001, 57:727–32.
68. Samson DJ, Seidenfeld J, Schmitt B, Hasselblad V, Albertsen PC, Bennett CL *et al.* Systematic review and meta-analysis of monotherapy compared with combined androgen blockade for patients with advanced prostate carcinoma. Cancer 2002, 95:361–76.

69. Sato N, Gleave ME, Bruchovsky N, Rennie PS, Goldenberg SL, Lange PH, Sullivan LD. Intermittent androgen suppression delays progression to androgen-independent regulation of prostate-specific antigen gene in the LNCaP prostate tumor model. J Steroid Biochem Mol Biol 1996, 58:139–46.
70. Klotz LH, Herr HW, Morse MJ, Whitmore WF Jr. Intermittent endocrine therapy for advanced prostate cancer. Cancer 1986, 58:2546–50.
71. Higano CS, Ellis W, Russell K, Lange PH. Intermittent androgen suppression with leuprolide and flutamide for prostate cancer: A pilot study. Urology 1996, 48:800–4.
72. Crook JM, Szumacher E, Malone S, Huan S, Segal R. Intermittent androgen suppression in the management of prostate cancer. Urology 1999, 53:530–4.
73. Kurek R, Renneberg H, Lubben G, Kienle E, Tunn UW. Intermittent complete androgen blockade in PSA relapse after radical prostatectomy and incidental prostate cancer. Eur Urol 1999, 35(Suppl 1):27–31.
74. Goldenberg SL, Bruchovsky N, Gleave ME, Sullivan LD, Akakura K. Intermittent androgen suppression in the treatment of prostate cancer: A preliminary report. Urology 1995, 45:839–44.
75. Horwich A, Huddart RA, Gadd J, Boyd PJ, Hetherington JW, Whelan P, Dearnley DP. A pilot study of intermittent androgen deprivation in advanced prostate cancer. Br J Urol 1998, 81:96–9.
76. Grossfeld GD, Chaudhary UB, Reese DM, Carroll PR, Small EJ. Intermittent androgen deprivation: Update of cycling characteristics in patients without clinically apparent metastatic prostate cancer. Urology 2001, 58:240–5.
77. Basaria S, Lieb J, 2nd, Tang AM, DeWeese T, Carducci M *et al*. Long-term effects of androgen deprivation therapy in prostate cancer patients. Clin Endocrinol 2002, 56:779–86.

Chapter 14

STRATEGIES FOR THE IMPLEMENTATION OF CHEMOTHERAPY AND RADIOTHERAPY

Paula Scullin[1], Joe M. O'Sullivan[1] and Christopher C. Parker[2]
[1]*Northern Ireland Cancer Centre and Queen's University Belfast, Belfast, Northern Ireland, UK*
[2]*Unit of Academic Urology, Institute of Cancer Research/Royal Marsden NHS Trust, Sutton, Surrey, UK*

Abstract: The traditional roles of cytotoxic chemotherapy and radiotherapy in metastatic prostate cancer have been in the palliation of symptoms of the disease. Two recent phase 3 randomised controlled trials have demonstrated for the first time a survival benefit for men with metastatic hormone refractory prostate cancer treated with decotaxel and steroids. This has generated a remened interest in the systemic management of the disease.

This chapter describes the evolution of the role of cytotoxic chemotherapy for patients with hormone refactory prostate cancer, from the early studies demonstrating improved symptom control, to a discussion on novel agents currenty under investigation.

The role of ionising radiation therapy, both external beam radio therapy and bone - seeking radio nuclide therapy, in the palliation of disease related symptom particularly bone pain is also discussed.

Key words: radiotherapy; chemotherapy; palliation; prostate cancer; bone metastases; radionuclide therapy

1. INTRODUCTION

This chapter reviews the role of chemotherapy and radiotherapy in metastatic prostate cancer. Until recently, this role was restricted to the palliation of symptoms in men with androgen-independent disease. However recent randomised trial evidence, demonstrating that docetaxel prolongs the survival of men with metastatic prostate cancer, has renewed interest in developing new treatment strategies for this disease.

2. CHEMOTHERAPY

This section reviews the use of conventional chemotherapy in metastatic prostate cancer. The use of immunotherapy, gene therapy and bisphosphonates are discussed elsewhere. Strategies for the implementation of chemotherapy that have been evaluated in clinical trials during the prostate-specific antigen (PSA) era will be reviewed. Pre-clinical studies of novel agents, and clinical trials for which there are no PSA data are not covered in detail.

For many years, chemotherapy had a relatively minor role in the management of prostate cancer. A review of 17 prostate cancer chemotherapy trials prior to 1985 found an overall response rate of less than 5% (1). With the development of new agents and new outcome measures, more recent studies have established a role for conventional chemotherapy, both in improving overall survival and in the palliation of symptomatic androgen-independent metastatic disease.

2.1 Methodological Considerations

Chemotherapy studies in metastatic prostate cancer are made difficult by the small proportion of patients with measurable soft-tissue disease (2), the difficulty in distinguishing progressive bone metastases from the disease 'flare' associated with treatment response (3), and the uncertain significance of changes in serum PSA levels. Bubley et al. for the Prostate-Specific Antigen Working Group have published guidelines concerning patient eligibility and methods for assessing response, with a view to standardising trial methodology in patients with androgen-independent disease (4). In summary, eligibility requirements should include castrate testosterone levels (<50 ng/ml), continued androgen suppression, no anti-androgen treatment in the previous six weeks, and evidence of disease progression, either on imaging or on PSA testing. In this context, PSA progression is defined as 2 consecutive rising PSA levels, with the last value >5 ng/ml. The criteria specified for a PSA response are a decline in PSA level of at least 50%, confirmed at least 4 weeks later, with no clinical or imaging evidence of progression during that time.

The natural history of androgen-independent metastatic prostate cancer varies widely, and trial reports should include a description of the distribution of known prognostic factors. Factors which are reliably found to predict outcome are haemoglobin level, PSA level, alkaline phosphatase level, lactate dehydrogenase level, and previous treatments (5, 6). In particular, a distinction should be drawn between androgen-independent prostate cancer, which is characterised by disease progression after castration, and hormone-independent prostate cancer, which is no longer sensitive to any conventional hormonal manipulation, including anti-androgens, oestrogens and corticosteroids. Most prostate cancer chemotherapy studies have been performed in androgen-independent, rather than hormone-independent, disease. Many of these studies have used some form of hormonal manipulation in addition to chemotherapy, which, in the absence of treatment randomisation, makes it impossible to discern the efficacy of the chemotherapy agent over and above that of the hormonal manipulation.

2.2 Chemotherapy for Hormone Refractory Prostate Cancer: A Brief History

Phase II studies of agents that have demonstrated activity in the setting of androgen-independent metastatic prostate cancer during the PSA era are listed in Table 1. While the demonstration of activity, as judged using PSA criteria, may be valuable in selecting agents, or combinations of agents, for further studies, trial methodology has varied so widely that comparisons of response rates between the different studies are not valid.

Many of the agents listed in Table 1 are conventional cytotoxic drugs, which have activity against a range of different cancers. However, two agents, namely suramin and estramustine, are used almost exclusively in prostate cancer. The mechanism of action of suramin against prostate cancer is not well understood, but may include suppression of adrenal hormone production (7), binding of growth factors including basic fibroblast growth factor (7), disruption of cellular respiration (8), and inhibition of topoisomerase II (9). Estramustine consists of an oestrogen, estradiol, attached to an alkylating agent by a carbamate bridge. While it has long been known that oestrogens have activity against prostate cancer, an *in vitro* study suggests that estramustine has a cytotoxic effect on estradiol-resistant human prostate cancer cell lines (10). It is thought that this cytotoxic effect is mediated via inhibition of microtubule assembly (11), and it has been postulated that estramustine may interact synergistically with other cytotoxics which target microtubules, such as the vinca alkaloids and the taxanes. While the high response rates seen in several phase II studies of drug combinations involving estramustine are encouraging (see references 12–15 & 17–18 in Table 1), it remains possible that similar results could be obtained using an oestrogen alone. These trials (12–18) were all conducted in androgen-independent, rather than hormone-independent, disease. Stilboestrol alone

Table 1. Phase 2 studies of chemotherapy in androgen independent metastatic prostate cancer in the PSA era

Combination	Ref.	Cases	PSA response rate	Imaging response rate	Median survival (m)
docetaxel	(84)	25	46%	2/5	
epirubicin	(85)	39		24%	
paclitaxel	(86)	23	0%	4%	
suramin	(87)	43	19%		
vinorelbine	(88)	47	17%	0/3	
5-FU + interferon	(89)	51	15%		8.3
Epirubicin + cisplatin	(90)	21	32%	14%	
estramustine + docetaxel	(12)	34	63%	5/18	
estramustine + vinorelbine	(91)	25	24%	0/5	14.1
estramustine + vinblastine	(18)	31	46%	3/13	
estramustine + vinorelbine + etoposide	(17)	25	56%	8/25	
estramustine + epirubicin	(13)	24	54%	0/9	
estramustine + paclitaxel	(14)	34	53%	4/9	15.9
estramustine + docetaxel + hydrocortisone	(15)	47	68%	12/24	20
estramustine + etoposide + paclitaxel	(92)	37	65%	10/22	12.8
estramustine + etoposide	(93)	55	22%		
ixabepilone	(37)	48	33%		18

has been reported to have a response rate of up to 62% in androgen-independent prostate cancer (19), and so it could be argued that drug combinations involving estramustine are simply a more toxic alternative to stilboestrol. In support of this argument, several large randomised trials performed during the 1980's demonstrated that estramustine was no more effective than stilboestrol alone as first line treatment of metastatic prostate cancer (20, 21), and that both estramustine and oestrogens were associated with a clinically significant, and comparable, degree of cardiovascular morbidity (22).

2.2.1 Mitoxantrone

The standard drug treatment for androgen-independent prostate cancer is second-line hormonal therapy, either with an anti-androgen (e.g., bicalutamide or flutamide), a corticosteroid (e.g., hydrocortisone, prednisolone or dexamethasone) or with an oestrogen (e.g., stilboestrol). The first randomised study in the PSA era to evaluate the addition of chemotherapy to second-line hormonal therapy in androgen-independent prostate cancer was reported by Tannock et al. in 1996 (23). Eleven Canadian centres recruited 161 men with progressive, symptomatic androgen-independent metastatic prostate cancer between 1990 and 1994, who were randomised to receive prednisone 10 mg daily $+/-$ mitoxantrone 12 mg/m^2 at three-week intervals. The main endpoint was pain relief, defined as a 2-point reduction in the pain intensity scale of the McGill-Melzack Pain Questionnaire, maintained for at least 3 weeks, without increased analgesia. Chemotherapy was generally well tolerated with WHO Grade 3 or 4 nausea and vomiting observed in just 0.5% of cycles, and Grade 3 or 4 haematologic toxicity in 1.1%. Two patients receiving mitoxantrone developed symptomatic congestive cardiac failure. A significant advantage was seen for the use of chemotherapy, with pain relief response achieved in 23/80 men (29%) receiving mitoxantrone and prednisone, and in 10/81 men (12%) receiving prednisone alone ($p = 0.01$). There was no difference in overall survival, with a median figure of approximately 11 months. The lack of overall survival benefit is not surprising given that patients receiving prednisone alone were crossed over to receive mitoxantrone at the time of disease progression. Significant predictors of overall survival on multivariate analysis were performance status, pain score and serum alkaline phosphatase level. PSA outcome was evaluable in 111 men, with a PSA response rate ($>50\%$ decline) observed in 12 of 54 men (22%) receiving prednisone alone, and 19 of 57 men (33%) receiving prednisone + mitoxantrone ($p = 0.11$). This was an important study, being the first to demonstrate that the addition of chemotherapy could improve symptom palliation in androgen-independent prostate cancer compared with second-line hormone therapy alone.

Cancer and Leukemia Group B (CALGB) 9182 had a very similar design, and randomised 242 men with progressive, but not necessarily symptomatic, androgen-independent prostate cancer to hydrocortisone 30 mg mane and

10 mg nocte +/− mitoxantrone 14 mg/m² three-weekly (5). The higher dose of mitoxantrone used in this study was associated with significant myelosuppression, with Grade 3 or 4 haematologic toxicity observed in 70% of patients. Grade 3 or 4 cardiac dysfunction was seen in 5% of men receiving mitoxantrone, and 0% of controls. Of 228 evaluable patients, 42/112 (38%) men receiving mitoxantrone and hydrocortisone had a >50% decline in PSA, compared with 25/116 (22%) men receiving hydrocortisone alone (p = 0.008). However, no difference was seen in terms of overall survival, with a median survival of approximately 12 months, and a non-significant trend in favour of the hydrocortisone alone arm (p = 0.08). Independent predictors of poor survival were LDH >227 U/l, haemoglobin <13 g/dl, alkaline phosphatase >165 U/l and PSA >150 ng/ml. Collection of quality of life data was incomplete, and so it is unknown whether the advantage in biochemical response translated into improved symptom palliation. However, the 70% risk of Grade 3 or 4 haematologic toxicity is probably not acceptable for a treatment that is given with palliative intent. Taken together with the results of the Tannock study, the starting dose for mitoxantrone in men with androgen-independent prostate cancer should be 12 mg/m² three-weekly.

2.2.2 Suramin

A randomised study in androgen-independent prostate cancer investigated the addition of suramin to second-line hormonal therapy with hydrocortisone (24). Four hundred and sixty men with progressive androgen-independent prostate cancer and painful bone metastases requiring opioid analgesics received hydrocortisone 40 mg daily and were randomised to receive suramin or placebo, which were given by intravenous infusion daily during week 1, twice weekly during weeks 2 and 3, and weekly from week 4 to week 12. Treatment was generally well tolerated with 24/228 (11%) of patients receiving suramin and 6/230 (3%) of patients receiving placebo discontinuing treatment because of an adverse event. Palliative response, defined as either a 3-point reduction in pain assessed using the Brief Pain Inventory, or a 33% reduction in opioid analgesic requirement, maintained for at least 3 weeks, was seen in 43% of men receiving suramin compared with 28% of men receiving placebo (p = 0.001). An advantage was also seen for suramin in terms of biochemical response with 33% achieving a reduction in PSA >50% compared with 16% of men in the placebo arm (p = 0.01). No difference was seen in terms of overall survival (median 9.5 months v 9.3 months), but 71% of patients in the placebo arm crossed over at disease progression and then received suramin. Thus suramin appears to have comparable efficacy to mitoxantrone, albeit with a less convenient dosing schedule.

2.2.3 Docetaxel

Two recently reported phase III trials have established that docetaxel is the chemotherapy of choice for men with metastatic hormone refractory prostate cancer (HRPC). Prior to this no significant survival benefit had been demonstrated with chemotherapy in this setting (Tables 2 & 3).

In the Taxotere (TAX) 327 study, men with progressive HRPC were randomised to receive either docetaxel or mitoxantrone (25). The standard regimen of mitoxantrone 12mg/m^2 three-weekly was compared to two different schedules of docetaxel, either 30mg/m^2 weekly for 5 weeks of a 6 week cycle, or 75mg/m^2 three-weekly. Patients in all treatment groups received prednisolone 5mg twice daily and patients in the two docetaxel groups had additional steroid pre-medication with dexamethasone. The trial recruited 1006 patients internationally. The primary end point was overall survival and secondary end points were PSA response, pain response, objective tumor response and quality of life (QoL).

Table 2. Randomised trials of chemotherapy versus none in androgen-independent metastatic prostate cancer in the PSA era

Trial	Cases	Randomisation	PSA Response (>50% decline)	Median Overall survival
Tannock (23)	161	Mitoxantrone + prednisone vs prednisone	33% vs * 22%	~11 m vs ~ 11 m
Kantoff (5)	242	Mitoxantrone + hydrocortisone vs hydrocortisone	38% vs * 22%	12.3 m vs 12.6 m
Small (24)	460	Suramin + hydrocortisone vs placebo + hydrocortisone	33% vs * 16%	9.5 m vs 9.3 m
Sternberg (39)	50	Satraplatin + prednisolone vs prednisolone	33% vs * 9%	
Carducci (48)	288	Atrasentan vs placebo		

* p = <0.05

Table 3. Randomised trials comparing different chemotherapy regimens in androgen-independent metastatic prostate cancer in the PSA era

Trial	Cases	Randomisation	PSA response	Median overall survival
Francini (94)	72	Epirubicin vs doxorubicin	38% vs 33%	12.5 m vs * 8 m
Daliani (89)	50	5 FU vs 5 FU + interferon	12% vs 17%	7.8 m vs 9 m
Albrecht (95)	92	Estramustine vs Estramustine + vinblastine	32% vs 32%	11.8 m vs 10.1 m
Hudes (14)	201	Vinblastine vs Vinblastine + estramustine	3% vs * 25%	9.2 m vs 11.9 m
TAX327 (25)	1006	Docetaxel + prednisolone vs Mitoxantrone + prednisolone	45% vs * 32%	18.9 m vs * 16.4 m
SWOG9916 (26)	674	Docetaxel + estramustine vs Mitoxantrone + prednisolone	50% vs * 27%	17.5 m vs * 15.6 m
Galsky (36)	92	Ixabepolilone vs Ixabepolilone + estramustine	48% vs 69%	
Dahut (44)	75	Docetaxel vs Docetaxel + thalidomide	37% vs 63%	

* p = <0.05

When results from the docetaxel arms were compared to the mitoxantrone arm there was a statistically significant improvement in survival for patients treated with docetaxel. The median survival in the three weekly treated docetaxel arm was 18.9 months, compared to 16.4 months in the mitoxantrone arm (p = 0.009). There was no statistically significant difference between mitoxantrone and the weekly docetaxel arm (17.3 months; p = 0.3). The three weekly treated docetaxel arm was also superior to mitoxantrone with respect to pain response (35% v 22%; p = 0.01) and PSA response rate (45% v 32%; p = 0.0005). Finally, improvement in QoL, as defined by at least a 16-point improvement from baseline in the FACT-P score on two measurements obtained at least 3 weeks apart, was significantly better in the docetaxel treated groups (Table 4).

Table 4. Efficacy outcomes from the TAX327 trial

	Three weekly docetaxel n = 335	**Weekly docetaxel** n = 334	**Mitoxantrone** n = 337
Median survival (months)	18.9 $p = 0.009$	17.4 $p = 0.036$	16.5
PSA response	45% (131/291) $p < 0.001$	48% (135/282) $p < 0.001$	32% (93/300)
Pain response rate	35% (54/153) $p = 0.01$	31% (48/154) $p = 0.08$	22% (35/157)
Tumor response rate	12% (17/141) $p = 0.11$	8% (11/134) $p = 0.59$	7% (10/137)
QoL response rate	22% (61/278) $p = 0.009$	23% (62/270) $p = 0.005$	13% (35/267)

All p values are for comparison with mitoxantrone.

Adverse events were more common in the docetaxel treated patients but febrile neutropenia was rare (not reported with weekly docetaxel, 3% with three weekly docetaxel, and 2% with mitoxantrone). The rate of left ventricular ejection fraction impairment was significantly higher with mitoxantrone (22% v 10% with three weekly docetaxel and 8% with weekly docetaxel; $p = 0.0015$).

The Southwest Oncology Group (SWOG) 9916 trial compared the combination of docetaxel and estramustine to mitoxantrone and prednisolone in men with progressive HRPC (26). The trial recruited 674 patients with progressive metastatic disease despite androgen ablative therapy and cessation of antiandrogen treatment. Eighteen percent of the patients had a rising PSA as the only manifestation of disease. Overall survival favoured docetaxel combined with estramustine (18.9 v 16 months; $p = 0.01$). Both disease-free survival and PSA response were significantly higher in the docetaxel/estramustine group (Table 5).

Toxicities were significantly higher in the docetaxel/estramustine group with 16% v 10% of patients discontinuing as a result of adverse events. Febrile neutropenia (5% v 2%; $p = 0.01$), gastrointestinal, neurological, metabolic and cardiovascular events were also significantly more common with docetaxel/estramustine. Halfway through the trial, prophylactic

Table 5. Efficacy outcomes from the SWOG9916 trial

	Docetaxel plus estramustine n = 338	Mitoxantrone plus prednisolone N = 336
Median survival(months)	17.5 p = 0.02	15.6
Median time to progression(months)	6.3 p<0.001	3.2
PSA response	50% p<0.001	27%
Objective tumor response rate	17% p = 0.3	11%

warfarin and aspirin were added to the treatment regimen for patients in the docetaxel/estramustine arm, based on the release of data demonstrating a significant reduction in estramustine-related coagulopathies with such therapy. However, the addition of warfarin and aspirin did not appear to reduce the incidence of severe thromboembolic complications.

These two phase III trials demonstrate the superiority of docetaxel over mitoxantrone for the treatment of patients with progressive HRPC. While the overall survival and secondary outcome measures were similar in the TAX 327 and SWOG 9916 trials, the docetaxel and prednisolone was the better tolerated regimen. Docetaxel 75mg/m^2 three weekly in combination with prednisolone 10 mg daily has now become the standard 1st line chemotherapy in the treatment of progressive HRPC.

While the trials discussed above demonstrate that chemotherapy is of benefit in improving overall survival as well as in the palliation of symptomatic, metastatic prostate cancer, some caution should be exercised in extrapolating these findings to clinical practice (27). Firstly, the role of chemotherapy in the treatment of asymptomatic, but biochemically progressive, metastatic prostate cancer is not established. Secondly, the benefit of chemotherapy was observed in patients meeting trial eligibility criteria, and may not be generalisable to, for example, those with poorer performance status.

2.3 Chemo-Endocrine Therapy as First-Line Treatment of Metastatic Disease

The standard first-line treatment of metastatic prostate cancer is castration, which may be surgical (bilateral orchidectomy) or medical (luteinising hormone-releasing hormone agonist). Eventual progression to androgen-independent disease is inevitable, and, in an attempt to target any androgen-independent sub-clones present at the time of diagnosis, first-line treatment with combined chemotherapy and castration has been investigated. Seven randomised studies, involving a total of over 1100 patients, have investigated the addition of chemotherapy to castration, and none has shown a survival benefit (28–34). Indeed, one of these studies, European Organization for Research and Treatment of Cancer (EORTC) 30893, in which 189 men were randomised to orchidectomy +/− mitomycin C 15 mg/m^2 six-weekly, reported a statistically significant detriment in overall survival for the use of chemotherapy (28). The only study to provide any encouragement for further investigation was that of Pummer *et al.* who randomly allocated 145 previously untreated patients with either metastatic or locally advanced prostate cancer to treatment with total androgen blockade +/− weekly epirubicin 25 mg/m2 i.v. for 18 weeks (31). The median progression-free survival for total androgen blockade alone was 12 months, compared with 18 months for the combined chemo-hormonal therapy ($p < 0.02$). Overall survival did not differ significantly between the treatment arms ($p = 0.12$), suggesting that delayed chemotherapy for androgen-independent disease may be as effective as early chemotherapy at presentation. There is at present no proven role for chemotherapy in the first-line treatment of metastatic prostate cancer, however a number of randomised trials are underway to address this question including the Systemic Therapy in Advancing or Metastatic Prostate Cancer: Evaluation of Drug Efficacy (STAMPEDE) trial in the UK (35).

2.4 Novel Approaches

2.4.1 Ixabepilone

Ixabepilone is an epothilone B analogue. The epothilones are a new class of tubulin-polymerizing agents with activity in taxane-sensitive and resistant tumor models (36). Ixabepilone has been used in chemotherapy naïve patients with HRPC in a phase II trials and has been associated with a PSA response rate of 33% (37, 38). In a phase II trial, a combination of ixabepilone plus estramustine was compared to ixabepilone alone as first-line treatment for patient with progressive HRPC (36). Patients received ixabepilone 35mg/m^2 three-weekly with or without estramustine 280mg three times daily days 1-5. Prophylactic warfarin was given in the combination arm. PSA response was achieved in 48% (21/44) patients in the ixabepilone arm, and in 69% (31/45) patients in the combination arm. Peripheral neuropathy and neutropenia were the most common adverse events. Toxicity was more common in the estramustine arm with 9% of patients having a grade 3-4 thrombotic event. Ongoing studies are evaluating ixabepilone as second line treatment for patients with HRPC both as a single agent and in combination with mitoxanthrone.

2.4.2 Satraplatin

Satraplatin is an oral, third generation platinum analogue with in vitro efficacy against taxane-resistant cell lines. A randomised, open-label, phase III trial comparing prednisolone alone or in combination with satraplatin as first-line treatment for patients with HRPC was terminated early for commercial reasons (39). The combination of satraplatin and prednisolone resulted in a significant increase in PSA response (33% v 9%; $p=0.046$) when compared to prednisolone alone. Progression free survival was also improved with the combination (5.2 v 2.5 months; $p=0.023$). The SPARC (Satraplatin and Prednisolone Against Refractory Cancer) trial is a multinational phase III trial which will compare progression-free survival in patients with HRPC after failure of one prior chemotherapy regimen. Patients will be randomised to receive prednisolone combined with either satraplatin or placebo. The trial has recruited over 900 patients and will report in 2007.

2.4.3 Anti-Angiogenesis Agents

As in other malignancies, abnormal angiogenesis is a feature of prostate cancer. In localised disease, measures of angiogenesis, such as microvessel density, correlate with prognosis (40). Serum levels of vascular endothelial growth factor (VEGF), an important angiogenic factor, are elevated in patients with metastatic prostate cancer (41), and in the Dunning rat model of advanced prostate cancer, systemic administration of anti-VEGF antibodies inhibit metastatic progression (42). The use of anti-angiogenesis agents, either alone, or in combination with conventional chemotherapy, is therefore a strategy that merits clinical investigation. Figg et al. have reported a phase II study of the anti-angiogenesis agent, thalidomide, in which a PSA response $\geq$ 50% decline was seen in 9 of 63 (14%) patients with androgen-independent metastatic disease (43). In a randomized phase II trial, 75 patients with chemotherapy naïve progressive HRPC were randomized to receive docetaxel or docetaxel combined with thalidomide (44). PSA response was 53% in the combination arm and 37% in the single agent arm, with progression-free survival of 5.9 and 3.7 months, respectively ($p=0.32$). Toxicity was manageable in both arms after the addition of prophylactic low-molecular-weight heparin to the combination group.

Bevacizumab is a humanized monoclonal antibody that targets VEGF. In a single arm phase II trial, patients with chemotherapy naïve progressive

HRPC were treated with a combination of bevacizumab, docetaxel and estramustine. PSA response rate was 65% (45). Ongoing phase II and III trials are evaluating bevacizumab in combination with chemotherapy in this setting.

2.4.4 Endothelin Receptor Antagonists

Endothelin-1, which was originally identified as a potent vasoconstrictor, is commonly expressed in human prostate cancers, and plasma endothelin-1 levels are significantly elevated in men with metastatic disease (46). Exogenous endothelin-1 induces prostate cancer proliferation directly and enhances the mitogenic effects of other tumor growth factors *in vitro* (47). These observations provided the basis for investigating endothelin receptor antagonists as potential therapeutic agents in metastatic prostate cancer. In a randomised, placebo-controlled trial of the endothelin receptor antagonist, atrasentan (ABT-627), in 288 asymptomatic men with metastatic HRPC median time to PSA progression was 155 days in the atrasentan group and 71 days in the placebo group ($p = 0.002$). Side effects were typically of mild to moderate severity and QoL was not adversely affected by atrasentan (48). Further clinical studies of this agent are ongoing in trials such as the SWOG S0421 study which will compare docetaxel and prednisolone to docetaxel, prednisolone and atrasentan in men with advanced HRPC.

2.4.5 Somatostatin Receptors as a Therapeutic Target

Androgen-independent metastatic prostate cancer has been shown to express somatostatin receptors (49). Studies are underway in an attempt to exploit this finding by using somatostatin analogues either as therapeutic agents (50), or as a means to target radioisotopes or cytotoxic drugs. For example, a doxorubicin derivative has been linked to the somatostatin analogue, RC-121, and has been shown to cause marked growth inhibition of prostate cancer in the Dunning rat model (51).

2.4.6 Chemo-Immunotherapy

At present, the role of immunotherapy in the treatment of prostate cancer remains investigational. The most encouraging clinical trial evidence to date comes from the placebo-controlled phase III trial of APC8015 (Provenge), which consists of autologous dendritic cells that have been exposed to a recombinant protein of prostatic acid phosphatase and granulocyte-macrophage colony-stimulating factor (GM-CSF). The primary end-point was not reached (time to progression) but on further analysis a median survival benefit was seen in the patients treated with the vaccine at 36 months (25.9 v 22 months; p = 0.02) (52). In the light of these findings, the strategy of combining chemotherapy with immunotherapy is now being explored. A single randomized phase II study of concurrent docetaxel plus vaccine targeted at PSA versus vaccine alone showed that specific T cell responses to the vaccine were maintained in patients receiving docetaxel (53). A 600 patient phase III trial is underway studying the addition of GVAX, an allogeneic cell line based vaccine genetically modified to express GM-CSF, to standard chemotherapy with docetaxel.

3. RADIOTHERAPY

The role of ionising radiation therapy in metastatic prostate cancer predominantly concerns the palliation of pain from skeletal involvement. Radiotherapy can also contribute to control of symptoms from non-skeletal disease, particularly pelvic nodal metastases. Ionising radiation is delivered either by external beam treatment, or with bone-seeking radionuclide therapy.

3.1 External Beam Radiotherapy

3.1.1 Indications and Efficacy

External beam radiotherapy is effective in the palliation of painful bone metastases with response rates in the order of 70% (54). The timing of pain relief varies between 2 days and 6 weeks after radiation with an average of 4 weeks (55). Spinal cord compression secondary to vertebral metastatic disease is an important indication for urgent radiotherapy, with about 50% of patients achieving improvement in leg weakness (56). External beam radiotherapy is also used to alleviate problems caused by pelvic and para-aortic nodal metastases such as pain, ureteric obstruction, and lymphoedema. Locally progressive prostate cancer may cause haematuria, or obstruction of the lower urinary tract or of the rectum, and external beam treatment can provide effective palliation.

Acute toxicity of palliative external beam radiotherapy depends on the area irradiated, but is usually minimal so that even men with a poor performance status may benefit from treatment. In view of the relatively short prognosis of men with androgen-independent metastatic prostate cancer, late toxicity of palliative radiotherapy is generally not a major consideration. However, particularly in men who have had previous external beam treatment, care must be taken not to exceed normal tissue tolerance of critical structures such as spinal cord (57).

3.1.2 Technique

Radiation is delivered using mega-voltage linear accelerators or Cobalt machines. Most commonly, parallel-opposed radiation fields with simple conventional treatment planning are used. The volume to be irradiated is chosen on the basis of the clinical history, physical examination and radiological assessment using isotope bone scans, plain x-rays, or cross-sectional imaging. Treatment fields are usually designed using a simulator, which is a diagnostic x-ray unit, designed to 'simulate' a radiotherapy treatment machine which can provide live fluoroscopic images of the patient, as well as hard copy record of the treated area for future reference.

A wide range of dose-fractionation schedules have been used, and controversy exists with regard to the optimum. In the UK, single fractions of 8 Gy are most commonly given for palliation of bone pain. This reduces the number of hospital visits and frees up machine time allowing more patients to be treated. Furthermore, randomised studies of dose fractionation have commonly been interpreted as providing support for the use of single fractions in this context.

Steenland et al. reported a Dutch multi-centre study in which 1171 patients (of whom 23% had prostate cancer) were randomized to receive either a single fraction of 8 Gy, or 6 fractions of 4 Gy (58). The main endpoint was pain response, as judged by a two point decrease on a 10-point pain scale. No difference in outcome was seen, with 71% of patients experiencing a response. There were four times as many re-treatments in the single fraction arm of the study, but it was postulated that there may have been a lower threshold for re-treatment in this group. Gaze et al. randomized 280 patients to receive either a single 10 Gy treatment or a course of 22.5 Gy in five daily fractions for the relief of localised metastatic bone pain (59). There was no statistically significant difference in response rates between the 2 arms with complete response rates of 38.8% for single treatment and 42.3% for five fractions. Quality of life parameters were the same for both groups. Nielsen et al. randomized 241 patients to receive a single fraction of 8 Gy or 20 Gy in 5 fractions (60). Prostate cancer was the primary site in 34% of patients. There was no difference in the degree or duration of pain relief, the number of new painful sites or the need for re-irradiation between the two treatment groups. Price et al. performed a prospective randomised trial of 288 patients with bone metastases (30% of whom had prostate cancer) comparing a single fraction of 8 Gy with 30 Gy in 10 daily fractions (61). There was no statistically significant difference in the speed of onset or duration of pain relief between the two treatment regimes.

There has only been one study directly comparing 2 single fraction dose schedules. Hoskin et al. randomized 270 patients with painful bone metastases to receive single fractions of 4 Gy or 8 Gy (62). Pain was assessed by patients on a four point graded scale using pain charts. Response was defined as an improved rating compared to the pretreatment value. There was a statistically significant difference in response rates in favour of 8 Gy at 4 weeks (69% versus 44%). There was no difference in complete response rates at 4 weeks, or duration of response between the two arms. The authors conclude that 8 Gy gives a higher probability of pain relief than 4 Gy, but that 4 Gy can be an effective alternative in situations of reduced tolerance.

A multicenter trial by the Radiation Therapy Oncology Group (RTOG) studied pain relief in 759 patients randomly assigned to a variety of dose-fractionation schedules: $2.7\,\text{Gy} \times 15$ fractions, $3\,\text{Gy} \times 10$, $3\,\text{Gy} \times 5$, $4\,\text{Gy} \times 5$, and $5\,\text{Gy} \times 5$ (55). Initially the low-dose, short-course schedules were shown to be as effective as the high-dose protracted programs. However subsequent re-analysis claimed that the protracted schedules were more effective in terms of complete combined relief i.e. absence of pain and cessation of the use of narcotics (63).

The use of multiple fractions for palliation of bone metastases is more common in North America and Australia than in Europe (64, 65). However, within Europe there are wide variations in practice. Lievens et al performed a survey of palliative radiotherapy practice for bone metastases, covering 565 radiotherapy centres in 19 Western European countries (66). Perhaps surprisingly, the most frequently used schedule was 30 Gy in ten daily fractions (50%), and single large fractions were used in just 11% of centres.

3.1.3 Hemi-Body Irradiation

In patients with large areas of the skeleton involved with prostate cancer, hemi-body irradiation is a therapeutic option. After steroid pre-medication, men receive either 6 Gy for the upper half of the body, or 8 Gy for the lower half. Potential toxicities include nausea, vomiting, lethargy and myelosuppression. Pain relief is achieved in 71–89% of patients, and maintained until death in approximately two thirds (67–69). Dearnaley et al. performed a retrospective analysis comparing the results of treatment using hemibody irradiation (HBI) with isotope therapy using the bone-seeking isotope strontium-89 (89Sr) in patients with prostate cancer metastatic to bone (67). There was no statistically significant difference in pain response between the 2 groups at 3 months. Transfusion requirements were higher for the HBI group than for the matched 89Sr group but other bone marrow toxicity was similar. Despite routine anti-emetic therapy, 37% of patients treated with HBI had some nausea or vomiting.

3.2 Bone Seeking Radionuclides

Bone seeking-radionuclides including strontium-89 (^{89}Sr), phosphorous-32 (^{32}P), Rhenium-186-Hydroxyethylene diphosphonate (^{186}Re-HEDP), and Samarium-153 (^{153}Sm) have been used for many years in the palliation of bone metastases in prostate cancer (70, 71). The characteristics of the most commonly used radionuclides are shown in Table 6. Radioisotopes can be attracted to areas of osteoblastic reaction in 2 ways. First, the isotope may have an inherent chemical affinity for bone as is the case for the calcium analogue ^{89}SrCl. Second, the isotope may be bound to a separate chemical with affinity for reactive bone such as hydroxyethylene diphosphonate (e.g., ^{186}Re-HEDP). Pain responses in the order of 70% have been reported with the most commonly used isotopes, ^{89}SrCl, ^{153}Sm and ^{186}Re-HEDP (72).

Bone seeking radionuclides are under-utilised in the treatment of painful bone metastases because of perceived lack of cost effectiveness and limited availability (70). However this treatment strategy has been shown to be cost-effective. McEwan et al. compared the costs of those receiving Strontium-89 with those receiving placebo in a Canadian trial of ^{89}Sr-chloride as adjunctive therapy in patients with prostate cancer metastatic to bone (73). The study suggested that treatment with ^{89}Sr- chloride could bring about meaningful reductions in lifetime management costs in patients with advanced prostate cancer. Malberg et al. used data from the same trial to assess the cost effectiveness of Strontium-89 in a Swedish setting (74). In a retrospective analysis, the average cost of a relapse treated with external beam radiotherapy (EBRT) alone was calculated from the actual care consumption of 79 consecutive patients who received EBRT because of skeletal pain due to prostate cancer metastatic to bone. They concluded that Strontium-89,

Table 6. Characteristics of the most commonly used radionuclides

Radionuclide	Pharmaceutical	Half-life (days)	β-max energy	Max range in Tissue (mm)	γ photon
Rhenium 186	HEDP	3.8	1.07	4.7	137(9)
Samarium 153	EDTMP	1.95	0.8	3.4	103(28)
Strontium 89	Chloride	50.5	1.46	6.7	0

as a supplement to EBRT for palliation of pain in androgen-independent metastatic disease was beneficial with regard to lifetime health service costs.

3.2.1 Strontium-89

Strontium-89 is an analogue of calcium, which concentrates in osteoblastic bone metastases. The isotope may remain in bone for 100 days and is excreted renally. Strontium is a beta-emitter with a range in tissue of 1.4 mm and a physical half-life of 50.5 days. Normal bone takes up a very small proportion of administered activity and bone marrow depression is transient with a nadir occurring at approximately 4 weeks. The usual administered activity is 150 MBq. An isolation room is not necessary and treatment is given as an outpatient by intra-venous infusion. The major contra-indications are bone marrow suppression and uncontrolled incontinence (because the isotope is excreted in urine and may cause contamination).

The role of treatment with strontium-89 has been investigated in several randomised studies. Lewington et al. performed a double-blind crossover study in 32 patients with prostate cancer metastatic to bone, in which men were randomised between strontium-89 chloride or non-radioactive strontium as a placebo (75). Complete pain relief was only seen in patients receiving the active compound, and there was a statistically significant improvement in pain control between the 2 groups. Quilty et al. randomized 284 patients with prostate cancer and painful bone metastases to receive either external beam radiotherapy or 200 MBq of strontium-89 (76). There was no significant difference in median survival and both treatments provided effective pain relief. There were statistically significantly fewer patients reporting new pain sites after strontium-89 than after local or hemibody radiotherapy. In the Canadian phase 3 trial mentioned above with respect to cost effectiveness, 126 patients with androgen-independent metastatic prostate cancer were randomized to receive local field radiotherapy and either strontium- 89 as a single injection or placebo (73, 77). There were no significant differences in survival or in relief of pain at the index site, although there was a significant benefit for the use of Strontium-89 in terms of analgesic intake, new sites of pain, need for further radiotherapy and physical activity. The authors concluded that the addition of strontium-89 is an effective adjuvant therapy to local field radiotherapy, reducing progression of disease and improving quality-of-life in this group of patients.

3.2.2 Rhenium-186 HEDP

Rhenium-186 emits gamma rays as well as beta rays, which allows for scintigraphic imaging of the isotope distribution (Figure 1). The usual admin-

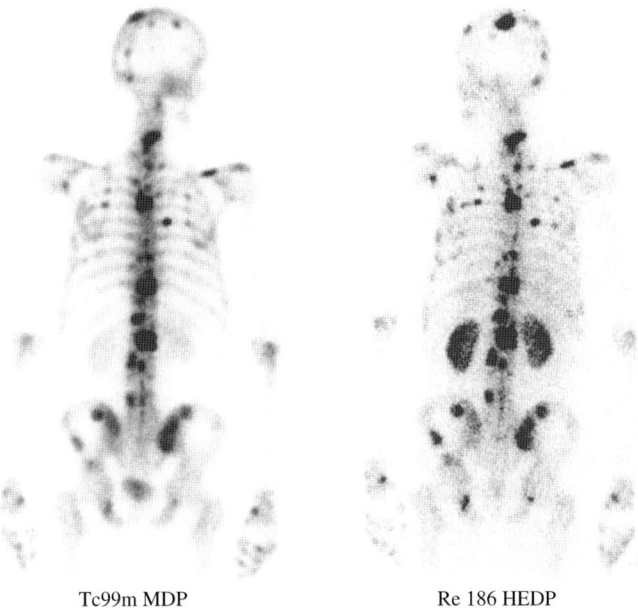

Tc99m MDP   Re 186 HEDP

Figure 1. This is a Technitium 99 labeled planar bone scan showing a very typical pattern of prostate cancer bone metastases and this is a scan of the same patient 4 days later using Rhenium-186 HEDP demonstrating a very close correlation of uptake.

istered activity of ^{186}Re-HEDP is between 1100 and 2500 MBq. Excretion is renal and the dose limiting toxicity is thrombocytopenia. Benefit over placebo has been shown in a randomised trial of 20 patients with prostate cancer metastatic to bone, using a double-blind crossover design with 99mTc-methylene diphosphonate (MDP) as placebo (78). A single intravenous administration of 1110–1295 MBq was associated with prompt pain relief in 80% of patients receiving the active isotope. In a phase 1 activity-escalation study using high activities of ^{186}Re-HEDP with peripheral blood stem cell support in patients with prostate cancer metastatic to bone, we have demonstrated an activity response with regard to PSA reduction using activities above 3500 MBq (79). Phase 3 studies are needed to fully evaluate the potential of this radionuclide.

3.2.3 Samarium-153 EDTMP

The distribution of Samarium-153 (^{153}Sm) mirrors that of ^{99m}Tc MDP on bone scintigraphy when injected. As with ^{186}Re-HEDP, ^{153}Sm emits gamma rays in addition to beta rays. Samarium-153 combined with ethylenediamine-tetra-methylene-phosphonate (EDTMP) was first described in 1987 (80). The maximum emitted beta energy is 0.81 MeV. The isotope also emits a gamma ray with an energy of 103 keV. The average beta particle energy is 233 keV with a maximum penetration of 3.1 mm in soft tissue and 1.0 mm in cortical bone. The physical half-life is 46.3 hours. Resche et al. randomized 114 patients with painful bone metastases to receive varying activities of 153Sm-ethylenediaminetetramethylenephosphonate (EDTMP) (81). Fifty-five patients received single doses of 0.5 mCi/kg and 59 patients received single doses of 1.0 mCi/kg. The physicians judged that approximately half of the patients in each dose group were experiencing some degree of pain relief by week 2. This value increased to 55% for the 0.5 mCi/kg group and 70% for the 1.0 mCi/kg group at week 4. The results suggest that the 1.0 mCi/kg dose of 153Sm-EDTMP is safe and effective for the treatment of painful bone metastases. In a double-blind, placebo-controlled study, 118 patients with painful bone metastases secondary to a variety of primary malignancies were randomized to receive 153Sm-EDTMP 0.5 or 1.0 mCi/kg, or placebo. Pain relief was observed in 62% to 72% of those who received the 1.O-mCi/kg dose during the first 4 weeks, with marked or complete relief noted in 31% by week 4. A significant correlation was observed between reductions in opioid analgesic use and pain scores only for those patients who received 1.0 mCi/kg 153Sm-EDTMP.

3.2.4 Radionuclides Plus Chemotherapy

Attempts have been made to enhance the effect of ^{89}SrCl by using concomitant chemotherapy, as a putative radiosensitiser. Cisplatin in low dose has been shown to improve pain palliation in patients treated with ^{89}SrCl in a randomised trial (82). Seventy patients with metastatic androgen-independent prostate cancer were randomized to 148 MBq Strontium-89 plus either 50 mg/m^2 cisplatin or placebo. Overall pain relief occurred in 91% of patients receiving Strontium-89 + cisplatin compared to 63% of patients receiving Strontium-89 + placebo ($P < 0.01$). Significantly less bone disease progression was observed in the experimental arm (27% versus 64%), with no clinically significant difference in toxicity between the arms.

Tu et al. have taken a different approach, and have studied the addition of strontium-89 to chemotherapy (83). Seventy-two patients with androgen independent prostate cancer responding to an induction regimen of ketoconazole and doxorubicin alternating with estramustine and vinblastine were randomised to receive further doxorubicin with or without strontium-89. There was a statistically significant difference in median survival for the group receiving strontium-89 (27.7 versus 16.8 months ($p = 0.0014$)).

While this strategy may not be generalisable to the majority of men with metastatic prostate cancer, it is encouraging to note that this is one of the few randomized trials in this setting to report a survival advantage.

REFERENCES

1. Eisenberger MA, Simon R, O'Dwyer PJ, Wittes RE, Friedman MA. A reevaluation of nonhormonal cytotoxic chemotherapy in the treatment of prostatic carcinoma. J Clin Oncol 1985, 3:827–41.
2. Figg WD, Ammerman K, Patronas N, Steinberg SM, Walls RG, Dawson N *et al*. Lack of correlation between prostate-specific antigen and the presence of measurable soft tissue metastases in hormone-refractory prostate cancer. Cancer Invest 1996, 14:513–7.
3. Pollen JJ, Witztum KF, Ashburn WL. The flare phenomenon on radionuclide bone scan in metastatic prostate cancer. AJR Am J Roentgenol 1984, 142:773–6.
4. Bubley GJ, Carducci M, Dahut W, Dawson N, Daliani D, Eisenberger M *et al*. Eligibility and response guidelines for phase II clinical trials in androgen-independent prostate cancer: Recommendations from the prostate-specific antigen working group. J Clin Oncol 1999, 17:3461–7.
5. Kantoff PW, Halabi S, Conaway M, Picus J, Kirshner J, Hars V *et al*. Hydrocortisone with or without mitoxantrone in men with hormone-refractory prostate cancer: Results of the cancer and leukemia group B 9182 study. J Clin Oncol 1999, 17:2506–13.
6. Petrylak DP, Scher HI, Li Z, Myers CE, Geller NL. Prognostic factors for survival of patients with bidimensionally measurable metastatic hormone-refractory prostatic cancer treated with single-agent chemotherapy. Cancer 1992, 70:2870–8.
7. La Rocca RV, Danesi R, Cooper MR, Jamis-Dow CA, Ewing MW, Linehan WM *et al*. Effect of suramin on human prostate cancer cells in vitro. J Urol 1991, 145:393–8.
8. Rago R, Mitchen J, Cheng AL, Oberley T, Wilding G. Disruption of cellular energy balance by suramin in intact human prostatic carcinoma cells, a likely antiproliferative mechanism. Cancer Res 1991, 51:6629–35.
9. Bojanowski K, Lelievre S, Markovits J, Couprie J, Jacquemin-Sablon A, Larsen AK. Suramin is an inhibitor of DNA topoisomerase II in vitro and in chinese hamster fibrosarcoma cells. Proc Natl Acad Sci USA 1992, 89:3025–9.
10. Hartley-Asp B, Gunnarsson PO. Growth and cell survival following treatment with estramustine nor-nitrogen mustard, estradiol and testosterone of a human prostatic cancer cell line (DU 145). J Urol 1982, 127:818–22.
11. Stearns ME, Tew KD. Antimicrotubule effects of estramustine, an antiprostatic tumor drug. Cancer Res 1985, 45:3891–7.
12. Petrylak DP, Macarthur RB, O'Connor J, Shelton G, Judge T, Balog J *et al*. Phase I trial of docetaxel with estramustine in androgen-independent prostate cancer. J Clin Oncol 1999, 17:958–67.
13. Hernes EH, Fossa SD, Vaage S, Ogreid P, Heilo A, Paus E. Epirubicin combined with estramustine phosphate in hormone-resistant prostate cancer: A phase II study. Br J Cancer 1997, 76:93–9.
14. Hudes GR, Nathan F, Khater C, Haas N, Cornfield M, Giantonio B *et al*. Phase II trial of 96-hour paclitaxel plus oral estramustine phosphate in metastatic hormone-refractory prostate cancer. J Clin Oncol 1997, 15:3156–63.

15. Savarese DM, Halabi S, Hars V, Akerley WL, Taplin ME, Godley PA *et al*. Phase II study of docetaxel, estramustine, and low-dose hydrocortisone in men with hormone-refractory prostate cancer: A final report of CALGB 9780. Cancer and Leukemia Group B. J Clin Oncol 2001, 19:2509–16.
16. Smith DC, Pienta KJ. Paclitaxel in the treatment of hormone-refractory prostate cancer. Semin Oncol 1999, 26(Suppl 2):109–1.
17. Colleoni M, Graiff C, Vicario G, Nelli P, Sgarbossa G, Pancheri F *et al*. Phase II study of estramustine, oral etoposide, and vinorelbine in hormone-refractory prostate cancer. Am J Clin Oncol 1997, 20:383–6.
18. Amato RJEJ, Bui C, Logothetis CJ. Estramustine and vinblastine for patients with progressive androgen-independent adenocarcinoma of the prostate. Urol Oncol Semin Orig Invest 1995, 1:168–172.
19. Smith DC, Dunn RL, Strawderman MS, Pienta KJ. Change in serum prostate-specific antigen as a marker of response to cytotoxic therapy for hormone-refractory prostate cancer. J Clin Oncol 1998, 16:1835–43.
20. Smith PH, Suciu S, Robinson MR, Richards B, Bastable JR, Glashan RW *et al*. A comparison of the effect of diethylstilbestrol with low dose estramustine phosphate in the treatment of advanced prostatic cancer: Final analysis of a phase III trial of the european organization for research on treatment of cancer. J Urol 1986, 136:619–23.
21. Hedlund PO, Jacobsson H, Vaage S, Hahne B, Sandin T, Kontturi M *et al*. Treatment of high-grade, high-stage prostate cancer with estramustine phosphate or diethylstilbestrol. A double-blind study. The SPCG-1 study group. Scandinavian prostate cancer group. Scand J Urol Nephrol 1997, 31:167–72.
22. Hedlund PO, Gustafson H, Sjogren S. Cardiovascular complications to treatment of prostate cancer with estramustine phosphate (estracyt) or conventional estrogen. A follow-up of 212 randomized patients. Scand J Urol Nephrol Suppl 1980, 55:103–5.
23. Tannock IF, Osoba D, Stockler MR, Ernst DS, Neville AJ, Moore MJ *et al*. With mitoxantrone plus prednisone or prednisone alone for symptomatic hormone-resistant prostate cancer: A canadian randomized trial with palliative end points. Chemotherapy 1996, 14:1756–64.
24. Small EJ, Meyer M, Marshall ME, Reyno LM, Meyers FJ, Natale RB *et al*. Suramin therapy for patients with symptomatic hormone-refractory prostate cancer: Results of a randomized phase III trial comparing suramin plus hydrocortisone to placebo plus hydrocortisone. J Clin Oncol 2000, 18:1440–50.
25. Tannock IF, de Wit R, Berry WR, Horti J, Pluzanska A, Chi KN *et al*. Docetaxel plus prednisone or mitoxantrone plus prednisone for advanced prostate cancer. N Engl J Med 2004, 351:1502–2.
26. Petrylak DP, Tangen CM, Hussain MH, Lara PN Jr, Jones JA, Taplin ME *et al*. Docetaxel and estramustine compared with mitoxantrone and prednisone for advanced refractory prostate cancer. N Engl J Med 2004, 351:1513–20.
27. Dowling AJ, Czaykowski PM, Krahn MD, Moore MJ, Tannock IF. Prostate specific antigen response to mitoxantrone and prednisone in patients with refractory prostate cancer: Prognostic factors and generalizability of a multicenter trial to clinical practice. J Urol 2000, 163:1481–5.
28. De Reijke TM, Keuppens FI, Whelan P, Kliment J, Robinson MR, Rea LA *et al*. De. J Urol 1999, 162:1658–64; discussion, 1664–5.
29. Osborne CK, Blumenstein B, Crawford ED, Coltman CA Jr, Smith AY, Lambuth BW *et al*. Combined versus sequential chemo-endocrine therapy in advanced prostate

cancer: Final results of a randomized southwest oncology group study. J Clin Oncol 1990, 8:1675–82.
30. Fontana D, Bertetto O, Fasolis G, Berruti A, Tarabuzzi R, Pagani G et al. Randomized comparison of goserelin acetate versus mitomycin C plus goserelin acetate in previously untreated prostate cancer patients with bone metastases. Tumori 1998, 84:39–44.
31. Pummer K, Lehnert M, Stettner H, Hubmer G. Randomized comparison of total androgen blockade alone versus combined with weekly epirubicin in advanced prostate cancer. Eur Urol 1997, 32:81–5.
32. Janknegt RA, Boon TA, van de Beek C, Grob P. Combined hormono/chemotherapy as primary treatment for metastatic prostate cancer: A randomized, multicenter study of orchiectomy alone versus orchiectomy plus estramustine phosphate. The dutch estracyt study group. Urology 1997, 49:411–20.
33. Boel K, Van Poppel H, Goethuys H, Derluyn J, Vandenbroucke F, Popelier G et al. Mitomycin C for metastatic prostate cancer: Final analysis of a randomized trial. Anticancer Res 1999, 19(3B):2157–61.
34. Miyake H, Hara I, Fujisawa M, Eto H, Okada H, Arakawa S et al. Comparison of hormonal therapy and chemohormonal therapy in patients with newly diagnosed clinical stage D prostatic cancer. Int J Urol 1996, 3:472–7.
35. James PN. PRO8: STAMPEDE – Systemic therapy in advancing or metastatic prostate cancer: Evaluation of drug efficacy. 2006 11/09/2006 [Cited].
36. Galsky MD, Small EJ, Oh WK, Chen I, Smith DC, Colevas AD et al. Multi-institutional randomized phase II trial of the epothilone B analog ixabepilone (BMS-247550) with or without estramustine phosphate in patients with progressive castrate metastatic prostate cancer. J Clin Oncol 2005, 23:1439–46.
37. Hussain M, Tangen CM, Lara PN Jr, Vaishampayan UN, Petrylak DP, Colevas AD et al. Ixabepilone (epothilone B analogue BMS-247550) is active in chemotherapy-naive patients with hormone-refractory prostate cancer: A southwest oncology group trial S0111. J Clin Oncol 2005, 23:8724–9.
38. Lee D. Activity of epothilone B analogues ixabepilone and patupilone in hormone-refractory prostate cancer. Clin Prostate Cancer 2004, 3:80–2.
39. Sternberg CN, Whelan P, Hetherington J, Paluchowska B, Slee PH, Vekemans K et al. Phase III trial of satraplatin, an oral platinum plus prednisone vs. Prednisone alone in patients with hormone-refractory prostate cancer. Oncology 2005, 68:2–9.
40. Borre M, Offersen BV, Nerstrom B, Overgaard J. Microvessel density predicts survival in prostate cancer patients subjected to watchful waiting. Br J Cancer 1998, 78:940–4.
41. Duque JL, Loughlin KR, Adam RM, Kantoff PW, Zurakowski D, Freeman MR. Plasma levels of vascular endothelial growth factor are increased in patients with metastatic prostate cancer. Urology 1999, 54:523–7.
42. Melnyk O, Zimmerman M, Kim KJ, Shuman M. Neutralizing anti-vascular endothelial growth factor antibody inhibits further growth of established prostate cancer and metastases in a pre-clinical model. J Urol 1999, 161:960–3.
43. Figg WD, Dahut W, Duray P, Hamilton M, Tompkins A, Steinberg SM et al. A randomized phase II trial of thalidomide, an angiogenesis inhibitor, in patients with androgen-independent prostate cancer. Clin Cancer Res 2001, 7:1888–93.
44. Dahut WL, Gulley JL, Arlen PM, Liu Y, Fedenko KM, Steinberg SM et al. Randomized phase II trial of docetaxel plus thalidomide in androgen-independent prostate cancer. J Clin Oncol 2004, 22:2532–9.

45. Picus JHS, Rini B, Vogelzang N, Whang Y, Kaplan E, Kelly W, Small E. 2003,:. The use of bevacizumab (B) with docetaxel (D) and estramustine (E) in hormone refractory prostate cancer (HRPC): Initial results of CALGB 90006. In: ASCO Annual Meeting; 2003: Proc Am Soc Clin Oncol; 2003.
46. Nelson JB, Hedican SP, George DJ, Reddi AH, Piantadosi S, Eisenberger MA *et al*. Identification of endothelin-1 in the pathophysiology of metastatic adenocarcinoma of the prostate. Nat Med 1995, 1:944–9.
47. Nelson JB, Chan-Tack K, Hedican SP, Magnuson SR, Opgenorth TJ, Bova GS *et al*. Endothelin-1 production and decreased endothelin B receptor expression in advanced prostate cancer. Cancer Res 1996, 56:663–8.
48. Carducci MA, Padley RJ, Breul J, Vogelzang NJ, Zonnenberg BA, Daliani DD *et al*. Effect of endothelin-A receptor blockade with atrasentan on tumor progression in men with hormone-refractory prostate cancer: A randomized, phase II, placebo-controlled trial. J Clin Oncol 2003, 21:679–89.
49. Nilsson S, Reubi JC, Kalkner KM, Laissue JA, Horisberger U, Olerud C *et al*. Metastatic hormone-refractory prostatic adenocarcinoma expresses somatostatin receptors and is visualized in vivo by [111in]-labeled DTPA-D-[PHE1]-octreotide scintigraphy. Cancer Res 1995, 55(23 Suppl):5805s–10s.
50. Kalkner KM, Nilsson S, Westlin JE. [111in-DTPA-D-PHE1]-octreotide scintigraphy in patients with hormone-refractory prostatic adenocarcinoma can predict therapy outcome with octreotide treatment: A pilot study. Anticancer Res 1998, 18(1B):513–6.
51. Koppan M, Nagy A, Schally AV, Arencibia JM, Plonowski A, Halmos G. Targeted cytotoxic analogue of somatostatin AN-238 inhibits growth of androgen-independent dunning R-3327-AT-1 prostate cancer in rats at nontoxic doses. Cancer Res 1998, 58:4132–7.
52. Small EJSPF, Higano CS, Neumanaitis J, Valone F, Hershberg R. 2005, Results of a Placebo-Controlled Phase III Trial of Immunotherapy with APC8015for Patients with Hormone Refractory Prostate Cancer (HRPC). In: ASCO Annual Meeting; 2005 June 1: Journal of Clinical Oncology, ASCO Annual Meeting Proceedings; 2005. p. 4500.
53. Arlen PM, Gulley JL, Parker C, Skarupa L, Pazdur M, Panicali D *et al*. A randomized phase II study of concurrent docetaxel plus vaccine versus vaccine alone in metastatic androgen-independent prostate cancer. Clin Cancer Res 2006, 12:1260–9.
54. Arcangeli G, Micheli A, Giannarelli D, La Pasta O, Tollis A, Vitullo A *et al*. The responsiveness of bone metastases to radiotherapy: The effect of site, histology and radiation dose on pain relief. Radiother Oncol 1989, 14:95–101.
55. Tong D, Gillick L, Hendrickson FR. The palliation of symptomatic osseous metastases: Final results of the study by the radiation therapy oncology group. Cancer 1982, 50:893–9.
56. Huddart RA, Rajan B, Law M, Meyer L, Dearnaley DP. Spinal cord compression in prostate cancer: Treatment outcome and prognostic factors. Radiother Oncol 1997, 44:229–36.
57. Schultheiss TE. Spinal cord radiation tolerance. Int J Radiat Oncol Biol Phys 1994, 30:735–6.
58. Steenland E, Leer JW, van Houwelingen H, Post WJ, van den Hout WB, Kievit J *et al*. The effect of a single fraction compared to multiple fractions on painful bone metastases: A global analysis of the dutch bone metastasis study. Radiother Oncol 1999, 52:101–9.

59. Gaze MN, Kelly CG, Kerr GR, Cull A, Cowie VJ, Gregor A et al. Relief and quality of life following radiotherapy for bone metastases: A randomised trial of two fractionation schedules. Pain 1997, 45:109–6.
60. Nielsen OS, Bentzen SM, Sandberg E, Gadeberg CC, Timothy AR. Randomized trial of single dose versus fractionated palliative radiotherapy of bone metastases. Radiother Oncol 1998, 47:233–40.
61. Price P, Hoskin PJ, Easton D, Austin D, Palmer SG, Yarnold JR. Prospective randomised trial of single and multifraction radiotherapy schedules in the treatment of painful bony metastases. Radiother Oncol 1986, 6:247–55.
62. Hoskin PJ, Price P, Easton D, Regan J, Austin D, Palmer S et al. A prospective randomised trial of 4 gy or 8 gy single doses in the treatment of metastatic bone pain. Radiother Oncol 1992, 23:74–8.
63. Blitzer PH. Reanalysis of the RTOG study of the palliation of symptomatic osseous metastasis. Cancer 1985, 55:1468–72.
64. Chow E, Danjoux C, Wong R, Szumacher E, Franssen E, Fung K et al. Palliation of bone metastases: A survey of patterns of practice among canadian radiation oncologists. Radiother Oncol 2000, 56:305–14.
65. Roos DE. Continuing reluctance to use single fractions of radiotherapy for metastatic bone pain: An australian and new zealand practice survey and literature review. Radiother Oncol 2000, 56:315–22.
66. Lievens Y, Kesteloot K, Rijnders A, Kutcher G, Van den Bogaert W. Differences in palliative radiotherapy for bone metastases within western european countries. Radiother Oncol 2000, 56:297–303.
67. Dearnaley DP, Bayly RJ, A'Hern RP, Gadd J, Zivanovic MM, Lewington VJ. Palliation of bone metastases in prostate cancer. Hemibody irradiation or strontium-89. Clin Oncol (R Coll Radiol) 1992, 4:101–7.
68. Hoskin PJ, Ford HT, Harmer CL. Hemibody irradiation (HBI) for metastatic bone pain in two histologically distinct groups of patients. Clin Oncol (R Coll Radiol) 1989, 1:67–9.
69. Salazar OM, Rubin P, Hendrickson FR, Poulter C, Zagars G, Feldman MI et al. Single-dose half-body irradiation for the palliation of multiple bone metastases from solid tumors: A preliminary report. Int J Radiat Oncol Biol Phys 1981, 7:773–81.
70. Lewington VJ. Therapy using bone-seeking isotopes. Cancer 1996, 41(10):2027–42.
71. Porter AT, Davis LP. Systemic radionuclide therapy of bone metastases with strontium-89. Oncology (Williston Park) 1994, 8:93–6; discussion 96, 99–101.
72. Mertens WC, Stitt L, Porter AT. Strontium 89 therapy and relief of pain in patients with prostatic carcinoma metastatic to bone: A dose response relationship. Am J Clin Oncol 1993, 16:238–42.
73. McEwan AJ, Amyotte GA, McGowan DG, MacGillivray JA, Porter AT. A retrospective analysis of the cost effectiveness of treatment with metastron (89sr-chloride) in patients with prostate cancer metastatic to bone. Nucl Med Commun 1994, 15:499–504.
74. Malmberg I, Persson U, Ask A, Tennvall J, Abrahamsson PA. Painful bone metastases in hormone-refractory prostate cancer: Economic costs of strontium-89 and/or external radiotherapy. Urology 1997, 50:747–53.
75. Lewington VJ, McEwan AJ, Ackery DM, Bayly RJ, Keeling DH, Macleod PM et al. A prospective, randomised double-blind crossover study to examine the efficacy of strontium-89 in pain palliation in patients with advanced prostate cancer metastatic to bone. Eur J Cancer 1991, 27:954–8.

76. Quilty PM, Kirk D, Bolger JJ, Dearnaley DP, Lewington VJ, Mason MD et al. A comparison of the palliative effects of strontium-89 and external beam radiotherapy in metastatic prostate cancer. Radiother Oncol 1994, 31:33–40.
77. Porter AT, McEwan AJ, Powe JE, Reid R, McGowan DG, Lukka H et al. Results of a randomized phase-III trial to evaluate the efficacy of strontium-89 adjuvant to local field external beam irradiation in the management of endocrine resistant metastatic prostate cancer. Int J Radiat Oncol Biol Phys 1993, 25:805–13.
78. Maxon HR, 3rd, Schroder LE, Hertzberg VS, Thomas SR, Englaro EE, Samaratunga R et al. Rhenium-186(sn)HEDP for treatment of painful osseous metastases: Results of a double-blind crossover comparison with placebo. J Nucl Med 1991, 32:1877–81.
79. O'Sullivan JM, McCready VR, Flux G, Norman AR, Buffa FM, Chittenden S et al. High activity rhenium-186 HEDP with autologous peripheral blood stem cell rescue: A phase I study in progressive hormone refractory prostate cancer metastatic to bone. Br J Cancer 2002, 86:1715–20.
80. Goeckeler WF, Edwards B, Volkert WA, Holmes RA, Simon J, Wilson D. Skeletal localization of samarium-153 chelates: Potential therapeutic bone agents. J Nucl Med 1987, 28:495–504.
81. Resche I, Chatal JF, Pecking A, Ell P, Duchesne G, Rubens R et al. A dose-controlled study of 153sm-ethylenediaminetetramethylenephosphonate (EDTMP) in the treatment of patients with painful bone metastases. Eur J Cancer 1997, 33:1583–91.
82. Sciuto R, Festa A, Rea S, Pasqualoni R, Bergomi S, Petrilli G et al. Effects of low-dose cisplatin on 89sr therapy for painful bone metastases from prostate cancer: A randomized clinical trial. J Nucl Med 2002, 43:79–86.
83. Tu SM, Millikan RE, Mengistu B, Delpassand ES, Amato RJ, Pagliaro LC et al. Bone-targeted therapy for advanced androgen-independent carcinoma of the prostate: A randomised phase II trial. Lancet 2001, 357:336–41.
84. Beer TM, Pierce WC, Lowe BA, Henner WD. Phase II study of weekly docetaxel in symptomatic androgen-independent prostate cancer. Ann Oncol 2001, 12:1273–9.
85. Brausi M, Jones WG, Fossa SD, de Mulder PH, Droz JP, Lentz MA et al. High dose epirubicin is effective in measurable metastatic prostate cancer: A phase II study of the EORTC genitourinary group. Eur J Cancer 1995, 31A:1622–6.
86. Roth BJ, Yeap BY, Wilding G, Kasimis B, McLeod D, Loehrer PJ. Taxol in advanced, hormone-refractory carcinoma of the prostate. A phase II trial of the eastern cooperative oncology group. Cancer 1993, 72:2457–60.
87. Dawson NA, Cooper MR, Figg WD, Headlee DJ, Thibault A, Bergan RC et al. Antitumor activity of suramin in hormone-refractory prostate cancer controlling for hydrocortisone treatment and flutamide withdrawal as potentially confounding variables. Cancer 1995, 76:453–62.
88. Oudard S, Caty A, Humblet Y, Beauduin M, Suc E, Piccart M et al. Phase II study of vinorelbine in patients with androgen-independent prostate cancer. Ann Oncol 2001, 12:847–52.
89. Daliani DD, Eisenberg PD, Weems J, Lord R, Fueger R, Logothetis CJ. The results of a phase II randomized trial comparing 5-fluorouracil and 5-fluorouracil plus alpha-interferon: Observations on the design of clinical trials for androgen-independent prostate cancer. J Urol 1995, 153:1587–91.
90. Huan SD, Stewart DJ, Aitken SE, Segal R, Yau JC. Combination of epirubicin and cisplatin in hormone-refractory metastatic prostate cancer. Am J Clin Oncol 1999, 22:471–4.

91. Smith MR, Kaufman D, Oh W, Guerin K, Seiden M, Makatsoris T *et al*. Vinorelbine and estramustine in androgen-independent metastatic prostate cancer: A phase II study. Cancer 2000, 89:1824–8.
92. Smith DC, Esper P, Strawderman M, Redman B, Pienta KJ. Phase II trial of oral estramustine, oral etoposide, and intravenous paclitaxel in hormone-refractory prostate cancer. J Clin Oncol 1999, 17:1664–71.
93. Pienta KJ, Fisher EI, Eisenberger MA, Mills GM, Goodwin JW, Jones JA *et al*. A phase II trial of estramustine and etoposide in hormone refractory prostate cancer: A southwest oncology group trial (SWOG 9407). Prostate 2001, 46:257–61.
94. Francini G, Petrioli R, Manganelli A, Cintorino M, Marsili S, Aquino A *et al*. Weekly chemotherapy in advanced prostatic cancer. Br J Cancer 1993, 67:1430–6.
95. Albrecht W, Van Poppel H, Horenblas S, Mickisch G, Horwich A, Serretta V *et al*. Randomized phase II trial assessing estramustine and vinblastine combination chemotherapy vs estramustine alone in patients with progressive hormone-escaped metastatic prostate cancer. Br J Cancer 2004, 90:100–5.

Chapter 15

IMMUNO-GENE THERAPY FOR METASTATIC PROSTATE CANCER

Takefumi Satoh, Terry L. Timme, Yehoshua Gdor, Brian J. Miles, Robert J. Amato, Dov Kadmon and Timothy C. Thompson
Scott Department of Urology, Baylor College of Medicine, Houston, TX, USA

Abstract: It has long been appreciated that a significant number of prostate cancers will not progress to clinical significance, yet some prostate cancers disseminate rapidly leading to lethal metastatic disease. Therefore, a reasonable goal of prostate cancer research is to develop novel alternative interventions and adjuvant therapeutic approaches that would suppress local tumor growth and/or impact pre-existing metastatic disease. This chapter will describe the potential for gene therapy to achieve this goal. We will review both pre-clinical and clinical studies using *in situ* gene therapy to generate a systemic immune response. These therapeutic strategies include a cytotoxic approach using the HSV-*tk* gene combined with the prodrug ganciclovir, the immune modulator gene for interleukin-12, and a novel gene that is both cytotoxic and immunomodulatory, Related to Testes-specific, Vespid and Pathogenesis proteins-1 (RTVP-1).

Key words: gene therapy, prostate cancer, immune therapy, metastasis

1. INTRODUCTION

Although the frequency of detection and treatment of prostate cancer has increased dramatically in recent years, this malignancy remains a serious threat to the lives of US men. During the last decade, a sharp increase was detected in the age-adjusted rate of mortality for prostate cancer, but fortunately this increase has begun to decline (1). However, mortality from prostate cancer remains at an unacceptably high rate. Currently available therapies for prostate cancer are limited, i.e., potentially curative localized therapy (radical prostatectomy or irradiation) or palliative androgen ablation therapy for advanced disease. The ability of radical prostatectomy or irradiation therapy to significantly reduce prostate cancer mortality must await the results of ongoing clinical trials, yet on the basis of current rates of biochemical, i.e., serum prostate-specific antigen (PSA), failure it appears that they will not be sufficient as single modalities. In patients treated with radical prostatectomy, increased serum PSA levels indicative of local tumor recurrence and/or metastases occurs within five years in 20% (2) to 57% (3) of the men. The apparent inadequacy of the treatment options for presumed localized disease appears to be related, in part, to the presence of occult micrometastases at the time of diagnosis and treatment. In general there is a relationship of tumor volume with metastatic progression, however, relatively small tumors that are confined to the prostate may also seed metastases (4, 5). These clinical observations have been supported by the results of *in vivo* experiments which indicate that metastases do not necessarily originate from the most abundant clone of malignant cells at the primary site (6). An additional confounding problem with prostate cancer is that the prevalence of histologic cancers with low malignant potential is high, about 40% in men over 50 (7, 8), suggesting that many of the cancers detected and treated may in fact be "clinically unimportant" (7). Indeed, data from some studies have shown that 10%-26% of nonpalpable cancers detected by PSA screening are "clinically unimportant" based on pathologic criteria, e.g., less than 0.5 cc, Gleason sum ≤6, and disease confined to the prostate (9–12). The detection of "clinically unimportant" cancers and their treatment with potentially harmful therapy, such as radical prostatectomy and irradiation therapy, may not be a reasonable therapeutic decision in many cases. It would be useful to have safe treatments that can supplement the current treatments for localized prostate cancer. In addition and perhaps more importantly, a treatment that provides effective anti-metastatic activity will be required to substantially reduce the mortality from this disease. Novel approaches, such as gene/immunotherapy, may provide this anti-metastatic activity. In this chapter we will review the preclinical studies which provide the rationale for anti-metastatic prostate cancer gene therapy and describe the ongoing clinical trials with these objectives in mind.

2. STRATEGIES FOR METASTATIC PROSTATE CANCER THERAPY

2.1 Conceptual Framework

Metastatic prostate cancer typically presents as disseminated multifocal disease. It is therefore often assumed that to achieve effective anti-metastatic activity against such disseminated lesions will require a systemic delivery approach. Systemic delivery of small molecules or antibodies has progressed rapidly for several cancers and has great potential as an anti-metastatic therapy. Systemic gene therapy must attain specificity for metastatic cells and several viral and non-viral strategies have been proposed to accomplish this. Various systemic immunotherapy approaches have been developed and tested in clinical trials with limited success for metastatic prostate cancer. As an alternative to systemic delivery we are of the opinion that immunomodulatory gene therapy delivered to localized prostate cancer lesions may achieve systemic antitumor effects that impact on disseminated disease. This *in situ* immunomodulatory gene therapy approach has been termed an "active vaccine."

2.2 Systemic Gene Therapy

Several groups have constructed adenoviral vectors for gene therapy that are prostate cancer selective (13–18) with the goal of using them systemically to transduce a cytotoxic gene or selectively replicate and lyse prostate cancer cells. Although this approach is attractive and very promising, the currently available vectors for gene therapy may not have the capacity to achieve complete infection of disseminated metastatic cell deposits within an acceptable toxicity profile. Indeed, it has been suggested that the systemic delivery of currently available adenoviral vectors may be inappropriate (19). Several investigators have used liposomes for systemic gene delivery in animal models (reviewed in 20, 21); however, it is unclear whether liposomes can successfully target genes to all sites where metastases develop.

2.3 Immunomodulation by Cytokine Gene Delivery

Enhancement of antigen presentation by stimulation of antigen presenting cells is exemplified by the use of granulocyte macrophage-colony stimulating factor (GM-CSF) gene modified cancer cell vaccination. A promising preclinical study with an anti-tumor vaccine comprised of irradiated autologous GM-CSF secreting-Dunning rat prostate carcinoma cells (22) led to a clinical trial. Eight of eleven patients with prostate cancer were treated with autologous GM-CSF-secreting, irradiated tumor cell vaccines prepared by *ex vivo* retroviral transduction of GM-CSF into surgically harvested cells (23). Insufficient cells were obtained from the other three patients. The treatment resulted in dendritic cell and macrophage infiltration at the injection site and activation of T-cells and B-cells against prostate cancer antigens, representing both Th1 and Th2 T cell response. No systemic side effects were reported. The major limitation of immunotherapy for prostate cancer using similar approaches is poor recovery and growth of cancer cells from clinical specimens.

Many immunomodulatory gene therapy approaches target the enhancement of the cellular response through the delivery of specific cytokine genes. In our opinion the *in situ* delivery of cytokine genes has several potential advantages and relatively few disadvantages. The presence of viable tumor cells at the site of treatment allows for viable tumor cells and peptides derived from these cells to act as the vaccine, thus this approach has been termed "*in situ* adenoviral vector-mediated gene-modified active vaccination." Below we discuss specific cytokines that are promising candidates for this therapeutic strategy.

2.4 Prostate Cancer as a Model System for Gene Therapy

As summarized at a recent conference on gene therapy and immunology, the choice of vector for a gene therapy trial should also take into account the delivery route, transcriptional regulation, target cell and clinical status of the patient in order to minimize toxicity and maximize efficacy (24). The selection of an appropriate gene delivery system is critical for treatment success. In theory the ideal gene delivery system for metastatic prostate cancer would transfer a therapeutic gene to all cancer cells while causing no adverse events and sparing healthy tissues. In practice, however, it is highly unlikely that such an ideal scenario can be achieved using currently available technologies. Fortunately some alternative approaches do not rely on achieving this level of initial targeting. Localized, *in situ*, prostate cancer gene therapy can have distant effects mediated by factors such a bystander effect or induction of host immunity. *In situ* gene therapy involving the direct injection of a viral vector into the tumor is well suited for prostate cancer for a number of reasons. Prostate cancer is highly accessible to gene transfer relative to many other tumor sites. Transrectal ultrasound guidance is a routinely used imaging modality that has proved exceedingly useful not only for biopsies but also for other clinical applications. Gene therapy can be administered through ultrasound guided needle injections directly into hypoechoic sites of presumed tumor foci and the spread of vector during injection monitored to a certain extent. The expendability of the prostate in older men and the relatively slow growth of local prostate tumors make the combined use of *in situ* gene therapy with neoadjuvant/adjuvant approaches such as surgery or irradiation therapy an attractive therapeutic option. *In situ* gene therapy for prostate cancer may result in anti-metastatic benefits since the generation of cytotoxic activities against localized prostate cancer may generate immunological activities affecting not only the primary tumor but also metastatic disease. We have pioneered a gene therapy approach using adenoviral vector delivery *in situ* for prostate cancer and will review the preclinical and clinical progress we have made with so-called "suicide gene therapy" using delivery of the Herpes Simplex Virus (HSV) thymidine kinase (*tk*) gene followed by a course of the pro-drug ganciclovir (GCV) or valacyclovir and our preclinical studies using immunomodulatory gene therapy.

3. *IN SITU* HSV-TK+GCV GENE THERAPY

3.1 Preclinical Evaluation

We developed and used preclinical mouse models of metastatic prostate cancer to demonstrate that extensive cytotoxic activity could be generated *in vivo* using adenoviral vector-mediated HSV-*tk* gene transfer followed by a course of systemic GCV. This gene therapy protocol established that a single vector injection not only suppressed the growth of local orthotopic mouse prostate cancer through necrotic and apoptotic activities, but also significantly reduced the size and number of pre-established metastatic lung foci (25–27) and reviewed in (28). Further preclinical studies demonstrated a satisfactory toxicological profile for this gene therapy protocol (29). We have recently developed additional vectors and compared the use of strong non-specific promoters such as the Rous Sarcoma Virus (RSV) or cytomegalovirus (CMV) promoters with one derived from the caveolin-1 (cav-1) gene that confers a unique specificity for prostate cancer and tumor associated endothelial cells (30). We have also expanded our toxicological evaluations to address the potential mechanisms of hepatoxicity of specific adenoviral vectors (31).

HSV-*tk* + GCV has also found to be effective when combined with other forms of therapy. In an androgen responsive prostate cancer model, castration therapy enhanced the effectiveness of HSV-*tk*+GCV gene therapy (27). *In vitro* and *in vivo* studies designed to evaluate the combination of gene therapy with radiation therapy demonstrated additive, if not synergistic, effects in cancer cell killing and in animal survival for the combined therapy when compared to either treatment alone (32, 33). Although the specific mechanism of action of systemic HSV-*tk*-stimulated anti-metastatic activity in prostate cancer models is still under investigation, it is believed that this involves a non-specific immune cell response of natural killer mainly (NK) cells (34, 35). Systemic depletion of NK cells in mice with orthotopic prostate tumors before and during the course of HSV-*tk*+GCV gene therapy confirmed the importance of this cell type in both local tumor control and control of pre-established lung metastases (35). In other models with retrovirus transduced cancer cells, systemic T cell responses have also been implicated (36–38).

3.2 Clinical Evaluation

Baylor College of Medicine conducted the first *in situ* gene therapy Phase I clinical trial for human prostate cancer and demonstrated safety of *in situ* HSV-*tk* gene therapy. In this clinical trial men with biochemical recurrence of localized prostate cancer following radiation therapy received a single injection of the adenoviral vector. Some toxicity was observed at the highest dose (1×10^{11} IU) and there were indications of efficacy as serum PSA levels in 3 of 18 patients were suppressed by 50% or more (39). This clinical trial was extended to an additional 18 patients with most receiving a dose of 1×10^{10} IU. Additional safety studies confirmed that this dose was safe even when administered at multiple sites or when repeated for up to three times (40). Further analysis of the patients in this gene therapy protocol indicated that this experimental treatment led to an increased PSA doubling time, a significantly increased mean percentage PSA reduction, and a significantly increased mean time to return to initial PSA following initial or repeat vector injections. An immune component in the response to this gene therapy protocol was evidenced by increased levels of activated (HLA DR+) CD8+ T cells in the peripheral blood following treatment, and interestingly, an increase in the density of CD8+ T cells in post-treatment biopsies. This latter observation was correlated with an increased number of apoptotic cells (41).

Having demonstrated the safety and potential efficacy of HSV-*tk* + GCV gene therapy in men with a biochemical recurrence of their prostate cancer after radiation therapy we expanded the clinical trial to a group of men with newly diagnosed prostate cancer with clinical markers that suggested high grade disease and who elected to undergo a radical prostatectomy. In this neo-adjuvant trial, the *in situ* gene therapy was delivered four to six weeks before surgery. The availability of the radical prostatectomy specimen allowed a clear demonstration that *in situ* gene therapy induced local inflammation within prostate cancer foci with an increased infiltration of CD4 and CD8 T cells (42). Remarkably, this form of therapy induced necrosis within prostate cancer lesions in preference to adjacent normal prostatic tissues (42). Further studies confirmed that HSV-*tk*+GCV gene therapy treatment led to increased numbers of HLA DR+ CD8$^+$ T cells in the peripheral blood of these men.

An additional Phase I-II trial in progress combines two to three doses of HSV-*tk* with standard of care radiotherapy and replaces intravenous GCV with the oral bioequivalent drug valacyclovir. Men in this trial were stratified to three groups, low stage disease (PSA <10 ng/ml, biopsy Gleason score <7 and clinical stage T1-T2a), high stage disease (PSA >10 ng/ml, biopsy Gleason score >7 and clinical stage T2b-T3), or stage D1 (regional lymph node metastases). The latter two groups also received concurrent hormonal therapy. Mild hematologic and hepatic abnormalities could be attributable to the gene therapy while genitourinary and gastrointestinal side effects were typical radiation-related side effects. There was no added toxicity attributable to the combination therapeutic approach (43).

4. *IN SITU* INTERLEUKIN-12 GENE THERAPY

4.1 Preclinical Evaluation

Based on our preliminary data from adenoviral vector-mediated HSV-*tk* + GCV clinical trials suggesting a role for Interleukin-12 (IL-12) in the immune response (unpublished data) and other promising results indicating the potential for IL-12 mediated cancer gene therapy we considered IL-12 as the next step in the development of gene/immunotherapy for prostate cancer. We have conducted preclinical studies using adenoviral vectors that overexpress IL-12 in a highly aggressive mouse model of prostate cancer. Orthotopic tumors were established by injecting only 5000 cells of the mouse prostate cancer cell line RM-9 directly into the prostate. One week later when the tumor has achieved a size of around 10 to 20 mm^3 it is injected with the adenoviral vector and the animals observed for the next two weeks. At the end of this period they are sacrificed and the treatment effects evaluated. Initial studies used doses ranging from 1×10^7 to 3×10^8 PFU per tumor. Systemic toxicity was not observed at doses of 1×10^8 or lower. However, in the 3×10^8 group some mice developed increased amounts of ascites but no lethality was observed. A dose-related splenomegaly was seen at the time of sacrifice in all treated animals. To further evaluate potential toxicity we performed a kinetic analysis with measurements of spleen weight and serum concentration of IL-12 during a period of ten days after vector injection. Serum IL-12 was maximal one day after vector injection and enlargement of the spleen was seen after a lag time of several days, with the maximum spleen size observed on day 7. No serum IL-12 or splenomegaly was seen in animals injected with a control vector (Adv/CMV/βgal) or PBS. The AdIL-12 induced splenomegaly was reversible, as a gradual decrease of the serum IL-12 strongly correlated with a return to normal spleen size (44).

Compared to controls AdIL-12 significantly suppressed localized tumor growth as well as spontaneous and experimental metastatic activities (35, 44, 45). Metastatic cells were detected in the pelvic lymph nodes in 50% of the animals with orthotopic tumors treated with AdIL12 compared to 83% of control animals (44). In the pre-established lung metastasis model 100,000 RM-9 mouse prostate cancer cells are injected into the tail vein at the same time that an orthotopic tumor is established. The orthotopic tumor is injected with adenoviral vector with either IL-12 or βgal six days later and the number of lung metastases evaluated eight days after that. Animals in the AdIL-12 treatment group had 16 ± 1 lung metastases compared to 62 ± 3 in the Adv/CMV/βgal treatment group (44). We also evaluated the ability of adenoviral vector-mediated IL-12 treatment of orthotopic prostate tumors to prolong survival. Mean survival for the control group injected with Adv/CMV/βgal (n=36) was 23.4 ± 0.8 days, while in the AdIL-12 treatment group (n=38) the mean survival was 28.9 ± 1.2 days. This survival advantage for the AdmIL-12 group was significant ($p < 0.0001$) and one animal that appeared to be a long term survivor was sacrificed on day 50 and found to have only microscopic tumor.

Several techniques were used to determine the immune effector cells that contributed to the antitumor and/or antimetastatic activity. We observed enhanced NK cell cytolytic activity during the first 7 days following AdIL-12 injection. Immunohistochemical analysis of tumor specimens revealed that antitumoral activities likely resulted to a large extent from 1) enhanced NK lytic activity during the shortly after virus injection, 2) enhanced macrophage activities such as NOS activation and 3) supportive cytokine production and possible cytolytic activities of $CD4^+$ and/or $CD8^+$ T cells. Multiple immune activities, that potentially could develop into a systemic anti-tumor immune response, involving the generation of memory T cells were evident, and the results of analysis of distant antimetastatic activity in response to local injection of AdmIL-12 further supported this notion.

4.2   Clinical Studies

These encouraging preclinical data led us to construct a replication-defective adenoviral vector containing the human IL-12 genes and evaluate it for clinical trials. The mRNA's for both IL-12 subunits (p35 and p40) were induced in the human lymphoblast cell line NC-37 (ATCC CCL 214) with phorbol 12,13-dibutyrate. The p35 and p40 cDNAs were used to construct an adenoviral vector with the encephalomyocarditis virus IRES. Single plaques were purified and used to generate an original virus preparation termed AdhIL-12. This virus was then used to manufacture a clinical grade version under GMP conditions by the Baylor Center for Cell and Gene Therapy Vector Core Facility. The seed vector and production lot to be used in the clinical trials was then extensively tested for quality control. Biological activity of the vector was confirmed by infection of cells in culture and evaluating the media after 48 hours for the presence of IL-12 by enzyme linked immunoassay.

Our IRB and FDA approved Phase I study involves direct intratumoral injection of a replication deficient adenoviral vector mediating expression of the human IL-12 gene in patients with prostate cancer who can be either hormone naïve or hormone refractory. Men who have a biopsy-proven recurrence of prostate cancer in association with a rising serum PSA level following radiotherapy will be eligible for enrollment. Men with a recurrence of their prostate cancer following radical prostatectomy will be eligible if they have metastatic disease either with the a soft tissue component suitable for vector injection. Patients with metastatic prostate cancer who are hormone refractory do not have any standard treatment available that has proven to be highly efficacious in eradicating the tumor with a reasonable degree of safety. For patients who are hormone naïve, hormonal ablation is only a palliative measure and hormone resistance develops over time in most patients. Therefore, the potential risks of the protocol seem justifiable and reasonable. The objective of the study is to assess the safety of direct intraprostatic injection of an adenoviral vector mediating expression of the IL-12 gene. Acute and long-term toxicity resulting from this treatment will be evaluated. The initial dose will be 1×10^{10} viral particles injected directly into the prostate under ultrasound guidance or into soft tissue metastases. This dose is essentially equivalent to the effective dose used in animal studies and below the maximal tolerated dose for mice. Since the human prostate weighs 20 to 50 g, whereas the mouse prostate is only 15 to 30 mg, we do not anticipate any toxic effects at this low dose. Doses will be increased by 1/2 log increments to a maximal dose of 5×10^{12} viral particles or until unacceptable toxicity is observed. Additional laboratory analyses such as detection of specific immune cells in the peripheral blood and evaluation of tissue samples for apoptosis, angiogenesis, and immune cell infiltrates will be performed for research purposes to evaluate potential mechanisms of action.

5. ADDITIONAL *IN SITU* IMMUNOMODULATORY GENE THERAPY APPROACHES

5.1 IL-12 + Co-stimulatory Molecules

Another immunomodulatory approach is to deliver genes encoding co-stimulatory molecules capable of promoting activation of T cells to a cytotoxic state (45). The enhancement of T-cell response using this approach is exemplified by experiments involving B7-1 gene therapy. B7-1 is poorly expressed on most tumor cells surface (46). The B7-1 gene combined with the IL-12 gene on an adenoviral vector (AdmIL-12/B7) was compared with IL-12 gene therapy alone in the RM-9 orthotopic murine prostate cancer model (45). Animals treated with AdmIL-12/B7 lived slightly longer 40 days versus 37 days with AdIL-12 alone at a dose of 1×10^8 PFU and a lower dose of AdmIL-12/B7 was even more effective with a mean survival time of 48 days with 20% having no evidence of tumor on day 50. Interestingly, the therapeutic benefits of the lower dose of AdmIL-12/B7 also appeared to extend to anti-metastatic activities. As depicted in Figure 1 both IL-12 and IL-12/B7 gene therapy led to suppression of pre-established metastases. The number of lung metastases in the animals treated with AdmIL-12/B7 at 5×10^7 was reduced to only 7.8 ± 3.7 whereas the higher dose (1×10^8) yielded slightly more metastases with 12.9 ± 2 and AdmIL-12 was the least effective with 17.2 ± 3.8 lung metastases. This suppression of lung metastases was significant in all treated mice compared to controls ($P \leq 0.001$)

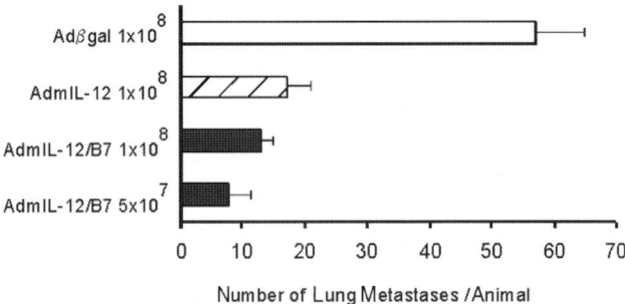

Figure 1. Anti-metastatic activity of *in situ* delivery of adenoviral vectors to orthotopic tumors. Lung metastases were established be tail vein injection at the time of orthotopic tumor establishment. Six days later the orthotopic tumors were transduced with the indicated adenoviral vector. Adapted from (69) .

but the differences between each treatment did not achieve significance (45). As with AdmIL-12 studies (Section 4.1), there was an increase in the number of immune cells in the tumor tissues with intratumoral CD4+ and CD8+ T lymphocyte infiltration similar seven days after injection but AdmIL-12/B7 treated tumors sustained the level of CD8+ cells longer after injection (45). Although a lower titer of AdmIL-12/B7 achieved a similar therapeutic response as AdmIL-12, a careful toxicological study of this vector is warranted; since higher doses tended to generate increased spleen weights compared to AdmIL-12.

The AdmIL-12/B7 vector may also be useful in cell-based vaccine approaches for prostate cancer. We tested a vaccination schedule with subcutaneous injections of transduced, irradiated cells every week for three weeks and were able to induce an immune response that led to rejection of an orthotopic tumor in one third of the mice which received the IL-12/B7 vaccine The IL-12 vaccine was also effective with one fifth of the mice protected from subsequent challenge with an orthotopic tumor (45). These studies are encouraging and suggest that both viruses may prove useful developing further optimized cell-based vaccines for prostate cancer.

5.2   IL-12 Combined with HSV-*tk*+GCV

AdIL-12 has also been directly compared with AdHSV-*tk*+GCV in the RM-9 mouse prostate cancer model (35). AdIL-12 alone had somewhat superior activity with in regard to local cytotoxicity, overall prolongation of survival time and antimetastatic effects. Combining both therapies at an optimal dose for each resulted in significantly increased suppression of orthotopic tumor growth but did not have any greater antimetastatic effects or improve survival time compared to AdIL-12 alone. HSV-*tk*+GCV therapy induced higher levels of necrosis in the orthotopic tumors compared to AdmIL-12 or combination therapy. Single and combination therapies all produced similar increases in apoptotic index in the local tumor. Quantitative immunohistochemical analysis of tumor-infiltrating immune cells indicated that HSV-*tk*+GCV therapy alone led to detectable increases in iNOS-positive cells, CD4+ and CD8+ T-cells and moderately increased numbers of F4/80 (macrophage selective)-positive cells. In contrast, AdmIL-12 elicited a highly robust pattern of tumor infiltration for all four immune cell markers. Combination therapy yielded results similar to AdIL-12 alone. Interestingly, local injection with AdHSV-*tk*+GCV induced splenocyte-derived NK cell cytolytic activities with a maximal response 6 days following treatment, whereas AdmIL-12 injection produced significantly higher NK activity with a maximal response 2 days following injection.

The combined treatment produced a higher systemic NK response over the entire 14-day treatment period. Depletion of NK cells *in vivo* demonstrated that this immune cell subpopulation was responsible for early locally cytotoxic activities induced by AdHSV-*tk*+GCV but not AdmIL-12 and that NK activities were largely responsible for activities against pre-established metastases demonstrated by both gene therapy protocols.

6. FUTURE DIRECTIONS - RTVP-1 GENE THERAPY

The overiding goal of our gene therapy program is to generate an "active vaccine" *in situ* through the cytotoxic effects acting either directly or indirectly. As discussed above there is preclinical and clinical evidence for the direct cytotoxic effects of HSV-*tk*+GCV gene therapy and the preclinical studies suggest that IL-12 gene therapy induces cytotoxicity indirectly through NK cell and T cell activities. It will likely be necessary to develop a greater understanding of the molecular basis of prostate cancer metastasis to design highly effective anti-metastatic therapies. The molecular changes that underlie stepwise development of malignancy from normal cells have been studied extensively during the last two decades (reviewed in 47). However, only recently have investigations been focused on genes that are specifically involved in regulation of the metastatic phenotype. Interestingly, numerous studies support a metastasis suppressor role for p53 in prostate cancer (reviewed in 48). Therefore p53-regulated genes or downstream targets of p53 may provide novel agents for future clinical trials.

To identify prostate cancer-related genes under the transcriptional regulation of p53, we used infected a p53 deficient mouse prostate cancer cell line (6) with an adenoviral vector that expresses wild-type p53 (49) used differential display-PCR to compare RNA expression with a control vector expressing β-galactosidase. Using this approach, we isolated numerous sequences that were known to be under p53 control including cyclin G, epoxide hydrolase, and MDM2. In addition, we isolated genes that had not been previously associated with p53 regulation. One of the sequences we identified encoded the mouse homologue for RTVP-1 (Related to Testes-specific, Vespid and Pathogenesis proteins) (50). In our efforts to understand the regulation of the mRTVP-1 gene by p53, we isolated genomic mRTVP-1 and sequenced a significant portion of this gene (~11 kb), including 3.5 kb of the promoter region, exon 1, intron 1, exon 2 and intron 2. Sequence analysis revealed four potential p53 binding sites that were located in exon 1 and intron 1. Co-transfection studies and electrophoretic mobility shift analyses led to the detection of site in intron 1 as the sole p53-specific binding site. Our results conclusively determined that mRTVP-1 is a direct p53 target gene.

We also evaluated expression of RTVP-1 in mouse and human cell lines. Northern blotting analysis of non-transformed and transformed mouse and human cell lines expressed relatively low levels of RTVP-1 mRNA. Three cell lines including two non-transformed cell lines (MEF p53 +/+ and HUVEC) and a transformed human cell line (CCD-11) that contains wild type p53 expressed significant levels of RTVP-1 mRNA. However, in general, there was no evidence for linkage between the expression of wild-type p53 and RTVP-1. Western blotting analyses revealed somewhat higher levels of RTVP-1 protein than expected from the northern blots and RTVP-1 protein levels were not related to p53 or p21 protein levels. These blotting studies and induction studies with γ-irradiation or doxorubicin indicate p53 independent regulation of RTVP-1.

Overexpression of mRTVP-1 resulted in apoptosis in multiple cancer cell lines, suggesting that mRTVP may play a role in inhibition of malignant growth and progression through its pro-apoptotic activities. In our initial report we overexpressed RTVP-1 by either transfection of a plasmid or by transduction with an adenoviral vector and induced apoptosis in various cancer cell lines *in vitro*. We further showed that the signal peptide was important for RTVP-1-mediated apoptosis suggesting that the secreted form of RTVP-1, in part, mediated these activities. Overall, our results indicated that RTVP-1 is a uniquely acting p53 effector gene with therapeutic potential. Although the human RTVP-1 cDNA was originally cloned from human glioma tissue (51, 52) and was subsequently reported to be expressed in differentiated macrophages (53) the functional significance of RTVP-1 expression and the potential for gene therapy applications of RTVP-1 have not been reported. Preliminary studies in an orthotopic model suggest that adenoviral vector mediated RTVP-1 transduction leads to suppression of tumor growth and lung metastasis and a prolongation of survival (54). These therapeutic responses may be associated with RTVP-1 mediated activities other than apoptosis as increased numbers of specific tumor-infiltrating immune cells were also observed in these studies (54). Thus, RTVP-1 may be considered as a potential therapeutic gene for prostate cancer and potentially other malignancies based on its pro-apoptotic and immunostimulatory properties.

7. CONCLUSIONS

An overiding concept/goal of our gene therapy program is to generate an "active vaccine" *in situ* through direct (e.g., HSV-*tk*+GCV) or indirect (e.g., NK activity via IL-12 stimulation) tumor cell cytotoxicity. Cytotoxicity combined with the capacity to induce the activation of a Th1 response (e.g., IL-12) may lead to a systemic antitumor response that impacts on metastatic disease. A novel gene we have identified, RTVP-1, may be an optimal therapeutic gene for use in "active vaccine" protocols based on its potential for direct (apoptosis induction) and indirect (immune cell recruitment and activation) activities. Because of the general difficulty of generating and maintaining specific antitumor immunity, we anticipate that combination gene(s) and vaccine(s) protocols will ultimately be required to generate therapeutically significant results. Therefore, the identification of novel tumor antigens that could be useful as vaccines alone or in combination with immunostimulatory gene therapy protocols should be actively pursued.

REFERENCES

1. Greenlee RT, Hill-Harmon MB, Murray T, Thun M. Cancer statistics, 2001. CA Cancer J Clin 2001, 51:15–36.
2. Ohori M, Wheeler TM, Kattan MW, Goto Y, Scardino PT. Prognostic significance of positive surgical margins in radical prostatectomy specimens. J Urol 1995, 154:1818–24.
3. Zietman AL, Edelstein RA, Coen JJ, Babayan RK, Krane RJ. Radical prostatectomy for adenocarcinoma of the prostate: The influence of preoperative and pathologic findings on biochemical disease-free outcome. Urology 1994, 43:828–33.
4. Sakr WA, Macoska JA, Benson P, Grignon DJ, Wolman SR, Pontes JE, Crissman JD. Allelic loss in locally metastatic, multisampled prostate cancer. Cancer Res 1994, 54:3273–7.
5. Qian J, Bostwick DG, Takahashi S, Borell TJ, Herath JF, Lieber MM, Jenkins RB. Chromosomal anomalies in prostatic intraepithelial neoplasia and carcinoma detected by fluorescence in situ hybridization. Cancer Res 1995, 55:5408–14.
6. Thompson TC, Park SH, Timme TL, Ren C, Eastham JA, Donehower LA *et al*. Loss of P53 function leads to metastasis in ras+myc-initiated mouse prostate cancer. Oncogene 1995, 10:869–79.
7. Stamey TA, Freiha FS, McNeal JE, Redwine EA, Whittemore AS, Schmid HP. Localized prostate cancer. Relationship of tumor volume to clinical significance for treatment of prostate cancer. Cancer 1993, 71:933–8.
8. Franks LM. Latent carcinoma of the prostate. J Pathol Bacteriol 1954, 68:603–16.
9. Epstein JI, Carmichael MJ, Partin AW, Walsh PC. Small high grade adenocarcinoma of the prostate in radical prostatectomy specimens performed for nonpalpable disease: Pathogenetic and clinical implications. J Urol 1994, 151:1587–92.

10. Ohori M, Wheeler TM, Dunn JK, Stamey TA, Scardino PT. The pathological features and prognosis of prostate cancer detectable with current diagnostic tests. J Urol 1994, 152:1714–20.
11. Goto Y, Ohori M, Arakawa A, Kattan MW, Wheeler TM, Scardino PT. Distinguishing clinically important from unimportant prostate cancers before treatment: Value of systematic biopsies. J Urol 1996, 156:1059–63.
12. Noguchi M, Stamey TA, McNeal JE, Yemoto CM. Relationship between systematic biopsies and histological features of 222 radical prostatectomy specimens: Lack of prediction of tumor significance for men with nonpalpable prostate cancer. J Urol 2001, 166:104–109; discussion 109–110.
13. Rodriguez R, Schuur ER, Lim HY, Henderson GA, Simons JW, Henderson DR. Prostate attenuated replication competent adenovirus (ARCA) CN706: A selective cytotoxic for prostate-specific antigen-positive prostate cancer cells. Cancer Res 1997, 57:2559–63.
14. Yu DC, Chen Y, Seng M, Dilley J, Henderson DR. The addition of adenovirus type 5 region E3 enables calydon virus 787 to eliminate distant prostate tumor xenografts. Cancer Res 1999, 59:4200–3.
15. Walker JR, McGeagh KG, Sundaresan P, Jorgensen TJ, Rabkin SD, Martuza RL. Local and systemic therapy of human prostate adenocarcinoma with the conditionally replicating herpes simplex virus vector G207. Hum Gene Ther 1999, 10:2237–43.
16. Koeneman KS, Kao C, Ko SC, Yang L, Wada Y, Kallmes DF et al. Osteocalcin-directed gene therapy for prostate-cancer bone metastasis. World J Urol 2000, 18:102–10.
17. Galanis E, Vile R, Russell SJ. Delivery systems intended for in vivo gene therapy of cancer: Targeting and replication competent viral vectors. Crit Rev Oncol Hematol 2001, 38:177–92.
18. Uchida A, O'Keefe DS, Bacich DJ, Molloy PL, Heston WD. In vivo suicide gene therapy model using a newly discovered prostate-specific membrane antigen promoter/enhancer: A potential alternative approach to androgen deprivation therapy. Urology 2001, 58:132–9.
19. Nasto B. Questions about systemic adenovirus delivery. Mol Ther 2002, 5:652–3.
20. Templeton NS. In liposomal gene delivery systems. Expert Opin Biol Ther Dev 2001, 1:567–70.
21. Pirollo KF, Xu L, Chang EH. Non-viral gene delivery for P53. Curr Opin Mol Ther 2000, 2:168–75.
22. Sanda MG, Ayyagari SR, Jaffee EM, Epstein JI, Clift SL, Cohen LK et al. Demonstration of a rational strategy for human prostate cancer gene therapy. J Urol 1994, 151:622–8.
23. Simons JW, Mikhak B, Chang JF, DeMarzo AM, Carducci MA, Lim M et al. Induction of immunity to prostate cancer antigens: Results of a clinical trial of vaccination with irradiated autologous prostate tumor cells engineered to secrete granulocyte-macrophage colony-stimulating factor using ex vivo gene transfer. Cancer Res 1999, 59:5160–8.
24. Steele FR, Aguilar-Cordova E. Cabo II: Immunology and gene therapy. Mol Ther 2002, 5:486–91.
25. Eastham JA, Chen SH, Sehgal I, Yang G, Timme TL, Hall SJ et al. Prostate cancer gene therapy: Herpes simplex virus thymidine kinase gene transduction followed by ganciclovir in mouse and human prostate cancer models. Hum Gene Ther 1996, 7:515–23.

26. Hall SJ, Mutchnik SE, Chen SH, Woo, SL, Thompson, TC. Adenovirus-mediated herpes simplex virus thymidine kinase gene and ganciclovir therapy leads to systemic activity against spontaneous and induced metastasis in an orthotopic mouse model of prostate cancer. Int J Cancer 1997:70: 183–187.
27. Hall SJ, Mutchnik SE, Yang G, Timme TL, Nasu Y, Bangma CH et al. Cooperative therapeutic effects of androgen ablation and adenovirus- mediated herpes simplex virus thymidine kinase gene and ganciclovir therapy in experimental prostate cancer. Cancer Gene Ther 1999, 6:54–63.
28. Thompson TC. In situ gene therapy for prostate cancer. Oncol Res 1999, 11:1–8.
29. Timme TL, Hall SJ, Barrios R, Woo SL, Aguilar-Cordova E, Thompson TC. Local inflammatory response and vector spread after direct intraprostatic injection of a recombinant adenovirus containing the herpes simplex virus thymidine kinase gene and ganciclovir therapy in mice. Cancer Gene Ther 1998, 5:74–82.
30. Pramudji C, Shimura S, Ebara S, Yang G, Wang J, Ren C et al. In Situ prostate cancer gene therapy using a novel adenoviral vector regulated by the caveolin-1 promoter. Clin Cancer Res 2001, 7:4272–9.
31. Ebara S, Shimura S, Nasu Y, Kaku H, Kumon H, Yang G et al. Gene therapy for prostate cancer: Toxicological profile of four HSV-tk transducing adenoviral vectors regulated by different promoters. Prost Can Prostatic Dis, 5:316–325, 2002.
32. Atkinson G, Hall SJ. Prodrug activation gene therapy and external beam irradiation in the treatment of prostate cancer. Urology 1999, 54:1098–104.
33. Chhikara M, Huang H, Vlachaki MT, Zhu X, Teh B, Chiu KJ et al. Enhanced therapeutic effect of HSV-tk+GCV gene therapy and ionizing radiation for prostate cancer. Mol Ther 2001, 3:536–42.
34. Hall SJ, Sanford MA, Atkinson G, Chen SH. Induction of potent antitumor natural killer cell activity by herpes simplex virus-thymidine kinase and ganciclovir therapy in an orthotopic mouse model of prostate cancer. Cancer Res 1998, 58:3221–5.
35. Nasu Y, Bangma C, Hull G, Yang G, Wang J, Shimura S et al. Combination gene therapy with adenoviral vector-mediated HSV-tk+GCV and IL-12 in an orthotopic mouse model for prostate cancer. Prost Cancer Prostatic Dis 2001:4: 44–55.
36. Yamamoto S, Suzuki S, Hoshino A, Akimoto M, Shimada T. Herpes simplex virus thymidine kinase/ganciclovir-mediated killing of tumor cell induces tumor-specific cytotoxic T cells in mice. Cancer Gene Ther 1997, 4:91–6.
37. Mullen CA, Anderson L, Woods K, Nishino M, Petropoulos D. Ganciclovir chemoablation of herpes thymidine kinase suicide gene-modified tumors produces tumor necrosis and induces systemic immune responses. Hum Gene Ther 1998, 9:2019–30.
38. Kuriyama S, Kikukawa M, Masui K, Okuda H, Nakatani T, Akahane T et al. Gene therapy with HSV-tk/GCV system depends on T-cell-mediated immune responses and causes apoptotic death of tumor cells in vivo. Cancer 1999, 83:374–80.
39. Herman JR, Adler HL, Aguilar-Cordova E, Rojas-Martinez A, Woo S, Timme TL et al. In situ gene therapy for adenocarcinoma of the prostate: A phase I clinical trial. Hum Gene Ther 1999, 10:1239–49.
40. Shalev M, Kadmon D, Teh BS, Butler EB, Aguilar-Cordova E, Thompson TC et al. Suicide gene therapy toxicity after multiple and repeat injections in patients with localized prostate cancer. J Urol 2000, 163:1747–50.
41. Miles BJ, Shalev M, Aguilar-Cordova E, Timme TL, Lee HM, Yang G et al. Prostate-specific antigen response and systemic T cell activation after in situ gene therapy in prostate cancer patients failing radiotherapy. Hum Gene Ther 2001, 12:1955–67.

42. Ayala G, Wheeler TM, Shalev M, Thompson TC, Miles B, Aguilar-Cordova E et al. Cytopathic effect of in situ gene therapy in prostate cancer. Hum Pathol 2000, 31:866–70.
43. Teh BS, Aguilar-Cordova E, Kernen K, Chou CC, Shalev M, Vlachaki MT et al. Phase I/II trial evaluating combined radiotherapy, in situ gene therapy with or without hormonal therapy in the treatment of prostate cancer–a preliminary report. Int J Radiat Oncol Biol Phys 2001, 51:605–13.
44. Nasu Y, Bangma CH, Hull GW, Lee HM, Hu J, Wang J et al. Adenovirus-mediated interleukin-12 gene therapy for prostate cancer: Suppression of orthotopic tumor growth and pre-established lung metastases in an orthotopic model. Gene Ther 1999, 6:338–49.
45. Hull GW, McCurdy MA, Nasu Y, Bangma CH, Yang G, Shimura S et al. Prostate cancer gene therapy: Comparison of adenovirus-mediated expression of interleukin 12 with interleukin 12 plus B7-1 for in situ gene therapy and gene-modified, cell-based vaccines. Clin Cancer Res 2000, 6:4101–9.
46. Chen L, Ashe S, Brady WA, Hellstrom I, Hellstrom KE, Ledbetter JA et al. Costimulation of antitumor immunity by the B7 counterreceptor for the T lymphocyte molecules CD28 and CTLA-4. Cell 1992, 71:1093–102.
47. Thompson T, Timme T, Bangma C, Nasu Y, Hull G, Hall S, Stapleton A. Molecular biology of prostate cancer, pp. 553–64. In: *Comprehensive Textbook of Genitourinary Oncology*. Coffey DS, Shipley WU, Vogelzang NJ, eds, Baltimore Md: Williams and Wilkins, 1999.
48. Thompson TC, Timme TL, Sehgal I. Oncogenes, growth factors, and hormones in prostate cancer, pp. 327–59. In: *Hormones and Growth Factors in Development and Neoplasia*. Dickson RB, Salomon DS, eds, New York: Wiley-Liss, Inc, 1998.
49. Eastham JA, Hall SJ, Sehgal I, Wang J, Timme TL, Yang G et al. In vivo gene therapy with P53 or P21 adenovirus for prostate cancer. Cancer Res 1995, 55:5151–5.
50. Ren C, Li L, Goltsov AA, Timme TL, Tahir SA, Wang J et al. MRTVP-1, a novel P53 target gene with proapoptotic activities. Mol Cell Biol 2002, 22:3345–57.
51. Murphy EV, Zhang Y, Zhu W, Biggs J. The human glioma pathogenesis-related protein is structurally related to plant pathogenesis-related proteins and its gene is expressed specifically in brain tumors. Gene 1995, 159:131–5.
52. Rich T, Chen P, Furman F, Huynh N, Israel MA. RTVP-1, a novel human gene with sequence similarity to genes of diverse species, is expressed in tumor cell lines of glial but not neuronal origin. Gene 1996, 180:125–30.
53. Gingras MC, Margolin JF. Differential expression of multiple unexpected genes during U937 cell and macrophage differentiation detected by suppressive subtractive hybridization. Exp Hematol 2000, 28:65–76.
54. Satoh T, Timme TL, Yang G, Wang J, Ren C, Kusaka N et al. Adenoviral vector mediated mRTVP-1 gene therapy for prostate cancer. Human Gene Therapy 2003, 14:91–101.

Chapter 16

DISTILLING THE PAST – ENVISIONING THE FUTURE

Richard J. Ablin[1] and Malcolm D. Mason[2]
[1]*Department of Immunobiology, University of Arizona College of Medicine and the Arizona Cancer Center, Tucson, AZ, USA*
[2]*Section of Oncology and Palliative Medicine, University of Wales College of Medicine, Velindre Hospital, Cardiff, Wales, UK*

The foregoing contributions make it patently clear there has and continues to be an "explosion" of burgeoning new technology and resulting information in cellular and molecular biology of prostate cancer. It is noteworthy that there is also a renewed interest in the under appreciated area of immunology with the immune response as a prospective biological marker and the use of immunotherapy. However, this knowledge has thus far out distanced our ability to assimilate and translate it to bring to bear on the complexities and dilemmas faced in meeting the "challenge" of the enigmatic face of prostate cancer. We are therefore of the opinion that the key to the "challenge" of prostate cancer is the translation of basic knowledge into more efficacious preventative, diagnostic and therapeutic end points.

1. NATURAL HISTORY

As a first priority, it must be acknowledged that the natural history of prostate cancer, as considered by Penson and Albertsen (1), remains as enigmatic as ever. Studies, cited by Penson and Albertson (1), and elsewhere in this Volume, have shown that a substantial proportion of men will survive long-term, and free of disease progression, even in the absence of any treatment. In the current era where, increasingly, men are diagnosed on the basis of a biopsy prompted by a marginally elevated level of prostate-specific antigen (PSA), it is likely that an even higher proportion of men diagnosed require no treatment (2). In the recently published study of Finasteride as a preventative agent for prostate cancer, the design anticipated a 6% incidence of prostate cancer in the control group of patients. What they actually found was a 24% incidence (3). On first thought this may appear to be a reflection surely, that we are getting better and better at picking up insignificant, or latent prostate cancer since it is obvious that 24% of the male population do not develop clinically significant prostate cancer. However, we would perhaps concur, as suggested by Welch et al. (4) that "...the cellular abnormality that pathologists call prostate cancer is far too prevalent to be consistently clinically important." And, "How much prostate cancer is found seems to be directly related to how hard it is looked for." (4). In addition, we have substantial uncertainties about the best treatment, even for patients with a higher likelihood of having "significant" disease; there is a conspicuous lack of high quality clinical trials in this area. Two ongoing studies – the European Randomised Trial of Screening for Prostate Cancer (ERSPC), and the UK ProtecT study (5), will shed light on the utility of screening and, perhaps on the optimum form of curative treatment. Analysis of the further follow up of a recent randomised trial conducted by the Scandinavian Prostate Cancer Study Group (6) reporting estimated 10-year results has shown an overall survival benefit for patients treated by radical prostatectomy rather than by watchful waiting, together with a significant difference in prostate cancer-specific mortality and in the rate of developing metastatic disease in favour of patients treated by surgery. The significance of this is, at the moment, unclear particularly as its magnitude could not easily be translated into the expected benefits of treatment in today's patient population.

And so, the time, if not already past due, has come to recognize and change the standard of care for patients with prostate cancer to reflect the facts that:

- Aggressive treatment for localized low-grade disease is not usually warranted.
- Prostate cancer beyond localized low-grade disease is potentially a systemic disease and must be managed with that in mind and that,
- Therein treatment should ideally include attention not only to the location of the tumor at detection, but to its biological properties.

Therefore, having set "metastasis as a therapeutic target" let us in that which follows endeavour to bring into perspective ongoing observations within each of the topics covered.

2. GENES AND METASTASIS

Initially, we can directly attack the tumor cell genotype. A greater understanding of the molecular basis of metastasis will itself generate a range of new targets (7). In addition to CpG methylation, pointed out by Maitland (7) as the most commonly recognized and observed mechanism for selective gene silencing, histone modifications, a second prominent type of epigenetic regulatory mechanism, is closely related. By way of example the Vitamin D receptor by which 1, 25 $(OH)_2$-vitamin D_3 acts to exert cell-cycle regulatory antiproliferative effects, is regulated by histone modification. Indeed, clinical trials with histone deacetylation inhibitors are now underway. The significance of epigenetic silencing of select genes can contribute to cancer initiation, progression, invasion and metastasis.

Of a number of methylated genes in prostate cancer which correlate with clinicopathological features and may be critical to the ability of tumor cells to invade and metastasize, E-cadherin may be selected as a prototypical example. The role of E-cadherin in the biology of the prostate, its partners, signalling mechanisms and implications in the progression and metastasization of prostate cancer have been meticulously covered in respective overviews by Hendrix et al. (8) and Davies et al. (9).

Of further interest in relation to the E-cadherin/catenin complex considered by Davies et al (9), is that in addition to its known immunohistochemical expression in the prostate, recent studies by Kuefer et al. (10) have reported the identification of an 80 kDa fragment of E-cadherin in the serum of patients with prostate cancer. Although not disease-specific, nor related to tumor burden, the highest serum levels were observed in patients with advanced hormone refractory metastatic prostate cancer. Parenthetically, at an optimized cutoff, high expression of the 80 kDa serum fragment at the time of diagnosis was associated with a significantly increased risk of late biochemical failure at 3 years after radical prostatectomy.

For those interested in CpG hypermethylation and alterations during the progression of prostate cancer to metastasis, the reader is referred to the recent review by Yegnasubramanian and Nelson (11).

Mention and, albeit brief, comment on the following genes and proteins identified through the technique of gene expression profiling described by Maitland (7), is appropriate given their potential to identify tumors that are on an aggressive path toward the development of metastasis and given that, in select instances, they may in themselves serve as potential therapeutic targets.

Metastasis-associated gene 1 (MTA1), is involved in transcriptional silencing and is overexpressed in metastatic compared to localized prostate cancer, suggesting it plays a role in cancer progression to the metastatic state (12). MTA1 silencing is mainly dependent on histone deacetylases and is another example of epigenetic silencing via histone modifications.

Expression of JAGGED1, a NOTCH receptor ligand, which plays a role in epithelial to mesenchymal transitions (requisite for the migration of cancer cells) in cancer is significantly increased in metastatic vs. localized prostate cancer or BPH (13). JAGGED1, as well as other genes is increased in other cancers, and, therefore, its role, as suggested by Santagata et al. (13) in distinguishing indolent from aggressive prostate cancer must be viewed with caution.

Survivin, an inhibitor of the apoptosis gene family and overexpressed in numerous cancers, has been linked to accelerated relapses, hormone refractory disease and unfavorable outcome. Given the association of differentiation of neuroendocrine (NE) cells in relationship to the growth and progression of prostate cancer, notably hormone refractory tumors, the identification of survivin and its overexpression in NE cells (14) is noteworthy.

In maintaining homeotic gene expression, two groups of proteins referred to as polycomb and trithorax play a key role in the transcriptional maintenance or memory system of the host. Dysregulation of this system can lead to malignancy. Among the polycomb proteins, there are genes involved in control of cell growth and division. Therein expression of Enhancer of Zeste homolog 2 (EZH2), a transcriptional repressor, has been found to be significantly higher in hormone-refractory, metastatic vs. localized prostatic tumors or normal prostate (15) suggesting that overexpression "portends aggressiveness and metastasis" (15). Studies of EZH2 to date have shown it to be the best predictor of clinical outcome; and have demonstrated EZH2 has a role in mediating cell proliferation and transcriptional repression contributing to the lethal progression of prostate cancer (15). Within this context, it may, pending further evaluation, be considered as a marker to distinguish indolent from aggressive prostate cancer.

In searching for further proteins influencing metastasis of prostate cancer, hedgehog – a cell signalling molecule that drives normal development and regeneration in the prostate (and in several other tissues) is significantly upregulated in prostate cancers that have been observed to metastasize (16, 17). Development of methods to selectively target hedgehog may prove useful in inhibiting the progression of prostate cancer.

Among investigations toward understanding the role of serine proteases upregulated by androgens in the metastatic process of prostate cancer, several recent studies have looked at the TMPRSS2 gene. *In situ* hybridization studies showed localization of TMPRSS2 to basal cells (18). However, given its presence in the normal, as well as the malignant prostate and in other tissues, e.g., colon and lung, the initial hopes for diagnostic and therapeutic targeting of TMPRSS2 in the absence of its other interacting macromolecules would seem to be questionable. It is noted however, that as TMPRSS2 is expressed on the cell membrane, as well as being released therefrom, it could function as a receptor for other proteins and/or act in an autocrine manner. In this regard, TMPRSS2 has been observed to activate the protease activated receptor (PAR)-2 expressed in the prostate which increases the levels of matrix metalloproteinases (MMPs)-2 and -9 –key proteases contributing to the metastization of tumor cells (19).

With up to 35% of prostate cancer patients treated for organ confined disease having a local recurrence which may eventually lead to metastatic disease, a key question is whether the metastasis comes from pre-existing micrometastasis or from persistent disease remaining locally. Therefore, in addition to the identification of tumors that are on an aggressive path toward metastasis, the ability to detect micrometastatic disease is critical. From this perspective, Kufer et al. (20) have described a novel sensitive multimarker nested RT-PCR capable of detecting individual expression of human melanoma-associated antigens (MAGE [also named cancer-testis antigens])-A genes. Members of the MAGE-A gene family, MAGE-1, -2, -3/6, -4 and –12 have been observed in rare disseminated tumor cells in the blood and bone marrow of patients with prostate cancer. Patients with an exceptionally high risk of metastatic disease, defined by clinical prognostic factors, were significantly more MAGE positive than lower risk patients (20).

Further, within the context of predicting clinical outcome, increased phosphorylation of the serine/threonine kinase Akt (Ser^{473}) [phosphorylated Akt (pAkt)] and decreased phosphorylation of extracellular signal-related kinase (ERK; Thr^{202}/Tyr^{204}) [phosphorylated ERK (pERK)] have been shown by Kreisberg et al. (21) to be an excellent predictor of poor clinical outcome. In terms of distinguishing an indolent vs. a would-be aggressive cancer, phosphorylation of Akt alone or together with ERK may, pending further study, be a useful biological marker of a clinically aggressive cancer.

In commenting on various signaling pathways and signaling elements, we should make brief mention of toll-like receptors (TLR) (22). TLR, which activate innate and adaptive immune responses are, in addition to being present on immune cells, expressed on tumor cells from a variety of tissues. Recent studies by Zheng et al. (23) have demonstrated sequence variants of the TLR4 gene in association with the risk of prostate cancer. The association of sequence variants in TLR4 and risk for prostate cancer is particularly interesting when placed in context with observations that chronic infection and inflammatory processes, hallmarks of several diseases, including prostatitis, prone to progress to cancer, are mediated in part by the recoginition of various stimuli by TLR (24). The significance of this in relation to evasion of immunosurveillance and metastasis may be seen from studies in which activation of TLR4 signaling in tumor cells has been observed to induce the synthesis of soluble factors which protect tumor cells from cytotoxic T-lymphocytes (CTL [25]).

As noted, there are a number of genes overexpressed in prostate cancer. However the majority of genes identified are also expressed in several common malignancies and thereby not specific for prostate cancer. Additionally, many of the genes identified may be reflective of the "output of hyperactive cells rather than the molecular machinery driving (the) metastasis" (26) and/or in themselves induce no or only a modest response, however when co-expressed with other genes be highly relevant. Therefore, as the question has been raised by Eccles and Paon (26): "How can we use gene profiling to find genes casually linked to metastasis?"

Recent observations, e.g., with vimentin by Singh et al. (27), in studies of its overexpression in an androgen-independent model of prostate cancer, provide an example of the role of the necessity for co-expression with other genes. In the case in point, transfected induced overexpression of vimentin needed the co-expression of cytokeratins intermediate filaments to confer the invasive and metastatic phenotype.

3. THERAPEUTIC TARGETS

3.1 Gene Therapy

Against this backdrop, Eccles and Paon (26) have suggested that from approaches investigating gene-expression profiles in combination, "we might eventually move closer to the ultimate goal of individualized targeted therapy". Additionally, and as logical as it may be, we must remember that while it is one thing for a gene to be expressed, we must also pose the questions: is the protein there and is it functional?

Gene therapy has yet to overcome the formidable problems of delivery, particularly in patients with disseminated disease, but there may, nonetheless, be other ways of using it in prostate cancer, for example by preventing disease progression in patients with localised disease (28). Nonetheless, using gene therapy as a means of recruiting the immune system is a strategy with inherent advantages in this respect, although data which suggests that tumors produce a cytokine repertoire that induces tolerance, or indeed apoptosis in cytotoxic T-cells, might yet defeat this approach (29, 30, 31), unless as suggested herein by Satoh et al. (32), the object of gene therapy itself is to reverse this (32).

3.2 Dietary Supplements

In continuing, one might target specific aspects of prostate cancer cell biology. Herein, initial thoughts perhaps turn to diet and hormone sensitivity.

The link between diet and prostate cancer, initially suggested by Armstrong and Doll (33) based on international differences in mortality rates and the national average intake of fats, has been considered herein by Jiang (34). In the interim of the observations by Armstrong and Doll (33) some case-control studies have shown a significant association between various measures of fat intake, most notably saturated fat, monounsaturated fat and alpha-linolenic acid with advanced prostate cancer, while others have not.

With the focus on the metastatic process, Jiang (34) has provided a meticulous look at the role of polyunsaturated fatty acids (PUFA) by examining their effect on the essential steps in the metastatic cascade toward the formation of tumor metastases. This analysis has illustrated the impact of PUFA and their potential therapeutic value on the metastatic process.

In keeping with the observations of Jiang (34), but with a focus on the general parameter of prostate cancer risk vs. metastasis, Bidoli et al. (35), in one of the largest case-control studies of diet and prostate cancer to date, have shown a decreased risk of prostate cancer (OR 0.8) in association with PUFA.

Not related to PUFA, but a possible *caveat* from the study by Bidoli et al. (35), for further investigation, was the association of high starch intake and an increased risk for prostate cancer (OR 1.4). As a possible explanation, Bidoli et al. (35) suggest the glycemic overload may be compensated by an increase in insulin-like growth factor-1 (IGF-1) known to be associated with prostate cancer. Within the context of IGF-1 and diet, the recent study by Kelavkar and Cohen (36) has shown overexpression of the fat-metabolizing enzyme, 15-lipoxygenase in prostate cancer, which contributed to cancer progression by regulating IGF-1 receptor expression and activation.

3.3 Molecular Mechanisms of Hormone Resistance and Optimization of Hormone Therapy

With reference to hormone sensitivity, there is an urgent need to understand the mechanisms whereby prostate cancers become hormone refractory (37). This might result from the recruitment of alternative "rescue" signal transduction pathways (38, 39, 40, 41, 42) or by subversion of androgen receptor (AR)-mediated signalling, e.g., using a different repertoire of co-activators and co-repressors (43, 44), including the cytokine IL-6 (45). Additionally, autocrine and/or paracrine mechanisms may, in lieu of, or in concert with mutations and/or amplifications of the AR, activate pathways, producing responses of the AR downstream (46), e.g., studies by Yeh et al. (47) and Wen et al. (48) have reported that overexpression of the tyrosine kinase, HER-2/neu (ErbB-2) in prostate cancer promotes androgen-independent survival and growth of prostate cancer cells and activated AR transcriptional function through the downstream mitogen-activated protein kinase or Akt pathway. Given the role of HER-2/neu signaling, it is a natural target to disrupt AR function. However, clinical trials using humanized monoclonal antibodies to HER-2/neu (Herceptin) only and in combination with docetaxel have been problematical due to the variable overexpression of HER-2/neu (49). In an attempt to obviate this problem a humanized monoclonal antibody, referred to as Pertuzumab, that targets the role of HER2 as coreceptor has been developed (50). Pertuzumab binds to a different epitope of the HER2 ectodomain than Herceptin and sterically hinders ligand-dependent heterodimerization of HER2 with other HER receptors. This results in inhibition of signaling by HER2-based heterodimers in cells with low and HER2 expression. Pertuzumab has shown antitumor activity in preclinical models of prostate cancer. However, a recently reported phase II study with this agent was negative (51).

Reviewed by Shelley et al. (52), the full potential of our existing modalities of hormone therapy has yet to be completely determined, and this deserves continued attention (53, 54, 55). Herein, the naturally occurring pathway of RNA interference (RNAi), a unique form of post-transcriptional gene silencing, may have application. Utilizing a prostate-specific vector expressing small interfering RNAs (siRNAs) from the PSA promoter –a RNA polymerase II promoter, Song et al. (56) recently demonstrated androgen-dependent and tissue-specific siRNA-mediated gene silencing in the androgen-dependent prostate cancer cell line, LNCaP. Biologically, the significance of this was evidenced by alteration of apoptotic activity via inhibition of the apoptosis-related regulatory gene. Additionally, by way of further example of siRNA interference, inactivation of TWIST, a highly conserved basic helix-loop-helix transcription factor, levels of which correlate with Gleason grade and metastasis in androgen-independent prostate cancer cells resulted in increased chemodrug-induced apoptosis and suppression of invasiveness (57). These observations provide impetus for further study of the potential effectiveness of siRNA-mediated gene silencing for the treatment of prostate cancer.

3.4 Proliferation

Concurrently there are many approaches, simply directed against proliferation, which may be of benefit in prostate cancer, just as they may be in many other cancers (58, 59, 60).

In addition to the loss of the tumor suppressor –PTEN, as considered by Newman and Zetter (58) and subsequent constitutive activation of the Akt pathway leading to activation of mitogenic and pro-survival signaling molecules (as one of the ways of undermining cell cycle control in the control of the progression of prostate cancer to androgen-independence), the pivotal transcriptional factor, nuclear factor kappaB (NFκB) has been shown to prevent cell death by apoptosis in PC-3 and DU-145 cell lines (61), Interestingly, blockade of NFκB activity in PC-3 xenografts in nude mice inhibited angiogenesis, invasion and regional lymph node metastasis (62). The observation that NFκB is constitutively activated in the bone metastasis-derived PC-3 cell line (63) further implicates its role in bone metastasis as also considered previously herein by Hoffman (64) and Clarke and Fleisch (65).

Of particular further interest with reference to the role of NFκB in metastasis are observations by Ayala et al. (66) in perineural invasion (PNI) in prostate cancer. A key process for the extracapsular spread of prostate cancer, studies of PNI in an *in vitro* model of PNI and of human prostate cancer tissue microarrays prepared from patients who underwent radical prostatectomy, demonstrated increased proliferation and decreased apoptosis of perineurally localized cancer cells in association with up-regulation of NFκB and its downstream targets, PIM-2 and defender against death 1.

The foregoing and related observations by others supports the rationale for inhibitors of NFκB presently in development and/or in clinical trials for the prevention and/or treatment of prostate cancer (67).

In addition to the cell cycle markers considered by Newman and Zetter (58) shown to have a direct role in dysregulation leading to metastatic prostate cancer, one of the earlier noted oncogenes, c-myc (also mentioned by Maitland [7]) exhibits increasing amplification with transition through PIN to metastatic prostate cancer (68) and with increasing Gleason score (69) and mortality. However, as several genes are also located at the 8q24 amplicon, which is amplified, the role of c-myc in prostate cancer has been unclear. However, recent studies have shown that: i) transgenic models overexpressing c-myc in the prostate have a concentration related progression towards malignancy and ii) c-myc in a model of human prostate cancer is sufficient to induce carcinogenesis (70).

4. TUMOR MICROENVIRONMENT

One area, which is proving to be of particular importance in prostate cancer, and in understanding mechanisms of invasion and metastasis, is the dynamic relationship between the tumor and the host, i.e., the tumor microenvironment (71, 72, 73, 74, 75, 76, 77).

Observation of the plasticity of tumor cells by Hendrix et al. (8), whereby the dynamic interplay between tumor cells and their microenvironment may determine their function and fate, *ergo*, vasculogenic mimicry and the acquisition of the malignant phenotype further demonstrates that: i) tumor cells do not grow in isolation and ii) that the inter- and/or intratumoral microenvironment are important to modulation of gene expression and the phenotypic properties of tumor cells and tumor-derived factors in extension and refinement of earlier studies pointing to the role of the microenvironment and factors therein in tumorigenesis (78). The environment, while not inducing malignancy, may permit activation of quiescent tumor and/or compromise the hosts control, i.e., immunosurveillance of tumor, thereby being permissive (78).

With the objective of looking into select aspects of these interactions in the microenvironment, but confronted with the challenge of the heterogeneous characteristics of prostate cancer, Hendrix et al. (8) utilized, as they have described, an integrated *in vitro* and *in vivo* strategy permitting development of a series of new Dunning R3327 Copenhagen rat cell lines. Ongoing studies of these cell lines are revealing expression of multiple molecular phenotypes by aggressive tumor cells and that their co-operation is necessary for the successful progression of prostate cancer (8).

Within the framework of the progression of prostate cancer, Wilson and Sinha (79) have, in their Chapter "Matrix Degradation in Prostate Cancer", provided a superbly detailed overview, with a specific focus on proteases, of the means by which prostate cancer cells proceed from the primary prostatic tumor promoting growth of the tumor and passage from one biological compartment to another to their subsequent colonization at distant sites. Inclusive of the diverse proteases permitting passage of malignant cells are the MMPs. In addition to their role in contributing to the cleavage of the basement membrane (BM) and extracellular matrix (ECM) proteins of prostate tissues, tumor-derived MMPs also react with host immune cells in the primary tumor facilitating the escape of tumors from immunosurveillance, e.g., by inducing proteolytic cleavage of IL-2Rα (a receptor essential for the proliferation of T-cells) they suppress the proliferative capability of cancer encountered T-cells (80). Also, increased numbers of immune system cells, i.e., macrophages, neutrophils, known to contain MMPs, may under select environmental conditions contribute to passage of tumor cells by proteolysis of the BM (80).

Turning briefly to the serine proteases, and PSA, Wilson and Sinha (79) have provided a brief comment on the clinical significance of serum PSA, the subject of which has also been considered herein by Penson and Albertson (1). For further specifics of current PSA assays the interested reader is referred to a brief communication by one of us (81) laying out the culpability of these assays (82). With an appreciation of the functionality of PSA as a serine protease, continuing investigations of its important role in the normal prostate and its pathophysiology (82) are further significantly considered (82).

Also of importance in the tumor microenvironment, are the presence of tumor-associated macrophages (TAMs). Contrary to general opinion, there is considerable recent evidence that TAMs not only fail to kill tumor cells, but contribute to tumor progression through enhanced invasiveness of tumor cells by the secretion of factors such as cytokines and MMPs (83). TAMs further inhibit lymphocytic activity at the tumor site via the production of immunosuppressive macromolecules.

Identified in TAMs and elsewhere in the normal and pathologic prostate and secretions (84), the calcium-dependent family of enzymes – transglutaminases (TGases), which include the thrombin-independent and – dependent, tissue and Factor(F) XIII (found in plasma and cells) forms, respectively, are noteworthy (84). Intriguingly: i) tissue and plasma TGases modulate the activity of select parameters of immune responsiveness and ii) significantly increased concentrations of plasma TGase have been found in association with prostate cancer vs. normal and benign prostate (84). The close association of TAMs and plasma TGase suggest it is involved in the binding of host proteins to tumor cells forming a stabilized intratumoral fibrin that facilitates tumor matrix generation, angiogenesis and a barrier to mechanisms of host defense. The localization of plasma TGase to prostatic histiocytes expressing monocyte/macrophage differentiation markers, providing a means for TGase in the regulation of antigen presentation and induction of immune responses, portends to the permissive, if not direct, role of TGase in the hosts regulation of invasion and metastasis of tumor cells (84, 85)

Of further interest regarding the role of TGase in regulation of the invasiveness of prostate cancer are studies of its effect on S100 protein function.

Members of the S100 family of Ca^{2+}-binding proteins have been implicated in a variety of cellular processes, e.g., calcium signal transduction, cytoskeletal-membrane interactions, cellular growth and differentiation. Referred to as psoriasin from its original association with abnormally differentiating keratinocytes in psoriasis (86), the gain or loss of S100 protein expression has been linked to various disease states, wherein, e.g., as cited by Maitland (7), S100A4 has been linked directly to metastatic disease.

Based on psoriasin as a candidate substrate for TGases (87), Davies et al. (88) observed that at the mRNA level, TGase-4 (prostate TGase) was strongly expressed in the low invasive CA-HPV-10 prostate cancer cell line and its substrate psoriasin was increased in TGase-4 knock-out cells, accompanied by increased immunocytochemical staining at regions of cell-cell contact. Requisite of further study, these observations suggest that through its effect on the cytoskeletal-membrane properties of psoriasin, TGase may modify the invasiveness of prostate cancer.

Enhanced invasiveness correlates with induction of NFκB and *c-Jun*-NH_2-kinase (JNK), wherein NFκB promotes migration of tumor cells by inducing the expression of the chemokine receptor CXCR4 (89).

In a somewhat over-simplification of a complex process, prostate cancer cells showing a propensity to metastasize to the skeleton express the CXCR4 chemokine receptor and are attracted by the CXCL12 (also known as stromal-derived factor-1) [SDF-1] chemokine ligand to secondary sites, where they form metastases (90). The binding of CXCR4/CXCL12 leads to the activation of multiple signaling pathways, e.g., PI3K/Akt, with differential secretion of various cytokines and MMPs, particular MMP-9, into the local environment and ensuing events. Migration studies show that antibodies to CXCR4 inhibit chemotaxis of metastatic cell lines of prostate cancer (90). Similarly, pharmacological inhibition of PI3 kinase and MAP kinase pathways abrogates CXCL12-induced MMP-9 expression (91). These observations suggest inhibition of the CXCR4/CXCL12 pathway may prove therapeutically beneficial. In fact, this approach has already been pursued in the instance of breast cancer (92).

Additionally, we note that some chemokines may enhance innate and specific host immunity against tumors, but at the same time other chemokines may contribute to escape from the immune system by recruiting Th_2 effectors and regulatory T cells.

A final point on this lengthy, but we do believe pertinent commentary on the microenvironment is recent attention to the importance of recognizing the "microenvironment of the circulation" (93). Referred to as the "third" microenvironment, with the primary tumor site being the "first" and the metastatic or secondary tumor site constituting the "second", the circulatory system, from the perspective of its importance to metastasis, has according to Loberg et al. (93) been "under appreciated." Analysis therein of circulating tumor cells and factors permitting their passage and survival, avoiding destruction by among other factors, e.g., the immune system, may disclose means for the therapeutic targeting of tumor cell survival.

The foregoing observations emphasize the importance of studying the tumor microenvironment. These observations suggest the biological behaviour of malignant cells are intimately related to the surrounding milieu, which in itself may be mutagenic and an important source of genetic instability.

With recognition of the critical importance of the microenvironment and advent and continuing refinement of today's technology, it should be possible to integrate molecular profiles of gene expression in the tumor microenvironment with the histological features of the tumor. This integration will permit a much-needed modification of the current tumor grading systems, i.e., in the case of prostate cancer – the Gleason score from static histopathology. The Gleason score cannot, in guiding treatment, presently distinguish an indolent from an aggressive cancer in more than 66% of newly diagnosed cancers with Gleason scores of 5–7. The significance of this is exemplified by innumerable observations where, biopsy specimens from two patients with prostate cancer may be histologically identical, but one may remain indolent, while the other may be aggressive.

Elucidation and understanding of interactions between the tumor and the microenvironment will also provide new opportunities for adjunct and new methods of diagnosis and treatment.

5. MODELS OF METASTASIS

A model whereby factors such as hepatocyte growth factor (HGF), produced by stromal cells, may induce tumor cells to metastasize is one that may be of importance (94). As well as introducing the possibility that antagonists of factors such as HGF might be useful in preventing metastases, it also serves to refocus attention on the "normal" stroma surrounding a tumor, to ask the question as to whether there may be interventions that might affect the natural history of the disease. This might fall exclusively into the realms of prevention, itself an important and worthy goal, but there is also evidence of cross-talk between receptors such as *c-met*, and the epidermal growth factor receptor family. Such treatments might, therefore, apply to established disease and maybe even to established metastatic disease. The development of appropriate orthotopic models is absolutely crucial for the further exploration of this area and we continually need to refine these in order to render them as realistic a model as possible, and free from the artificialities that such an approach can all too often engender (64).

From this perspective Hoffman (64) has provided a valuable overview of the background and description of orthotopic metastatic animal models of prostate cancer and their application for the study of the progression and metastasis of prostate cancer. Included, is an extremely useful narrative on materials and methods of implantation and evaluation of tumor growth and metastasis.

Surgical orthotopic implantation of human tumor to an animal host provides a more realistic model of human cancer. When used in concert with the introduction (via transfection) of a green fluorescent protein gene to tumor cells, this enables metastasis to be visualized throughout the skeletal system and to other important organs. The approach permits important insight into mechanisms of prostate cancer metastasis. With this in mind, and from the perspective of treatment, Hoffman (64) has considered the application of selected gene and other types of therapy in the metastasis models presented.

There may, however, be quite specific mechanisms which drive proliferation in prostate cancer cells, e.g., ornythine decarboxylase (95) and tissue-specific mechanisms, if they exist, would further open up new therapeutic avenues.

6. IMPACT OF BONE METASTASIS

A natural extension of this line of argument is to consider the impact of bone as a specific site of metastases, on the development of new methods of diagnosis, prediction of metastasis and treatments. In this regard, we are reminded from the chapter by Clarke and Fleisch (65) that with the axial skeleton involved in 85% of patients dying from prostate cancer, bone metastasis is the hallmark of metastatic prostate.

With reference to new methods of diagnosis and prediction of metastasis, use of fluorodeoxyglucose as a tracer to detect abnormal metabolism in invaded tissues, single-photon emission CT and positron emission tomography have improved sensitivity (96). For early prediction of bone metastasis, two promising osteoblastic markers –P1NP and P1CP are suggested as particularly promising (96).

Bone metastasis factors which encourage prostate cancer cell growth in bone, such as transferin, might themselves be amenable to manipulation. In addition, the use of bisphosphonates as a means of switching off osteoclast-mediated bone destruction, is already well established, at least in clinical trials (65). The optimum use of such agents remains to be determined, and as with almost every other possible therapeutic, is likely to be most useful in combination i.e., in multimodality therapy. There is also an issue about the timing of therapy. The published data on bisphosphonates in clinical use is heavily weighted towards patients with established metastatic disease. The Medical Research Council (MRC) PR04 Study which, was a double blind randomised trial of adjuvant clodronate in patients with non-metastatic cancer, was an attempt to see whether bisphosphonate treatment earlier in the natural history might be of benefit. The first results of this trial have shown no improvement in time to onset of symptomatic bone metastases, in stark contrast to similar trials in breast cancer and myeloma (97), and one wonders what the effect might have been with a more potent, newer generation bisphosphonate.

On the subject of the use of bisphosphonates in combination with other agents, systemic administration of zoledronate combined with STI571 (imatinib mesylate, Gleevec [an inhibitor of phosphorylation of the platelet-derived growth factor receptor]) and paclitaxel in experimental prostate cancer bone and lymph node metastasis, produced a significant decrease in tumor incidence and size accompanied by significant preservation of bone structure and a decrease in lymph node metastasis (98).

Although the efficacy of treatment with bisphosphonates in inhibiting bone resorption has been clearly demonstrated, several secondary and undesirable side-effects have also been noted ranging from, e.g., from the recent FDA safety warning on Aredia (pamindronate disodium) and Zometa (zoledronic acid) injection after cases of osteonecrosis, particularly of the jaw (http://www.fda.gov/medwatch/SAFETY/2004/safety04.htm#zometa) to nephrotoxicity. Within this context, alternate treatments to bisphosphonates based on knowledge of osteoclast biology have been proposed. These include strategies based on cytokines, peptidomimetics and inhibitors of specific signaling pathways.

Before leaving these comments on bisphosphonates, we should mention recently reviewed preclinical studies have shown bisphosphonates exhibit antitumor activity (99).

7. OTHER BIOLOGICAL AGENTS

Other biological agents are also finding their way into clinical trials. The importance of prostaglandin synthesis in the development of prostate cancer has been highlighted earlier in this book. Whether or not inhibitors of COX-2 might be useful therapeutically is an open question (95). In this regard, recent concerns of COX-2 inhibitors have arisen due to their association with an increased risk of mortality from cardiovascular complications (100).

In the interim, studies in human prostate cancer cells, i.e., LNCaP and PC3, and PC3 xenografts in nude mice have shown celecoxib (Celebrix) not only targets COX-2, but reduces levels of cyclin D1 (impacting on the progression of cells from G_1 to S) and caused approximately a 50% decrease in proliferation and microvascular density (101). Although still an investigational product in prostate cancer, given confirmation and extension of the foregoing results, one may have to eventually balance the toxicity issues with celecoxib with those of chemotherapy.

This and other questions, are being addressed in the ongoing MRC "STAMPEDE" (Systemic Therapy in Advancing or Metastatic Prostate Cancer: Evaluation of Drug Efficacy) study, which is a 5 arm study randomising patients beginning hormone therapy to either standard hormone therapy alone, or to hormone therapy plus docetaxal, zoledronic acid, a COX-2 inhibitor, to a combination of chemotherapy and bisphosphonate, and to a combination of COX-2 plus bisphosphonate (Figure 1). This study is aiming to recruit 3000 patients in the next 6 years, and is currently in its pilot phase of patient recruitment (Figure 1).

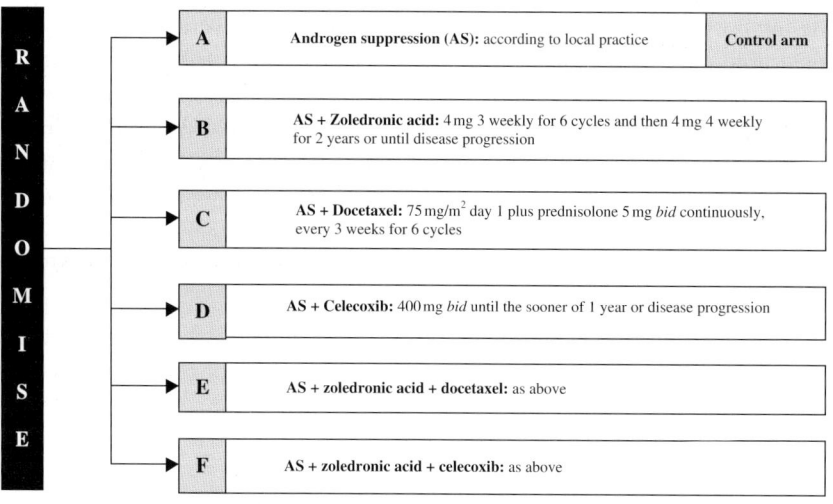

AS = Androgen suppression as in Arm A

Figure 1. Schema of the Medical Research Council STAMPEDE Trial. Patients beginning long-term hormone therapy, for either metastatic or non-metastatic prostate cancer, are randomised as above. Following a pilot phase to establish feasibility and safety, the trial will proceed to a first analysis with failure-free survival as the primary endpoint. Arms not showing a benefit will then be dropped, and the trial will proceed to a second phase, using the successful arms, with overall survival as the primary endpoint.

In concert with the known capabilities and limitations of chemo- and radiotherapy considered by Scullin et al. (102), various approaches have been undertaken toward augmenting their effects. Within the obvious limitations of a complete discussion here of all of these approaches, mention and a brief comment is made on selected potentially promising approaches.

Evidence of the repopulation of surviving tumor cells between courses of chemotherapy and an increase of their rate of proliferation has suggested the use of short acting agents selectively inhibiting tumor cells may be beneficial (103). Toward this end, Wu et al. (103) have shown the use of the rapamycin analogue CCI-779 given between courses of mitoxantrone or docetaxel increased growth delay of PC-3 xenografts.

Coupling cytotoxic agents to specific monoclonal antibodies to target tumor antigens has been applied in prostate cancer. Based on the expression of prostate-specific membrane antigen (PSMA) on the surface of prostate epithelial cells, monoclonal antibody to PSMA coupled to maytansinoid 1, a microtubule-depolymerizing compound, demonstrated antitumor activity in the CWR22 xenograft model of osteoblastic prostate cancer metastasis (104).

With further reference to the earlier mentioned use of siRNA-mediated gene silencing (55), siRNA silencing of p53 mutant PC-3 prostate cancer cells and the caffeine target, ataxia telangiectasia mutated (ATM) gene (a member of the phosphatidylinositol 3-kinase [PI3K] family of proteins, that activates DNA repair and cell cycle checkpoint pathways) selectively increased the sensitivity of PC-3 cells vs. normal cells to doxorubicin (105). Within the context of silencing select checkpoint pathways toward the selective killing of tumor cells, the use of an antisense RNA to ATM also increased the radiosentivitivity of prostate cancer cells (106).

8. RADIATION THERAPY AND BEYOND

Toward clarifying the ion beam-specific biological effects, comparison of the metastatic capabilities of tumor cells following irradiation with photon, proton and ion carbon beams has demonstrated preclinical evidence that particle radiation best suppresses metastatic potential of tumor cells (107), at least in this experimental model. Whether this observation has clinical application or not may require a renewed effort to develop further studies of proton beam therapy in prostate cancer (108).

Looking toward expanding the use of radiation therapy to metastasis, several investigators have applied radioimmunotherapy. Here a radiolabeled antibody specific for a component of the primary tumor and metastatic cells is used to deliver radiation to the target. Radiolabeled antibody to

PSMA, represents one popularized approach (109). Most recently, Zhao et al. (110) have utilized an antibody to tomoregulin, a transmembrane protein selectively expressed in the brain, prostate and prostate cancer (primary tumor and metastatic tissues, i.e., in lymph nodes and bone), but not in other normal tissues or a wide range of tumors of other major organs, to deliver radiation to inhibit the growth of LNCaP xenografts in nude mice in the absence of any overt toxicity. As noted, the presence of tomoregulin protein in metastases portends that tomoregulin is a potentially excellent target for radioimmunotherapy.

In an attempt to target occult metastatic disease (presumptively suggested by many) as an explanation for biochemical failure, which occurs in 30–40% of patients treated by surgery or radiation for localized prostate cancer, Gulley et al. (111) demonstrated in a randomized Phase II Clinical Trial that a poxviral vaccine encoding PSA induced a PSA-specific T-cell response when combined with definitive external beam radiation therapy in patients with localized prostate cancer. The trial has demonstrated the feasibility of combination therapy, its effect on the immune system and that radiotherapy to the prostate is not broadly immunosuppressive. However, even though the authors state the foregoing was the purpose of the study, there is no reference to the identification of the supposed occult metastasis in the patients and thus no demonstrated clinical effect of the antibodies. Furthermore, two patients who received vaccine plus radiation therapy and previously had lymph node positive disease developed metastatic disease (to the liver and adrenals, respectively) and went on to receive chemotherapy! So much for the proposed synergistic effect of the vaccine plus radiation and the beneficial clinical effect of the immune response, at least in these two patients.

9. NOVEL THERAPEUTIC APPROACHES

Scullin et al. (102) have further given consideration, albeit brief, to "Novel (therapeutic) approaches".

On the subject of anti-angiogenesis agents, it is noted bevacizumab (Avastin), currently used in combination with taxane-based therapies is the recombinant humanized version of the murine antihuman vascular endothelial growth factor (VEGF) monoclonal antibody A4.6.1 referred to by Scullin et al. (102) in the studies by Melnyk et al. (112).

With further reference to VEGF, a *caveat* perhaps to regulation of angiogenesis in the prostate is appreciation that there are at least four isoforms of VEGF, i.e., A, B, C and D, each with different physiological roles and receptor affinities (113). Therefore, a greater understanding of the differential role of VEGF receptors and whether therapies designed to target these specific molecules will prove efficacious. Presently, decreased VEGFR1 and increased VEGFR2 are associated with the transition from a differentiated cancer to more poorly differentiated state (114). Equally, different angiogenic mechanisms may be differentially expressed at various stages of tumor progression.

With reference to variation in angiogenic mechanisms in general and in accord with various stages of disease, there are in addition to VEGF, as recently reviewed by Lissbrant et al. (115), a variety of blood flow and angiogenesis regulatory factors. These include among others, fibroblast growth factor, transforming growth factor-beta1 (TGF-β1) and endoglin –a receptor for TGF-β1 on endothelial cells. A particularly interesting angiogenesis factor associated with a metastatic phenotype is pigment epithelium-derived factor (PEDF [116]). Independent studies by Halin et al. (116) and Filleur et al. (117), to which the interested reader is referred, provide evidence that decreased expression of PEDF contributes to tumor progression possibly through increased tumor cell proliferation and angiogenesis.

Buoyed by the increased incidence of prostate cancer and number of patients who fail local therapy for "presumed to be" localized disease, presenting with a recurrence of their cancer, the number of therapeutic agents and clinical trials have increased significantly over the past decade. A search, e.g., of the Pharmaceutical Research and Manufacturers of America for New Medicines in Development for Prostate Cancer 2005 (http://www.phrama.org, 5 October 2005) disclosed 50+ drugs under development. From these and others, we mention in brief the following which appear within Scullin et al.'s (102) category of "Novel (therapeutic) approaches".

Identification of unique or metastasis specific signal transduction pathways in prostate cancer may provide insight into development of small molecule inhibitors with clinical utility. Therapeutic small molecules that inhibit components of such signal transduction pathways have the potential to specifically target metastatic cancer.

Studies suggesting the epidermal growth factor receptor (EGFR) signaling pathways may be involved in angiogenesis and invasion in prostate cancer prompted investigations of targeting it as a potential therapeutic approach.

Early preclinical studies of Cetuximab, an anti-EGFR monoclonal antibody, directed toward prevention of activation of the tyrosine kinase receptor in an orthotopic model of androgen-independent prostate cancer - PC-3M-LN4, demonstrated activity alone and in combination with paclitaxel

(118) and based on stabilization of PSA in a small group of patients with androgen-independent prostate cancer (119). However, subsequent studies of an EGFR anatagonist, Iressa (Gefitinib, ZD1839) in androgen-independent prostate cancer were marked by inconsistent PSA responses and early progression of disease (120). These mixed results await further clarification of the role of EGFR in prostate cancer.

Another growth factor implicated in the progression of prostate cancer is platelet-derived growth factor (PDGF) and its receptor (PDGF-R). Binding of PDGF to PDGF-R and its activation stimulates cell division, migration and angiogenesis. Activation of PDGF-R also has been shown to inhibit pathways leading to apoptosis. Observations that Gleevec (STI157, imatinib mesylate) a specific inhibitor of the oncogene Bcr-Abl associated with chronic myloid leukemia (121) also inhibits PDGF-R, prompted investigation of its effect on prostate cancer. Therein studies by Uehara et al. (122) of the effects of Gleevec alone or in combination with paclitaxel in the androgen-independent PC-3MM2 mouse model of bone metastasis in prostate cancer, disclosed Gleevec, particularly in combination with paclitaxel resulted in significant inhibition of tumor growth, increased apoptosis, decrease in lymph node metastases and bone lesions and preservation of bone structure. While suggestive that PDGF-R would be a promising therapeutic target in prostate cancer, clinical trials of Gleevec in combination with the bisphosphonate Zometa or alone have thus far shown no (123) or at best a limited response (124). A current study is looking at Gleevec in combination with docetaxel.

The use of antisense oligonucleotides have been used to target the antiapoptotic proteins Bcl-2 and clusterin.

Preclinical studies of models of prostate cancer have shown that antisense Bcl-2 inhibits expression of Bcl-2 and delays the transition from an androgen-dependent to androgen-independent growth (125). A Phase II trial of Genasense (G3139, Oblimersen) and docetaxel by the European Organization for Research and Treatment of Cancer is ongoing.

Observations of increased expression of clusterin in association with high Gleason scores and high levels in tumor cells surviving androgen ablation therapy, suggests follow up to an initial Phase 1 clinical trial in prostate cancer of the second-generation antisense drug OXG-011 (which compared to the 1st generation, has a longer half-life and fewer side effects) may be of importance. OXG-011 may, in the trend of the multi-drug approach, i.e., a "cocktail" of drugs vs. a stand-a-lone drug, prove efficacious not only in treating localized but in hormone-refractory disease (126).

Ansamycin antibiotics, often referred to as "antineoplastic antibiotics," can inhibit the function of heat shock protein 90 (hsp90), a chaperone protein for select signaling proteins, such as AR, HER2 and Akt. This leads to destabilization and degradation of the complexes, which is frequently mediated by the ubiquitin-proteasome pathway. In response to appropriate signals, a chain of ubiquitin molecules covalently attaches to a protein that targets it for destruction by the proteasome which controls the regulated turnover of proteins (127). The potential use of ansamycin antibiotics, for which geldanamycin (GA) (128) is an example of one such agent for prostate cancer, has been evaluated in preclinical studies (129). In addition to degradation of the AR, Mabjeesh et al. (130) have shown GA induces degradation of hypoxia-inducible factor 1α (HIF1α). HIF1α plays an essential role in the adaptation of tumor cells to hypoxia and in promoting angiogenesis. Inhibition of HIF1α blocks tumor angiogenesis and tumor cell growth (130).

Perhaps also broadly within the category of "antineoplastic antibiotics", studies by Lokeshwar et al. (131) and ongoing studies by one of us (RJA) have demonstrated the potential efficacy of chemically-modified tetracyclines in inhibiting metastasis in preclinical models of prostate cancer.

Another promising approach involves inhibition of the ubiquitin-proteasome pathway. Preclinical studies of the proteasome inhibitor, bortezomib (PS-341, Velcade) in LNCaP cells show it blocks the AR signaling pathway, inhibits tumor growth and induces apoptosis (132). Phase II studies of bortezomib alone and in combination with docetaxel are in progress.

10. ANTIOXIDANTS, PHYTOCHEMICALS AND OTHER NATURAL PRODUCTS

In recent years an interest in complementary and alternative medicine (CAM) not considered part of conventional medicine, has gained considerable popularity to the extent that upwards of 60% of cancer patients use one form or another of substances found in nature such as vitamins and herbs. In taking a cursory look at approaches within the broad category of CAM, select dietary antioxidants and natural products are suggestive of having potentially varying degrees of efficacy for metastatic prostate cancer.

Dietary antioxidants as vitamin E, lycopene and selenium have primarily been evaluated as potential chemopreventative agents. However, reviewed by Venkateswaran et al. (133), independent studies have shown each to have effects ranging from induction of cell arrest to inhibition of tumor progression in preclinical models of prostate cancer, with lycopene having an effect by reducing the odds of patients with prostate cancer developing advanced and aggressive disease. Of particular interest are recent studies carried out by Venkateswaran et al. (133) in the *Lady* transgenic model of prostate cancer of the mouse prostate. This is a less aggressive version of the original model, which in spontaneously developing metastatic prostate cancer, mimics progressive forms of human prostate cancer. Therein, vitamin E, selenium and lycopene in the diet in proportion to the human equivalent dramatically reduced the incidence of prostate tumors and increased disease free survival.

Recently, vitamin D_3 (cholecalciferol) alone (134) and in combination with the synthetic retinoid N-(4-hydroxyphenyl) retinamide (135) have been observed to inhibit growth and invasion and the expression of vimentin and MMP-2 associated with tumor progression, respectively, in human prostate cancer cells.

It is important to note that studies have shown that antioxidants may have negative effects by promoting or protecting cancer cells (136, 137) and/or reducing the oncologic effectiveness of cytotoxic therapies (138). Therefore, the use of antioxidants concurrently during chemo- and radiotherapy may be contraindicated.

Several phytochemicals, exemplified by genistein –a prominent isoflavonoid found in soy products, have been shown to possess substantial anticancer activities in prostate cancer, and clinical trials not only for prevention, but for treatment of prostate cancer and its metastases are ongoing (139).

Proceeding with genistein as an example, several mechanisms have been suggested for its effects. Genistein is an inhibitor of protein tyrosine kinases which play key roles in cell growth and apoptosis. Studies have demonstrated genistein can inhibit cancer cell growth, induce apoptosis and inhibit the activation of NFκB and Akt in prostate cancer. Cognizant genistein is a phytoestrogen, the relationship of the foregoing effects to its oestrogenic content, as well as its potential to induce adverse effects associated with the earlier prevalent use of DES, remain to be determined. The interested reader is referred to two recent excellent studies by Li et al. (140) and Huang et al. (141) on the role of genistein in the invasion and metastasis of prostate cancer.

Logical as it is, as long as the AR is functional irrespective of AR-dependent or –independent status, the growth of prostate cancer continues.

Potentially effective as genistein may be, pending the outcome of clinical trials (139), emodin –a natural compound extracted from the plant, *Rheum palmatum* (commonly known as Chinese rhubarb), has been reported by Cha et al. (142) to be more potent and to directly target the AR. Specifically, emodin induces degradation of the AR through the proteasome-mediated pathway by decreasing the association of AR and heat shock protein 90 (hsp90) (142). This results in inhibition of cell proliferation and tumor growth of prostate cancer cells with increased survival of PC-3 xenografts of prostate cancer (142). Pending the outcome of clinical trials, emodin could be a novel and vastly needed therapeutic for directly targeting the AR.

The earlier *caveat* regarding the possible adverse effects given for the use of antioxidants applies equally well for the foregoing natural products.

11. IN TRANSITION

Despite advances in the detection of localized disease, there is no effective treatment for patients who develop recurrent disease following surgery or radiation therapy or for those with metastatic disease. And, while hormonal therapy may be temporarily palliative for patients with advanced disease, the progression to incurable hormone refractory prostate cancer is inevitable. Furthermore, with the: earlier diagnosis; questionable treatment of prostate cancer; substantial number of patients with recurrent disease and the earlier institution of hormonal therapy, patients are becoming hormone refractory earlier in their course of disease while still having a reasonable remaining life expectancy, but with no further effective therapeutic options available.

Therefore, although it may appear to the newly interested basic- and clinical-investigators of prostate cancer that there has been an improvement in the treatment of this disease, if there has, it has been marginal at best. By way of example, the present management of patients with advanced prostatic cancer exemplified by the recent studies with docetaxel based regimens, i.e., docetaxel + prednisone (143) or docetaxel + estramustine (144) have been met with laudable enthusiasm. However, they unfortunately do not result in curing patients and the survival benefit has been on the order of 2–3 months compared with standard therapy, modest at best.

While it may too severe of a statement, the effective treatment of prostate cancer within the current accepted "standard of care," and overall survival for metastatic disease have not significantly changed since the introduction of hormonal therapy by Huggins et al. (145). Therefore, the urgent need to develop more effective treatments with the appreciation that prostate cancer requires localized as well as systemic therapy. The development and implementation of "novel therapeutic" approaches, some of which have already been considered, as well as those to follow, have recently emerged and/or are in development.

12. IMMUNOTHERAPY

Waxing and wanning since the time of Ehrlich's "magic bullet" (146) and the introduction of "immunosurveillance" by Burnet (147), the concept of immunotherapy (including vaccination) based on the exquisite sensitivity and specificity of the immune response presents a formidable means for the destruction of localized tumor and metastases. However, a deeper appreciation and understanding of how immunologic responsiveness may play a fundamental role in prostate cancer is slowly becoming a reality.

With one of us (RJA) perhaps the first to introduce and review possible immunotherapeutic approaches for prostate cancer (148), it is particularly gratifying to see the recent and continued development of the use gene therapy and other vehicles to generate a systemic immunologic response as a therapeutic strategy for this disease.

Considered in a recent overview of viral gene therapy by Hawkins et al. (149), oncolytic viruses continue to receive widespread attention as novel therapeutic agents for the treatment of malignancies, including prostate cancer. *Herpes simplex* virus thymidine kinase (HSV—tk) has been one of the most widely used "suicide genes" to date, particularly because of its "bystander effect." In fact, the initial therapeutic strategy described for metastatic prostatic cancer herein by Satoh et al. (32) employed a direct cytotoxic approach using the HSV-tk gene combined with the prodrug ganciclovir (GCV). This strategy was further modified and expanded, as described by Satoh et al. (32), to include additional immunomodulatory gene therapeutic approaches.

In looking at other approaches, Kaminski et al. (150) and Markiewicz and Kast (151), have provided excellent reviews of immunotherapy for prostate cancer. Lest we be redundant, further and albeit brief comment here, will be reserved in the main, to what are viewed as potentially noteworthy approaches for metastatic prostate cancer not included in the referenced reviews.

Using active specific immunization, major histocompatibility complex (MHC) Class I and non-restricted CD8+ cytotoxic T lymphocytes (CTL) to PSA and specific residues of PSA have been demonstrated *in vitro* by a number of investigators (152, 153). In an extension of their initial study (152), Perambakam et al. (153) induced PSA peptide-specific CTL from two patients with hormone-refractory prostate cancer (Stage D_3). The T cells obtained from these patients were of a Tc2 (Type 2 $CD8^+$ T cells) as opposed to a Tc1 (Type 1 $CD8^+$ T cells), cytokine profile response, i.e., primarily IL-4 rather than IFNγ.

In an extension of an earlier study demonstrating PSA-specific CTL responses *in vitro* to monocyte-derived dendritic cells (DC) transfected with PSA mRNA (154), Hesiser et al. (155) have reported PSA-specific CTL responses in a Phase 1 study in 13 patients with metastatic prostate cancer (Stages D_1-D_3). Therein, the immune response was associated with a: i) significant decrease in PSA velocity and ii) transient clearing of circulating tumor cells in the peripheral blood of some patients. Albeit limited to 13 patients, an important concern is whether the immune response demonstrated using PSA RNA-transfected DC as a "surrogate target" in cytotoxic assays, will show lysis of autologous tumor cells? Given resolution of the foregoing, of particular significance for the further application of this approach is that in contrast to peptide-based vaccines, which are limited in use to select patient subsets based on their MHC Class I type, DC transfected with RNA-encoded antigens permits stimulation of PSA-specific CTL from all prostate cancer patients.

Mentioned earlier, the MAGE family of genes have been detected in disseminated tumor cells in the blood and bone marrow of patients with prostate cancer (20). As MAGE antigens can induce autologous CTL *in vivo*, it seems appropriate to redirect attention to them within the context of immunotherapy. The determination of MAGE expression patterns and their selected activation may play a role in immunosurveillance and provide a venue for immunotherapy.

A novel form of active immunization, which in addition to inducing a specific immune response, destroys the primary tumor, is known as "cryoimmunotherapy." (156). Likened to an autoimmune response and associated immunopathology, the response following cryosurgery (cryoablation) is characterized by the development of local and systemic tumor-specific immunity. The systemic immunity is critical to the destruction of tumor cells beyond the freezing site, i.e., metastases. This approach is particularly attractive because of the specificity of the immune response to destroy malignant cells while sparing, for the most part, normal tissue. Furthermore, the immune response may leave behind a long-term memory serving to protect the patient from subsequent disease. To our knowledge, there is presently no treatment regimen for cancer that can claim such specificity of memory.

Axiomatic to the success of cryoimmunotherapy is the necessity to augment its tumoricidal effectiveness. The use of immunomodulators (156, 157) in concert with re-attention to changes in the microcirculation following freezing permitting improved delivery of select chemotherapeutic agents (158), have provided initial observations toward maximizing the synergistic effects of cryosurgery, immunological responsiveness and chemotherapy in patients with metastatic prostatic cancer (159). Whether this success in concert with the use of cryosurgery for the treatment of bone tumors (recently reviewed by Veth et al. [160]) irrespective of its immunological aspects (for which there is limited and conflicting observations [156]) can be directly applied to the treatment of bone metastasis in prostate cancer remains to be determined. Of note in this regard, is the recent report of the successful use of percutaneous cryosurgery for treatment of metastatic bone lesions and the resulting reduction in pain (161).

Albeit appealing, with early reports of remission of metastases (162), cryoimmunotherapy has, at best, received limited clinical application. This has been due, in part to: i) earlier reports of enhancement (progression) of metastases following cryosurgery of atypical (highly specialized) experimentally-induced tumors not comparable to other animal or human tumors which portended to an unfavorable clinical outcome (see Ablin [163] for further discussion) and ii) the need for technological improvements in cryosurgery itself and thereafter the absence of longterm follow up.

Observations that there is a gradual decrease in the presence of HLA molecules with the progression of prostate cancer, suggests that active immunotherapy may have its limitations. A reasonable alternative is passive immunotherapy via adoptive transfer. Here tumor specific antibodies or immunocytes, e.g., T cells, are adoptively transferred into the recipient. Two approaches using adoptive transfer of immunocytes are noteworthy.

The *first,* is essentially an extension of the *in situ* adenoviral-vector immunomodulatory gene therapy approaches considered herein by Satoh et al. (32). Here, adoptive transfer of splenocytes from an orthotopic mouse model of prostate cancer (178-2BMA) treated with adenoviral-vector-mediated interleukin 12 (AdIL-12) gene therapy or AdIL-12 in combination with the costimulatory gene B7-1 (AdlL-12/B7) resulted in significant suppression of tumor growth and spontaneous lung metastases, respectively, and improved survival of newly generated orthotopic tumors and pre-established metastases (164).

In consideration of a *second* approach of adoptive transfer, Pinthus et al. (165) have directed attention that a major limitation in its use for immunotherapy in cancer is the inefficient homing of the transferred immunocytes to their target, i.e., the site of metastasis. A pivotal factor according to Pinthus et al. (166) is mediated by the interaction between tissue-secreted chemokines and their corresponding receptor on the membrane of the transferred immunocytes, e.g., T cells. With this in mind, Pinthus et al. (166) have advocated the use of the "T body" ("chimeric-immune receptor") approach. This approach (166) "...combines effector functions of T and natural killer cells with the ability of antibodies to recognize a pre-selected antigen with high specificity and without MHC Class restriction." Stated another way, "The chimeric receptor (CR) combines the antitumor specificity of antibodies with the ability to activate lymphocytes" (167). The ability for immunological activity without MHC Class restriction is of particular significance as it enables elimination of tumor cells that have lost cell surface HLA expression.

Applying the principles of the "T body" approach, Pinthus et al. (165) initially demonstrated that direct intratumoral administration of erbB2 (HER-2) specific, CR-bearing human lymphocytes in xenograft models of prostate cancer (CWR22 and WISH-PC14) in SCID mice resulted in significant retardation of tumor growth, decrease in PSA levels and prolonged survival. Against this backdrop, Pinthus et al. (166) subsequently established an *in vivo* system extending the therapeutic scope of T bodies to metastatic prostate cancer. Therein, they demonstrated that induction of the chemokine, SDF-1 with low dose radiation or cyclophosphamide plus IL-2, within the bone marrow enhanced the homing of erbB2-specific human T bodies resulting in eradication of the tumor cells.

These preclinical studies point to the further importance of the tumor microenvironment and suggest implementation of clinical trials of the application of the T body approach for metastatic prostate cancer in man.

Based on their novelty, the foregoing are but two approaches of adoptive immunotherapy. Compared with active immunization (vaccine) strategies, adoptive therapy may overcome, as mentioned above, some of constraints effecting the magnitude and avidity of a targeted response. Additionally, through the transfer, e.g., of CTL of defined specificity and reactivity for tumor, the cells can be expanded for infusion to the patient.

The foregoing has illustrated with selected approaches and examples the role immunotherapy may play in the treatment of patients with advanced prostate cancer. Inherent to these and/or other approaches, is the necessity to give due consideration to the:

- Endogenous immunosuppressive microenvironment of the prostate (78, 84, 156, 168)
- Expression of membrane-bound complement regulatory proteins (CD35, CD46, CD55 and CD59), which are linked to the cell membrane via a glycosylphosphatidylinositol (GPI) linkage (169).

Prostate cancer cells also utilize sialic acid residues and intracellular protein phosphorylation cascades to resist attack by complement (170)

It is therefore important in terms of immunotherapeutic strategies to consider the use of agents that either block or down-regulate the foregoing factors.

13. EMERGING THEMES

In drawing to the conclusion, we believe it appropriate to direct attention to what we will refer to as "emerging themes." These for the purpose of comment fall into two broad areas: i) Clinical Biomarkers and ii) Targeted

Therapeutics, on which we have by necessity limited our discussion to the most pertinent points.

Parallel to our perceived importance for the re-attention to biomarkers, there is a re-interest by-an-large by the cancer community, including and specifically for prostate cancer by National Cancer Institute (171), for their use in identifying and analyzing primary tumors and metastases. This re-interest is perhaps nowhere better exemplified than in prostate cancer where the gradual, but eventual realization of the less-than-definitive nature of the PSA test as a marker for prostate cancer (81) is ever so slowly becoming a reality. Concomitant with this re-interest in biomarkers and the realization of the role of the tumor microenvironment in contributing to invasion and metastasis, biomarkers may further provide a means by which to elucidate the interplay between tumor cells and their microenvironment.

Emerging clinical biomarkers, for which brief comment follows are: telomerase, "a death-from cancer signature" and "antibody signature."

Telomerase and "A Death-From Cancer Signature". Knowledge of telomerase as a potentially useful biomarker for early detection, prognosis and monitoring of residual disease in prostate cancer is not new (172). However, perhaps with other potentially useful markers, the oversell and literally "ad campaign" by the manufacturers and their urological consultants of the PSA test virtually, until recently, obscured rightful attention to other biomarkers for prostate cancer.

Several studies have generated enthusiasm for the use of telomerase as a prognostic indicator for metastatic prostatic cancer. In one approach, Botchkina et al. (173) have shown that quantitative real-time PCR may be used to measure telomerase expression levels in exfoliated epithelial cells from the urine of patients after digital rectal examination of the prostate. One-hundred per cent of the patients with prostate cancer showed high telomerase expression in the assay, while 90% of patients with benign prostatic hyperplasia (BPH) showed low or no telomerase expression. Intriguingly, 10% of patients with BPH showed high levels of telomerase expression, which might indicate BPH in the very early stages of transition to cancer, or the presence of occult foci of cancer.

Rather than a single biomarker like telomerase, detecting a set of biomarkers may also prove useful. Using micro-array profiling Glinsky et al. (174) recently showed that in 10 different types of cancer, including prostate, metastatic cells displayed a conserved BMI-1 oncogene-driven 11-gene signature expression pathway. BMI-1 is one of the genes in the polycomb group (mentioned earlier) that determines the proliferative potential of normal and leukemic stem cells. Overexpression of BMI-1 causes neoplastic transformation of lymphocytes. Reports of the expression of BMI-1 in non-small lung and breast cancer have suggested an oncogenic role for BMI-1 beyond leukemia and perhaps in epithelial malignancies. In the 100 patients analyzed, expression of the BMI-1 11-gene signature expression pathway was a consistent powerful predictor of a short interval to disease recurrence, distant metastasis, and death after therapy, *ergo*, "a death-from cancer signature."

It is of significance to note that both of these examples of new putative biomarkers for prostatic metastatic cancer are also expressed in normal somatic stem cells. The idea that tissue stem cells may be involved in cancer development has been vigorously pursued in recent years (175), with experimental data accumulating that shows stem cell involvement in dozens of solid tissue cancers, including prostate cancer (176, 177, 178, 179, 180). Other groups have shown that the Wnt and Notch signaling pathways, which are known to be crucial in maintaining stem cell self-renewal capabilities, are also active in metastatic cancers – consistent with stem cells being involved in the origin of the cancers (181, 182). Recently, Schmelz et al. (183) have proposed a new candidate prostate stem cell population within the basal epithelium, which is positive for cytokeratin 6a (Ck6a+) expression and Collins et al (184) have identified and characterized a cancer stem cell population from human prostate tumors. Further findings of novel prostatic cancer biomarkers may continue to be simply stem cell biomarkers.

"Antibody Signature." The exquisite sensitivity and specificity of the immune response make it an ideal biomarker. In principle, a malignant neoplasm may be diagnosed immunologically by detecting: i) Circulating tumor antigens (markers) in blood, secretions and/or tissue fluids and ii) An immune response – humoral or cellular, of the host against tumor (185). In applying this principle, prostate tumor-associated antigens and an immune response, the latter demonstrating autoantibodies, in patients with prostate cancer have previously been reported some 25+ years ago (185). With a renewed interest in the immune response and the urgent necessity to identify more exacting markers for prostate cancer, Wang et al. (186) have reported the use of a phage-display library derived from prostate cancer tissues in a phage protein microarray in which they have identified what they refer to as "autoantibody signatures" in the serum of patients with prostate cancer. Of particular significance pending follow up and the ability of the "autoantibody signatures" to differentiate BPH from prostate cancer (surprisingly not assessed in the study) was its positivity in PSA ranges of 2.5–10.0 ng/ml, where the PSA test is particularly inaccurate.

Screening for an immune response to prostate-specific antigens using protein microarrays could lead to improved biomarkers of disease. Whether the "autoantibody signatures" defined by Wang et al. (186) can distinguish between indolent and aggressive tumors, a distinction urgently needed, remains to be determined. Additionally, the "autoantibody signatures" may permit identification of select antigens to be utilized in immunotherapeutic approaches.

Targeted Therapeutics. If prostate cancer originates from abnormal stem cells, the implications for future therapy are far reaching as this small proportion of the cancer cell population, <1% of the total (187), may be driving the disease. It is also true that this group of cells are fundamentally resistant to most types of chemotherapy and radiotherapy. These existing therapies have been developed to work against the bulk of cancer cells in a tumor and in many cases they are successful. However, in most solid tumors such as prostate cancer, relapse often occurs after a relatively short interval. It is therefore important to take into consideration the notion that whilst conventional treatments may destroy a large number of cancer cells in a tumor, the cancer stem cells, present in potentially very small numbers, will often survive (188). Future therapies which selectively target cancer stem cells may be necessary. Indeed, studies have already begun which target a normal stem cell associated characteristic, the expression of telomerase, in order to treat metastatic prostate cancer (189), including hormone-refractory prostate cancer (190).

Studies of telomerase inhibitors, immunotherapy using telomerase as a tumor associated antigen, and telomerase promoter based gene therapy for cancer are all on-going. The extension of this idea is clear – cancer therapeutics which target stem cell-like biomarkers or phenotypes. The development of drugs which interfere in the BMI-1 pathway can be envisioned, along with drugs which stimulate stem cell differentiation pathways.

While more effective detection and treatment of prostate cancer, based on a stem cell view of cancer development, will be enormously valuable, new methods of preventing prostate cancer may follow from knowledge of the role of stem cells in cancer promotion. In a recent paper, He et al. (191) have proposed that the promotion of a benign tumor to malignant cancer could arise from fusing of local benign tumor cells with bone marrow derived stem cells. The fusion of the two cells gives rise to a hybrid cell with all of the phenotypic requisites of malignant cancer, including being poorly differentiated and telomerase positive. The model by He et al. (191), as well as another recent stem cell fusion cancer promotion model (192) suggests that stem cell fusion may be triggered by components of the inflammatory prostate microenvironment, in which case prevention of the development of prostate cancer could be effected by reducing chronic prostate inflammation (193).

14. CONCLUSION

The thrust of this volume has, rightly, been on adenocarcinoma of the prostate, the commonest histological type of prostate cancer, and the one which makes the disease the public health problem that it is. It should not, however, be forgotten that other histological variants also exist. The most noteworthy of these, small cell carcinoma of the prostate, is of neuroendocrine origin, and is characterized by a number of specific immunohistochemical and other markers (194). The interest in this rare subtype is, firstly, because of the presence of neuroendocrine cells in the prostatic epithelium, and the possible origin of such cells from prostatic epithelial cells may be some reflection of their behaviour, though they have their own distinct patterns of cell signaling and growth control (195). Like neuroendocrine tumors elsewhere, they are exquisitely chemo-sensitive, but there is a limit to how far conventional chemotherapy, e.g., with cisplatin and etoposide, can go in controlling the disease, with the addition of other drugs simply increasing treatment toxicity (196). The disease has a propensity for widespread dissemination and a poor prognosis in comparison with adenocarcinomas.

Last but not least, in consideration of metastasis of prostate cancer, we cannot omit brief mention to the female prostate. Within the wall of the urethra, recognition of the female prostate, first described and assigned the term by deGraaf in 1672, has been hindered by use of the historically acquired terminology "Skene's paraurethral glands and ducts", so named after Alexander Skene, who redescribed the female prostate in 1880 (197, 198).

With structural and functional parameters, including PSA and prostatic acid phosphatase (197, 198) and diseases, i.e., prostatitis, BPH, and cancer (albeit rare accounting for <0.003% of all female genital malignancies) of its male counterpart, metastasis of the female prostate have been observed (199).

Absence of knowledge and/or the vestigial concept of the female prostate, failure to distinguish carcinoma of the female urethra from that of the prostate and high frequency and long term persistence of undetected prostatitis in association with chronic inflammatory disease and the subsequent development of cancer, portends the frequency of cancer of the female prostate and metastasis may be greater than currently thought.

By the nature of the title of this closing Chapter "Distilling the Past, Envisioning the Future," the foregoing, inclusive of what we have referred to as "emerging themes," has endeavoured to capture the highlights of the topics covered and bring them into perspective and prospective relative to the biology and treatment of metastasis of prostate cancer. If we have succeeded, this in great measure may be attributed to the excellent and timely contributions by each of the authors. With further references to the contributors, we make special mention of appreciation to the late Gaynor Davies, who passed away during production of this volume.

Never has there been a greater need for communication between scientists and clinicians as there is today in the field of prostate cancer. The difficulties, on both sides, are formidable, but if this book has played its part, even in a small way, then it will have been worthwhile.

REFERENCES

1. Penson DF, Albertsen PC. The natural history of prostate cancer. This volume, 2008.
2. Kessler B, Albertsen P. The natural history of prostate cancer. Urol Clin North Am 2003, 30:219–6.
3. Thompson IM, Goodman PJ, Tangen CM, Scott Lucia M, Miller GJ, Ford LG. The influence of finasteride on the development of prostate cancer. N Eng J Med 2003, 349:215–4.
4. Welch HG, Schwartz LM, Woloshin S. Prostate-specific antigen levels in the united states: Implications of various definitions for abnormal. J Natl Cancer Inst 2005, 97:1132–37.
5. Donovan J, Hamdy F, Neal D, Peters T, Oliver S, Brindle L, et. A. Prostate testing for cancer and treatment (protect) feasibility study. Health Technol Assess 2003, 7:1–88.
6. Bill-Axelson A, Holmberg L, Ruutu M, Haggman M, Andersson SO, Bratell S *et al.* Radical prostatectomy versus watchful waiting in early prostate cancer. N Engl J Med 2005, 352:1977–84.
7. Maitland NM. The search for genes which influence prostate cancer metastasis: A moving target. This volume, 2008.
8. Hendrix MJC, Luo J, Seftor E, Sharma N, Heidger P, Cohen M *et al.* Epithelial-mesenchymal molecular interactions in prostatic tumor cell plasticity. This volume, 2008.
9. Davies G, Harrison G, Mason, M. β-Catenin, its binding partners, signalling mechanisms: Implications in prostate cancer. This volume, 2008.
10. Kuefer R, Hofer MD, Zorn CSM, Engel O, Volkmer BG, Juarez-Brito MA *et al.* Assessment of a fragment of e-cadherin as a serum biomarker with predictive value for prostate cancer. Br J Cancer 2005, 92:2018–3.
11. Yegnasubramanian S, Nelson WG. CpG hypermethylation changes during prostate cancer progression and metastasis, pp. 45–79. In: *DNA Methylation, Epigenetics and Metastasis*. Esteller M, ed., Dordrecht: Springer, 2005.
12. Hofer MD, Kuefer R, Varambally S, Li H, Ma J, Shapiro GI *et al.* The role of metastasis-associated protein 1 in prostate cancer progression. Cancer Res 2004, 64:825–9.
13. Santagata S, Demichelis F, Riva A, Varambally S, Hofer MD, Kutok JL *et al.* JAGGED1 expression is associated with prostate cancer metastasis and recurrence. Cancer Res 2004, 64:6854–57.

14. Xing N, Qian J, Bostwick D, Bergstrahl E, Young CY. Neuroendocrine cells in human prostate over-express the anti-apoptosis protein survivin. Prostate 2001, 48:7–15.
15. Varambally S, Dhanasekaran SM, Zhou M, Barrette TR, Kumar-Sinha C, Sanda MG. The polycomb group EHZ2 is involved in progression of prostate cancer. Nature 2002, 419:624–9.
16. Fan L, Pepicelli CV, Dibble CC, Catbagan W, Zarycki JI, Laciak R et al. Hedgehog signaling promotes prostate xenograft tumor growth. Endocrinology 2004, 145:3961–70.
17. Karhadkar SS, Bova GS, Abdallah N, Dhara S, Gardner D, Maltra A et al. Hedgehog signaling in prostate regeneration, neoplasia and metastasis. Nature 2004, 431:707–12.
18. Lin B, Ferguson C, White JT, Wang S, Vessala R, True LD et al. Prostate-localized and androgen-regulated expression of the membrane-bound serine protease TMPRSS2. Cancer Res 1999, 59:4180–84.
19. Wilson S, Greer B, Hooper J, Zijlstra A, Walker B, Quigley J et al. The membrane-anchored serine protease, TMPRSS2, activates PAR-2 in prostate cancer cells. Biochem J 2005, 388:967–72.
20. Kufer P, Zippelius A, Lutterbüse R, Mecklenburg I, Enzmann T, Montag A et al. Heterogeneous expression of MAGE-A genes in occult disseminated tumor cells: A novel multimarker reverse transcription-polymerase chain reaction for diagnosis of micrometastatic disease. Cancer Res 2002, 62:251–61.
21. Kreisberg JI, Malik SN, Prihoda TJ, Bedolla RG, Troyer DA, Kreisberg S et al. Phosphorylation of akt (SER473) is an excellent predictor of poor clinical outcome in prostate cancer. Cancer Res 2004, 64:5232–36.
22. Akira S, Takeda K. Toll-like receptor signaling. Nat Rev Immunol 2004, 4:499–511.
23. Zheng SL, Augustsson-Bälter K, Chang B, Hedelin M, Li L, Adami H-O et al. Sequence variants of toll-like receptor 4 are associated with prostate cancer risk: Results from the cancer prostate in sweden study. Cancer Res 2004, 64:2918–2.
24. Li L. Regulation of innate immunity signaling and its connection with human diseases. Curr Drug Targets Inflamm Allergy 2004, 3:81–6.
25. Huang B, Zhao J, Li H, He KL, Chen Y, Chen SH et al. Toll-like receptors on tumor cells facilitate evasion of immune surveillance. Cancer Res 2005, 65:5009–14.
26. Eccles SA, Paon L. Breast cancer metastasis: When, where, how. Lancet 2005, 365:1006–07.
27. Singh S, Sadacharan S, Su S, Belldegrun A, Persad S, Singh G. Overexpression of vimentin: Role in the invasive phenotype in an androgen-independent model of prostate cancer. Cancer Res 2003, 63:2306–11.
28. Martiniello-Wilks R, Dane A, Voeks DJ, Jeyakumar G, Mortensen E, Shaw JM et al. Gene-directed enzyme prodrug therapy for prostate cancer in a mouse model that imitates the development of human disease. J Gene Med 2004, 6:43–54.
29. Kacani L, Wurm M, Schennach H, Braun I, Andrle J, Sprinzl GM. Immunosuppressive effects of soluble factors secreted by head and neck squamous cell carcinoma on dendritic cells and T lymphocytes. Oral Oncol 2003, 39:672–9.
30. Kubsch S, Graulich E, Knop J, Steinbrink K. Suppressor activity of anergic T cells induced by IL-10-treated human dendritic cells: Association with IL-2- and CTLA-4-dependent G1 arrest of the cell cycle regulated by P27KIP1. Eur J Immunol 2003, 33:1988–97.

31. Mukherjee P, Ginardi AR, Madsen CS, Tinder TL, Jacobs F, Parker J et al. MUC1-specific CTLs are non-functional within a pancreatic tumor microenvironment. Glycoconj J 2001, 18:931–42.
32. Satoh T, Timme TL, Gdor Y, Miles BJ, Amato RJ, Kadmon D et al. Immuno-gene therapy for metastatic prostate cancer. This volume, 2008.
33. Armstrong B, Doll R. Environmental factors and cancer incidence and mortality in different countries, with special reference to dietary practices. Int J Cancer 1975, 15:617–31.
34. Jiang WG. Polyunsaturated fatty acid and prostate cancer metastasis. This volume, 2008.
35. Bidoli R, Talamini R, Bosetti C, Negri E, Maruzzi D, Montella M et al. Macronutrients, fatty acids, cholesterol and prostate cancer risk. Ann Oncol 2005, 16:152–57.
36. Kelavkar UP. Cohen C. 15-Lipoxygenase-1 expression upregulated, activates insulin-like growth factor-1 receptor in prostate cancer cells. Neoplasia 2004, 6:41–52.
37. Culig Z. Role of the androgen receptor axis in prostate cancer. Urology 2003, 62:21–6.
38. Bakin RE, Gioeli D, Bissonette EA, Weber MJ. Attenuation of ras signaling restores androgen sensitivity to hormone-refractory C4-2 prostate cancer cells. Cancer Res 2003, 63:1975–80.
39. Kiyama S, Morrison K, Zellweger T, Akbari M, Cox M, Yu D et al. Castration-induced increases in insulin-like growth factor-binding protein 2 promotes proliferation of androgen-independent human prostate LNCaP tumors. Cancer Res 2003, 63:3575–84.
40. Lee MS, Igawa T, Yuan TC, Zhang XQ, Lin FF, Lin MF. Erbb-2 signaling is involved in regulating PSA secretion in androgen-independent human prostate cancer LNCaP C-81 cells. Oncogene 2003, 22:781–96.
41. Leung HY, Mehta P, Gray LB, Collins AT, Robson CN, Neal DE. Keratinocyte growth factor expression in hormone insensitive prostate cancer. Oncogene 1997, 15:1115–20.
42. Murillo H, Huang H, Schmidt LJ, Smith DI, Tindall DJ. Role of PI3K signaling in survival and progression of LNCaP prostate cancer cells to the androgen refractory state. Endocrinology 2001, 142:4795–805.
43. Miyoshi Y, Ishiguro H, Uemura H, Fujinami K, Miyamoto H, Kitamura H et al. Expression of AR associated protein 55 (ARA55) and androgen receptor in prostate cancer. Prostate 2003, 56:280–6.
44. Rahman MM, Miyamoto H, Lardy H, Chang C. Inactivation of androgen receptor coregulator ARA55 inhibits androgen receptor activity and agonist effect of antiandrogens in prostate cancer cells. Proc Natl Acad Sci USA 2003, 100:5124–29.
45. Lee SO, Lou W, Hou M, deMiguel F, Gerber L, Gao AC. Interleukin-6 promotes androgen-independent growth in LNCaP human prostate cancer cells. Clin Cancer Res 2003, 9:370–76.
46. Jenster G. The role of the androgen receptor in the development and progression of prostate cancer. Semin Oncol 1999, 26:407–21.
47. Yeh S, Lin HK, Kang Thin HYTH, Lin MF, Chang C. From HER2/neu signal cascade to androgen receptor and its coactivators: A novel pathway by induction of androgen target genes through MAP kinase in prostate cancer cells. Proc Natl Acad Sci USA 1999, 96:5458–63.

48. Wen Y, Hu MC, Makino K, Spohn B, Bartholomeusz G, Yan DH, Hung MC. HER-2/neu promotes androgen-independent survival and growth of prostate cancer cells through the akt pathway. Cancer Res 2000, 60:6841–45.
49. Lara PN Jr, Chee KG, Longmate J, Ruel C, Meyers FJ, Gray CR *et al*. Trastuzumab plus docetaxel in HER-2/neu-positive prostate carcinoma: Final results from the california cancer consortium screening and phase II trial. Cancer 2004, 100:2125–31.
50. Albanell J, Codony J, Rovira A, Mellado B, Gascon P. Mechanism of action of anti-HER2 monoclonal antibodies: Scientific update on trastuzumab and 2C4. Adv Exp Med Biol 2003, 532:253–68.
51. de Bono J, Bellmunt J, Droz J, Miller K, Zugmaier G, Sternberg C. An open label, phase II, multicenter, study to evaluate the efficacy, safety of pertuzumab (P) in chemotherapy naïve patients (pts) with hormone refractory prostate cancer (HRPC). J Clin Oncol 2005, 23(Suppl):4609.
52. Shelley M, Bennett C, Nathan D, Sator O. Hormone treatment for prostate cancer. This volume, 2008.
53. Klotz L. Hormone therapy for patients with prostate carcinoma. Cancer 2000, 88:3009–14.
54. Medical Research Council Prostate Cancer Working Party Investigators Group. Immediate versus deferred treatment for advanced prostatic cancer; initial results of the medical research council trial. Br J Urol 1997, 79:235–46.
55. Sciarra A, Casale P, Colella D, Di Chiro C, Di Silverio F. Hormone-refractory prostate cancer? Anti-androgen withdrawal and intermittent hormone therapy. Scand J Urol Nephrol 1999, 33:211–6.
56. Song J, Pang S, Lu Y, Yokoyama KK, Zheng J-Y, Chiu R. Gene silencing in androgen-responsive prostate cancer cells from the tissue-specific prostate-specific antigen promotor. Cancer Res 2004, 64:7661–63.
57. Kei Kwok W, Ling M-T, Lee T-W, Lau TCM, Zhou C, Zhang X *et al*. Up-regulation of TWIST in prostate cancer and its implication as a therapeutic target. Cancer Res 2005, 65:5153–62.
58. Newman RM, Zetter BR. Cell cycle regulation. This volume, 2008.
59. Oudard S, Legrier ME, Boye K, Bras-Goncalves R, De Pinieux G, De Cremoux P *et al*. Activity of docetaxel with or without estramustine phosphate versus mitoxantrone in androgen dependent and independent human prostate cancer xenografts. J Urol 2003, 169:1729–34.
60. Schiller JH. New directions for ZD1839 in the treatment of solid tumors. Semin Oncol 2003, 30:49–55.
61. Sumitomo M, Tachibana M, Nakashima J, Murai M, Miyajima A, Kimura F *et al*. An essential role for nuclear factor kappa B in preventing TNF-alpha-induced cell death in prostate cancer cells. J Urol 1999, 161:674–79.
62. Huang S, Pettaway CA, Bucana CD, Fidler IJ. Blockage of NF-kappaB activity in human prostate cancer cells is associated with suppression of angiogenesis, invasion and metastasis. Oncogene 2001, 20:4188–97.
63. Suda T, Takahashi N, Udagawa N, Jimi E, Gillespie MT, Martin TJ. Modulation of osteoclast differentiation and function by the new members of the tumor necrosis factor receptor and ligand families. Endocr Rev 1999, 20:345–57.
64. Hoffman RM. Orthotopic metastatic mouse models of prostate cancer. This volume, 2008.

65. Clarke N, Fleisch H. The biology of bone metastases from prostate cancer and the role of bisphosphonates. This volume, 2008.
66. Ayala GE, Dai H, Ittmann M, Li R, Powell M, Frolov A et al. Growth and survival mechanisms associated with perineural invasion in prostate cancer. Cancer Res 2004, 64:6082–90.
67. Adis R&D Insight. NF-kappa B inhibitors in development. (file://C:\WINDOWS\ Temporary%20Internet%20Files\Content.IE5\CKO62R50\NF_Kappa_inhi_Drugs.htm) Accessed August 31, 2005.
68. Jenkins RB, Qian J, Lieber MM, Bostwick DG. Detection of c-myc oncogene amplification and chromosomal anomalies in metastatic prostatic carcinoma by fluorescence in situ hybridization. Cancer Res 1997, 57:524–31.
69. Buttyan R, Sawezuk IS, Benson MC, Siegal JD, Olsson CA. Enhanced expression of c-myc protooncogene in high-grade prostate cancers. Prostate 1987, 11:327–7.
70. Williams K, Fernandez S, Stein X, Ishii K, Love HD, Lau YF et al. Unopposed c-MYC expression in benign prostatic epithelium causes a cancer phenotype. Prostate 2005, 63:369–84.
71. Blaszczyk N, Masri BA, Mawji NR, Ueda T, McAlinden G, Duncan CP et al. Osteoblast-derived factors induce androgen-independent proliferation and expression of prostate-specific antigen in human prostate cancer cells. Clin Cancer Res 2004, 10:1860–69.
72. Garcia-Moreno C, Mendez-Davila C, de La Piedra C, Castro-Errecaborde NA, Traba ML. Human prostatic carcinoma cells produce an increase in the synthesis of interleukin-6 by human osteoblasts. Prostate 2002, 50:241–6.
73. Masuda H, Fukabori Y, Nakano K, Shimizu N, Yamanaka H. Expression of bone morphogenetic protein-7 (BMP-7) in human prostate. Prostate 2004, 59:101–6.
74. McAlhany SJ, Ressler SJ, Larsen M, Tuxhorn JA, Yang F, Dang TD et al. Promotion of angiogenesis by PS20 in the differential reactive stroma prostate cancer xenograft model. Cancer Res 2003, 63:5859–65.
75. Mohammad KS, Guise TA. Mechanisms of osteoblastic metastases: Role of endothelin-1. Clin Orthop Relat Res 2003, S67–74.
76. Nemeth JA, Cher ML, Zhou Z, Mullins C, Bhagat S, Trikha M. Inhibition of alpha(v)BETA3 integrin reduces angiogenesis, bone turnover, and tumor cell proliferation in experimental prostate cancer bone metastases. Clin Exp Metastasis 2003, 20:413–20.
77. Yonou H, Kanomata N, Goya M, Kamijo T, Yokose T, Hasebe T et al. Osteoprotegerin/osteoclastogenesis inhibitory factor decreases human prostate cancer burden in human adult bone implanted into nonobese diabetic/severe combined immunodeficient mice. Cancer Res 2003, 63:2096–102.
78. Ablin RJ, Gonder MJ, eds, Male accessory sexual glands secretions and their antithetical role in immunosurveillance, pp. 271–77. *Protides of the Biological Fluids*. Oxford: Pergamon Press, Ltd., Vol. 1985.
79. Wilson MJ, Sinha AA. Matrix degradation in prostate cancer. This volume, 2008.
80. Szabo KA, Ablin RJ, Singh G. Matrix metalloproteinases and the immune response. Clin Appl Immunol Rev 2004, 4:295–319.
81. Ablin RJ. PSA assays. Lancet Oncol 2000, 1:13.
82. Ablin RJ. A retrospective and prospective overview of prostate-specific antigen. J Cancer Res Clin Oncol 1997, 123:583–94.

83. Hagemann T, Wilson J, Kulbe H, Li NF, Leinster DA, Charles K et al. NF-κB and JNK. J Immunol 2005, 175:1197–205.
84. Ablin RJ, Bartkus JM, Gonder MJ, Polgar J. Factors contributing to suppression of tumor-host responsiveness, pp. 279–99. In: *Human Tumour Markers-Biology and Clinical Applications*. Cimino F, Birkmayer CD, Pimentel E, Klavins JV, Salvatore F, eds, Berlin: Walter de Gruyter, 1987.
85. Ablin RJ, Whyard TC. Immunobiological implications of select bioactive molecules in the prostate with A known and unknown target, pp. 148–72. In: *the Prostate as an Endocrine Gland*. Farnsworth WE, Ablin RJ, eds, Boca Raton, FL: CRC Press, 1990.
86. Madsen P, Rasmussen HH, Leffers H, Honore B, Dejgaard K, Olsen E et al. Molecular cloning, occurrence, and expression of a novel partially secreted protein "psoriasin" that is highly up-regulated in psoriatic skin. J Invest Dermatol 1991, 97:701–12.
87. Ruse M, Lambert A, Robinson N, Ryan D, Shon K-J, Eckert RL. S100A7, S100A10 and S100A11 are transglutaminase substrates. Biochemistry 2001, 40:3167–73.
88. Davies G, Watkins G, Sanders AJ, Harrison GM, Ablin RJ, Mason MD et al. A hammerhead ribozyme transgene to transglutaminase-4 increases the level of its substrate psoriasin and reduces the invasive capacity of prostate cancer cells *in viro* (abstract). Proc Am Assoc Cancer Res 2005, 46:5643.
89. Helbig G, Christopherson IIKW, Bhat-Nakshatri P, Kumar S, Kishimoto H, Miller KD et al. NF-κB promotes breast cancer cell migration and metastasis by inducing the expression of the chemokine receptor CXCR4. J Biol Chem 2003, 278:21631–38.
90. Ayra M, Patel HR, McGurk C, Tatoud R, Klocker H, Masters J et al. The importance of the CXCL12-CXCR4 chemokine ligand-receptor interaction in prostate cancer metastases. J Exp Ther Oncol 2004, 4:291–303.
91. Chinni SR, Sivalogan S, Dong Z, Filho JC, Deng X, Bonfil RD et al. CXCL12/CXCR4 signaling activates akt-1 and MMP-9 expression in prostate cancer cells: The role of bone microenvironment-associated CXCL12. Prostate 2006, 66:32–48.
92. Epstein RJ. The CXCL12-CXCR4 chemotactic pathway as a target of adjuvant breast cancer therapies. Nat Rev Cancer 2004, 4:901–09.
93. Loberg RD, Fridman Y, Pienta BA, Keller ET, McCauley LK, Taichman RS et al. Detection and isolation of circulating tumor cells in urologic cancers: A review. Neoplasia 2004, 6:302–09.
94. Davies G, Jiang WG, Mason MD. Hepatocyte growth factor/scatter factor and prostate cancer metastasis. This volume, 2008.
95. Badawi AF. Role of prostaglandin synthesis and cyclooxygenase-2 in prostate cancer and metastasis. This volume, 2008.
96. Thurairaja R, McFarlane J, Traill Z, Persad R. State-of-the-art approaches to detecting early bone metastasis in prostate cancer. BJU Int 2004, 94:268–71.
97. Mason M, Collaborators. MRCPR4. Of bone metastases from prostate cancer: First results of the MRC PR04 trial (ISCRTN 61384873). Development 2004, 22(Suppl):4511.
98. Kim S-J, Uehara H, Yazici S, He J, Langley RR, Mathew P et al. Modulation of bone microenvironment with zoledronate enhances the therapeutic effects of STI571 and paclitaxel against experimental bone metastasis of human prostate cancer. Cancer Res 2005, 65:3707–25.
99. Clézardin P, Ebetino FH, Fournier PGJ. Bisphosphonates and cancer-induced bone disease: Beyond their antiresorptive activitivity. Cancer Res 2005, 65:4971–74.

100. Vanchieri C. Vioxx withdrawal alarms cancer prevention researchers. J Natl Cancer Inst 2004, 96:1734–35.
101. Patel MI, Subbaramaiah K, Du B M, Yang P, Newman RA et al. Celecoxib inhibits prostate cancer growth: Evidence of cyclooxygenase-2-independent mechanism. Clin Cancer Res 2005, 11:1999–2007.
102. Scullin, P, O'Sullivan J, Parker C. Strategies for the implementation of chemotherapy and radiotherapy. This volume 2008.
103. Wu L, Birle DC, Tannock IF. Effects of the mammalian target of rapamycin inhibitor CCI-779 used alone or with chemotherapy on human prostate cancer cells and xenografts. Cancer Res 2005, 65:2825–31.
104. Henry MD, Wen S, Silva MW, Chandra S, Milton M, Worland PJ. A prostate-specific membrane antigen-targeted monoclonal antibody-chemotherapeutic conjugate designed for the treatment of prostate cancer. Cancer Res 2004, 64:7995–8001.
105. Mukhopadhyay UK, Senderowicz AM, Ferbeyre G. RNA silencing of checkpoint regulators sensitizes P53-defective prostate cancer cells to chemotherapy while sparing normal cells. Cancer Res 2005, 65:2872–81.
106. Fan Z, Chakravarty P, Alfieri A, Pandita TK, Vikram B, Guha C. Adenovirus-mediated ATM gene transfer sensitizes prostate cancer cells to radiation. Cancer Gene Ther 2000, 7:1307–4.
107. Ogata T, Teshima T, Kagawa K, Hishikawa Y, Takahashi Y, Kawaguichi A et al. Particle irradiation suppresses metastatic potential of cancer cells. Cancer Res 2005, 65:113–20.
108. Zietman AL, DeSilvio ML, Slater JD, Rossi CJ Jr, Miller DW, Adams JA et al. Comparison of conventional-dose vs high-dose conformal radiation therapy in clinically localized adenocarcinoma of the prostate: A randomized controlled trial. J Am Med Assoc 2005, 294:1233–9.
109. Milowsky MI, Nanus DM, Kostakoglu I, Vallabhajosula S, Goldsmith SJ, Bander NH. Phase I trial of 90y-labeled anti-prostate specific membrane antigen monoclonal antibody J591 for androgen-independent prostate cancer. J Clin Oncol 2004, 22:2522–31.
110. Zhao X-Y, Schneider D, Biroc SL, Parry R, Alicke B, Toy P et al. Targeting tomoregulin for radioimmunotherapy of prostate cancer. Cancer Res 2005, 65:2846–53.
111. Gulley JL, Arlen PM, Bastian A, Morin S, Marte J, Beetham P et al. Combining a recombinant cancer vaccine with standard definitive radiotherapy in patients with localized prostate cancer. Clin Cancer Res 2005, 11:3353–62.
112. Melnyk O, Zimmerman M, Kim KJ, Shuman M. Neutralizing anti-vascular endothelial growth factor antibody inhibits further growth of established prostate cancer and metastases in a pre-clinical model. J Urol 1999, 161:960–3.
113. Ferrara N. Vascular endothelial growth factor: Basic science and clinical progress. Endocr Rev 2004, 25:581–611.
114. Huss WJ, Hanrahan CF, Barrios RJ, Simons JW, Greenberg NM. Angiogenesis and prostate cancer: Identification of a molecular progression switch. Cancer Res 2001, 61:2736–43.
115. Lissbrant IF, Lissbrant E, Damber J-E, Bergh A. Blood vessels are regulators of growth, diagnostic markers and therapeutic targets in prostate cancer. Scand J Urol Nephrol 2001, 35:437–52.

116. Halin S, Wikström P, Rudolfsson SH, Stattin P, Doll JA, Crawford SE et al. Decreased pigment epithelium-derived factor is associated with metastatic phenotype in human and rat tumors. Cancer Res 2004, 64:5664–71.
117. Filleur S, Volz K, Nelius T, Mirochnik Y, Huang H, Zaichuk TA et al. Two functional epitopes of pigment epithelium-derived factor block angiogenesis and induce differentiation in prostate cancer. Cancer Res 2005, 65:5144–51.
118. Karashima T, Sweeney P, Slaton JW, Kim SJ, Kedar D, Izawa JI et al. Inhibition of angiogenesis by the antiepidermal growth factor antibody IMCLONE C225 in androgen-independent prostate cancer growing orthotopically in nude mouse. Clin Cancer Res 2002, 8:1253–64.
119. Slovin SF, Kelly WK, Cohen R. Epidermal growth factor receptor (egfr) monoclonal antibody (MOAB) C225 and doxorubicin (DOC) in androgen-independent (AI) prostate cancer (PC): Results of a phase ib/iia study (abstract). Proc Am Soc Clin Oncol 1997, 16:311a.
120. Rosenthal M, Toner GC, Gurney H. Inhibition of the epidermal growth factor receptor (EGFR) in hormone refractory prostate cancer (HRPC): Initial results of a phase II trial of gefitinib (abstract). Proc Am Soc Clin Oncol 2003, 22:416.
121. Griffin J. The biology of signal transduction inhibition: Basic science to novel therapies. Semin Oncol 2001, 28:3–8.
122. Uehara H, Kim SJ, Karashima T, Shepherd DL, Fan D, Tsan R et al. Effects of blocking platelet-derived growth factor-receptor signaling in a mouse model of experimental prostate cancer bone metastases. J Natl Cancer Inst 2003, 95:458–70.
123. Tiffany NM, Wersinger EM, Garzotto M, Beer TM. Imatinib mesylate and zoledronic acid in androgen-independent prostate cancer. Urology 2004, 63:934–39.
124. Rao KV, Goodin S, Capanna M. A phase II trial of imatinib mesylate in patients with PSA progession after local therapy for prostate cancer. (Abstract). Proc Am Soc Clin Oncol 2003, 22:409.
125. Gleave M, Tolcher A, Miyake H, Nelson C, Brown B, Beraldi E et al. Progression to androgen independence is delayed by adjuvant treatment with antisense bcl-2 oligodeoxynucleotides after castration in the LNCaP prostate tumor model. Clin Cancer Res 1999, 5:2891–98.
126. Kerr C. Second-generation antisense drug for prostate cancer. Lancet Oncol 2004, 5:646.
127. Hershko A, Ciechanover A. The ubiquitin system. Ann Rev Biochem 1998, 67:425–79.
128. Neckers L, Schulte TW, Mimnaugh E. Geldanamycin as a potential anti-cancer agent: Its molecular target and biochemical activity. Invest New Drugs 1999, 17:361–73.
129. Solit DB, Zheng FF, Drobnjak M, Munster PN, Higgins B, Verbel D et al. 17-Allylamino-17-demthoxygeldanamycin induces the degradation of androgen receptor and HER-2/neu and inhibits the growth of prostate cancer xenografts. Clin Cancer Res 2002, 8:986–3.
130. Mabjeesh NJ, Post DE, Willard MT, Kaur B, Van Meir EG, Simons JW et al. Geldanamycin induces degradation of hypoxia-inducible factor 1α protein via the proteasome pathway in prostate cancer cells. Cancer Res 2002, 62:2478–82.
131. Lokeshwar BL, MG Selzer, Zhu B, Block NL, Golub LM. Inhibition of cell proliferation, invasion, tumor growth and metastasis by an oral non-antimicrobial tetracycline analog (COL-3) in a metastatic prostate cancer model. Int J Cancer 2002, 98:297–309.
132. Ikezoe T, Yang Y, Saito T, Koeffler HP, Taguichi H. Proteasome inhibitor PS-341 down-regulates prostate-specific antigen (PSA) and induces growth arrest and

apoptosis of androgen-independent human prostate cancer LNCaP cells. Cancer Sci 2004, 95:271–75.
133. Venkateswaran V, Fleshner NE, Sugar LM, Klotz LH. Antioxidants block prostate cancer in *lady* transgenic mice. Cancer Res 2004, 64:5891–96.
134. Tokar EJ, Webber MM. Cholecalciferol (vitamin D3) inhibits growth and invasion by up-regulating nuclear receptors and 25-hydroxylase (CYP27A1) in human prostate cancer cells. Clin Exp Metastasis 2005, 22:275–84.
135. Tokar EJ, Ancrile BB, Ablin RJ, Webber MM. Cholecalciferol (vitamin D3) and the retinoid N-(4-hydroxyphenyl) retinamide (4-HPR) are synergistic for chemoprevention of prostate cancer. J Exp Ther Oncol 2006, 5:323–3.
136. Guaiquil VH, Vera JC, Golde DW. Mechanism of vitamin C inhibition of cell death induced by oxidative stress in glutathione-depleted HL-60 cells. J Biol Chem 2001, 276:40955–961.
137. Ablin RJ. Lycopene: A word of caution. Am J Health-Syst Pharm 2005, 62:899.
138. D'Andrea GM. Use of antioxidants during chemotherapy and radiotherapy should be avoided. CA Cancer J Clin 2005, 55:319–21.
139. Surh YJ. Chemoprevention with dietary phytochemicals. Cancer 2003, 3:768–80.
140. Li Y, Che M, Bhagat S, Ellis K-L, Kucuk O, Doerge DR *et al*. Regulation of gene expression and inhibition of experimental prostate cancer bone metastasis by dietary genistein. Neoplasia 2004, 6:354–63.
141. Huang X, Chen S, Xu L, Liu Y, Deb DK, Platanias LC *et al*. Genistein inhibits P39 map kinase activation, matrix metalloproteinases type 2, and cell invasion in human prostate epithelial cells. Cancer Res 2005, 65:3470–78.
142. Cha T-L, Qiu L, Chen C-T, Wen Y, Hung M-C. Emodin down-regulates androgen receptor and inhibits prostate cancer cell growth. Cancer Res 2005, 65:2287–95.
143. Tannock IF, de Wit R, Berry WR, Horti J, Pluzanska A, Chi KN *et al*. TAX 327 investigators. Docetaxel plus prednisone or mitoxantrone plus prednisone for advanced prostate cancer. N Eng J Med 2004, 351:1502–2.
144. Petrylak DP, Tangen CM, Hussain MH, Lara PN Jr, Jones JA, Taplin ME *et al*. Docetaxel and estramustine compared with mitoxantrone and prednisone for advanced refractory prostate cancer. N Eng J Med 2004, 351:1513–20.
145. Huggins CB, Stevens RE Jr, Hodges CV. Studies on prostate cancer. II. The effects of castration on advanced carcinoma of the prostate gland. Arch Surg 1941, 143:209–3.
146. Ehrlich P. Ueber den jetzigen stand der karzinomforschung. Ned Tijdschr Geneeskd 1909, 5:273–90.
147. Burnet FM. Cancer: A biological approach. Br Med J 1957, 1:779–86.
148. Ablin RJ. Immunotherapy for prostatic cancer. Previous and prospective considerations. Oncology 1975, 31:177–202.
149. Hawkins LK, Lemoinine NR, Kim D. Oncolytic biotherapy: A novel therapeutic platform. Lancet Oncol 2002, 3:17–26.
150. Kaminski JM, Summers JB, Ward MW, Huber MR, Minev B. Immunotherapy and prostate cancer. Cancer Treat Rev 2003, 29:199–09.
151. Markiewicz MA, Kast WM. Advances in immunotherapy for prostate cancer. Adv Cancer Res 2003, 87:159–94.
152. Xue B-H, Zhang Y, Sosman JA, Peace DJ. Induction of human cytotoxic T lymphocytes specific for prostate-specific antigen. Prostate 1997, 30:73–8.

153. Perambakam S, Xue B-H, Sosman JA, Peace DJ. Induction of TC2 cells with specificity for prostatate-specific antigen from patients with hormone-refractory prostate cancer. Cancer Immunol Immunother 2002, 51:263–70.
154. Heiser A, Dahm P, Yancey DR, Maurice MA, Boczkowski D, Nair SK *et al.* Human dendritic cells transfected with RNA encoding prostate-specific antigen stimulate prostate-specific CTL responses in vitro. J Immunol 2000, 164:5508–14.
155. Heiser A, Coleman D, Dannull J, Yancey D, Maurice MA, Lallas CD *et al.* Autologous dendritic cells transfected with prostate-specific antigen RNA stimulated CTL responses against metastatic prostate tumors. J Clin Invest 2002, 109:409–17.
156. Ablin RJ. An appreciation of the concept of cryoimmunology, pp. 136–54. In: *Percutaneous Prostate Cryoablation.* Onik GM, Rubinsky B, Watson G, Ablin RJ, eds, St. Louis, MO: Quality Medical Publishing, Inc, 1995.
157. Ablin RJ, Bradley PF. Immunological aspects of cryosurgery, pp. 77–99. In: *Cryosurgery of the Maxillofacial Region, Vol. 1.* Bradley PF, ed., Boca Raton, FL: CRC Press, 1986.
158. Ikekawa S, Ishihara K, Tanaka S, Ikeda S. Basic studies of cryochemotherapy in a murine tumor system. Cryobiology 1985, 22:477–83.
159. Mouraviev V, Prochorov G, Ablin RJ. Cryoimmunochemotherapy for advanced prostate cancer (abstract). Int J Mol Med 2000, 6(Suppl 1):S30.
160. Veth R, Schreuder B, van Beem H, Pruszczynski M, de Rooy J. Cryosurgery in aggressive, benign, and low-grade malignant tumours. Lancet Oncol 2005, 6:25–34.
161. Callstrom M.,Cryoablation treatment helps diminish pain of bone cancer (Abstract). Society of Interventional Radiology, 30th Annual Meeting. New Orleans, LA. 2005.
162. Ablin RJ, Soanes WA, Gonder MJ. Prospects for cryo-immunotherapy in cases of metastasizing carcinoma of the prostate. Cryobiology 1971, 8:271–76.
163. Ablin RJ. The current status and the prospect for cryoimmunotherapy. Low Temp Med 2003, 29:46–9.
164. Saika T, Kusaka N, Mouraviev V, Satoh T, Kumon H, Timme TL *et al.* Therapeutic effects of adoptive splenocyte transfer following *in situ* ADIL-12 gene therapy in a mouse model of prostate cancer. Cancer Gene Ther 2006, 13:91–8.
165. Pinthus JH, Waks T, Malina V, Kaufman-Francis K, Harmelin A, Aizenberg I *et al.* Adoptive immunotherapy of prostate cancer bone lesions using redirected effector lymphocytes. J Clin Invest 2004, 114:1774–81.
166. Pinthus JH, Waks T, Kaufman-Francis K, Schindler DG, Harmelin A, Kanety H *et al.* Immuno-gene therapy of established prostate tumors using chimeric receptor-redirected human lymphocytes. Cancer Res 2003, 63:2470–76.
167. Eshhar Z. Tumor-specific T bodies: Towards clinical application. Cancer Immunol Immunother 1997, 45:131–6.
168. Whiteside TL. Signaling defects in T lymphocytes of patients with malignancy. Cancer Immunol Immunother 1999, 48:346–52.
169. Gorter A, Meri S. Immune evasion of tumor cells using membrane-bound complement regulatory proteins. Immunol Today 1999, 20:576–82.
170. Donin N, Jurianz K, Ziporen L, Schultz S, Kirschfink M, Fishelson Z. Complement resistance of human carcinoma cells depends on membrane regulatory proteins, protein kinases and sialic acid. Clin Exp Immunol 2003, 131:254–63.
171. NCI Launches Biorepository for Prostate Cancer. NIH News, November 7, 2005. (http://spores.nci.hih.gov/current/prostate/prostate.html) Accessed November 7, 2005.

172. Kim NW, Piatyszek MA, Prowse KR, Harley CB, West MD, Ho PLC et al. Specific association of human telomerase activity with immortal cells and cancer. Science 1994, 266:2011–15.
173. Botchkina GI, Kim RH, Botchkina IL, Kirshenbaum A, Frischer Z, Adler HL. Noninvasive detection of prostate cancer by quantitative analysis of telomerase activity. Clin Cancer Res 2005, 11:3243–49.
174. Glinsky GV, Berezovska O, Glinskii AB. Microarray analysis identifies a death-from-cancer signature predicting therapy failure in patients with multiple types of cancer. J Clin Invest 2005, 115:1503–21.
175. Pipes BL, Ablin RJ. Cancer stem cells revisited. Curr Oncol 2005, 12:134–5.
176. Bonkhoff H, Remberger K. Differentiation pathways and histogenic aspects of normal and abnormal prostate growth: A stem cell model. Prostate 1996, 28:98–106.
177. Isaacs JT, Coffey DS. Etiology and disease process of benign prostatic hyperplasia. Prostate Suppl 1989, 2:33–50.
178. Van Leenders G, Schalken JA. Stem cell differentiation within the human prostate epithelium: Implications for prostate carcinogenesis. BJU Intl 2001, 8:35–42.
179. Collins AT, Habib FK, Maitland NJ, Neal DE. Identification and isolation of human prostate epithelial stem cells based on α2β1-integrin expression. J Cell Sci 2001, 114:3865–72.
180. Schalken JA, Van Leenders G. Cellular and molecular biology of the prostate: Stem cell biology. Urology 2003, 62:11–20.
181. Reya T, Clevers H. Wnt signalling in stem cells and cancer. Nature 2005, 434:843–50.
182. Taipale J, Beachy PA. The hedgehog and wnt signalling pathways in cancer. Nature 2001, 411:349–54.
183. Schmelz M, Moll R, Hesse U, Prasad AR, Gandolfi JA, Bartholdi M, Cress AE. Identification of a stem cell candidate in the normal human prostate gland. Eur J Cell Biol 2005, 84:341–54.
184. Collins AT, Berry PA, Hyde C, Stower MJ, Maitland NJ. Prospective identification of tumorigenic prostate cancer stem cells. Cancer Res 2005, 65:10946–51.
185. Ablin RJ, Bhatti RA. Tumor-associated immunity in prostate cancer, pp. 183–204. In: *Prostatic Cancer*, Ablin RJ, ed., New York: Marcel Dekker, Inc, 1981.
186. Wang X, Yu J, Sreekumar A, Varambally S, Shen R, Giacherio D et al. Autoantibody signatures in prostate cancer. N Eng J Med 2005, 353:1224–35.
187. Bhatt RI, Brown MD, Hart CA, Gilmore P, Ramani VA, George NJ et al. Novel method for the isolation and characterization of the putative prostatic stem cell. Cytometry 2003, A: 54:89–99.
188. Reya T, Morrison SJ, Clarke MF, Weissman IL. Stem cells, cancer, and cancer stem cells. Nature 2001, 414:105–1.
189. Su Z, Dannull J, Yang BK, Dahm P, Coleman D, Yancey D et al. Telomerase mRNA-transfected dendritic cells stimulate antigen-specific CD8+ and CD4+ T cell responses in patients with metastatic prostate cancer. J Immunol 2005, 174:3798–807.
190. Biroccio A, Leonetti C. Telomerase as a new target for the treatment of hormone-refractory prostate cancer. Endocr Relat Cancer 2004, 11:407–21.
191. He X, Tsang TC, Pipes BP, Ablin RJ, Harris DH. A stem cell fusion model of carcinogenesis. J Exp Ther Oncol 2005, 5:101–9.
192. Glinsky GV. Death-from-cancer signatures and stem cell contribution to metastatic cancer. Cell Cycle 2005, 4:1171–5.

193. Pipes BL, Ablin RJ. Cancer: Evasion of stem cell senescence. Submitted.
194. Yao JL, Madeb R, Bourne P, Lei J, Yang X, Tickoo S et al. Small cell carcinoma of the prostate: An immunohistochemical study. Am J Surg Pathol 2006, 30:705–12.
195. Slovin SF. Neuroendocrine differentiation in prostate cancer: A sheep in wolf's clothing. Nat Clin Pract Urol 2006, 3:138–44.
196. Papandreou CN, Daliani DD et al. Results of a phase II study with doxorubicin, etoposide, and cisplatin in patients with fully characterized small-cell carcinoma of the prostate. J Clin Oncol 2002, 20:3072–80.
197. Zaviacic M. *the Human Female Prostate. From Vestigial Skene's Paraurethral Glands and Ducts to Woman's Functional Prostate*. Bratislava: Slovak Academic Press, 1999. 171 p.
198. Zaviacic M, Ablin RJ. The female prostate and prostate-specific antigen. Immunohistochemical localization, implications of this prostate marker in woman and reasons for using the term "prostate" in the human female. Histol Histopathol 2000, 15:131–42.
199. Sloboda J, Zaviacic M, Jakubovsky J, Hammar E, Johnson J. Metastasizing adenocarcioma of the female prostate (skene's paraurethral glands). Pathol Res Pract 1998, 194:129–36.

Index

12 0 tetradecanylphorbol-13-acetate (TPA) 98
12-lipoxygenase (12-LOX) 153
153Sm-ethylenediaminetetramethylenephosphonate (EDTMP) 325, 327, 328
2D gel separation 49
3T12 embryonic mouse cells 27
3T3 embryonic mouse cells 27, 98, 201
3T6 embryonic mouse cells 27
5-lipoxygenase 76
5α-reductase 284
99mTc-methylene diphosphonate (MDP) 326, 327
α1-antichymotrypsin 49, 235, 237
α2-macroglobulin 227, 235
ABT-627 321
acanthoma 181
actin 28, 41, 129, 171–173
actomyosin 203
ADAMs (A Disintegrin And Metalloproteinase) 229
ADAMTS (ADAM with thrombospondin type I motifs) 229
adherens junction 129, 171, 172
AdhIL-12 345
adjuvant therapy 287, 290, 291, 326, 337
AdmIL-12 156, 344, 346–348
adrenal hormone 311
Aequorea victoria 147
Akt 116, 359, 362, 363, 366, 374, 376
AkT/PKB 116
alkaline phosphatase 100, 310, 313, 314
alkylating agents 311
alpha-1 antichymotrypsin 49, 235, 237
alphaII(b)beta3 integrin 154
aminopeptidase 89, 230
anaemia 260, 261
analgesia 313

adrogen ablation 113, 114, 143, 253, 260, 273, 291, 293, 294, 337, 374
androgen ablation therapy 113, 114, 294, 316, 337
androgen deprivation 273–275, 283, 284, 287, 291–296, 299–302
androgen receptor (AR) 25, 42, 52, 96, 111, 113, 186, 208, 284, 286, 296, 361
androgen-independent metastatic prostate cancerandrogens 310–313, 315, 321, 322, 326
androstenedione 186, 295
angiogenesis 23, 39, 63, 70, 72, 116, 136, 152–156, 201, 210, 211, 239, 270, 320, 345, 363, 365, 372–375
angiogenin 155
angiopoietin 136
ansamycin 374, 375
antigen presenting cells (APCs) 339
antisense oligodeoxynucleotide 155
antisense-oligonucleotide 205, 374
antizyme 111, 118–120
APC (adenomatous polyposis coli) 172, 173, 175–178, 180–182, 184, 187
APC2 177
APCL 177
apoptosis 32, 48, 51, 67, 75, 87, 94, 97–99, 114, 116, 180, 202, 207, 269, 270, 284, 285, 291, 345, 349, 350, 358, 360, 362, 363, 374–376
arachidonic acid 65, 66, 69, 74, 75, 87–89
armadillo 173, 174, 187
arsenic trioxide 157
AXIN1 176, 180, 181
AXIN2 176, 180, 181

ß-catenin 129, 171–187, 202, 207
β-galactosidase 348
ß-TRCP 175, 177

B7–1 156, 346, 380
Balb/c 3T3 cells 98
basement membrane (BM) 69, 70, 132, 133, 144, 146, 202, 204, 205, 206, 210, 221–224, 238, 253, 364
basic fibroblast growth factor 155, 311
Batsons' theory 254
bcl family 67
Bcr-Abl 374
benign prostatic hyperplasia (BPH) 12, 13, 73, 96, 225, 227, 230–232, 235–237, 273, 358, 382, 383, 385
Bevacizumab 320, 372
bFGF, see basic fibroblast growth factor
bicalutamide 186, 283, 286, 287, 290, 291, 301, 312
bisphosphonates 253, 262, 263, 265–275, 309, 368–370, 374
bladder cancer 100, 101, 146, 172
blastogenesis 100
bombesin 229
bone mineralisation 256
bone morphorgenetic protein (BMP) 40, 255
bone resorption 255–257, 260, 262, 265–270, 272
Bone Scintigraphy 327
breast cancer 23, 69, 77, 132, 136, 174, 181, 210, 260, 262, 265, 366, 369, 383
breast carcinoma 23, 128, 136
burserelin 296
bystander effect 340, 378

C_{19}-steriods 295
C57B116 101
cadherins 70, 171–175, 184–187, 202, 204
CA-HPV-10 184, 366
calcitonin 267
'calcium sink' effect 262
calciuria 268
CALGB 313
cAMP 98
canine prostate cancer 158
canine prostate cancer DPC-1 158
casein kinase1ε (CK1ε) 178
castration 227, 283, 284, 286, 287, 293, 296, 298, 301, 310, 318, 341
catenins (p120cas, plakoglobin) 129, 171–174, 184, 185, 207
cathepsin B 221, 226, 231–233, 238
cathepsin D 221, 230
cathepsins 230, 231, 238, 239
cav-1, see caveolin-1
caveolin-1 29, 157, 178, 179, 341

CBP (Creb-element binding protein) 178, 179
CCD-11 349
CD antigens 48
CD31 136, 156
CD4 156, 342, 344, 347
CD44 22, 29, 34, 48, 186
CD8 156, 342–344, 347, 378
cell cycle
    checkpoints 371
    M Phase 112
    G0 Phase 112
    G1 Phase 112, 119
cell cycle regulators 67, 112
cell motility 28, 201–205, 221, 222
cell surface carbohydrate/lectin 255
c-fos 90
chemo-endocrine therapy 318
chemotherapy 102, 265, 272, 274, 309–316, 138–321, 328, 370–372, 379, 384, 385
chlormadione acetate 286
chronic myeloid leukemia 374
cisplatin 312, 328, 385
c-jun 74, 90, 179, 366
clodronate 266–269, 272, 369
c-Met 199, 201, 204, 207, 210, 367
c-myc 33, 37, 38, 45, 52, 90, 179, 363
cobalt 322
collagen 27, 39, 41, 117, 133, 202, 224, 225, 233, 235, 256, 257
collagen IV 70, 71, 146, 155, 222–224, 227
collagenase 226
collagenase type IV 71, 155
combined androgen blockade 143, 260, 283–285, 287, 295–299, 302
comparative genomic hybridization (CGH) 34, 36–38, 41, 44, 152
conductin 175, 176
Connecticut Tumor Registry 14, 16
contact inhibition 115
corticosteroids 267, 310, 312
CpG methylation 25, 357
CTNNB1 180
CT-PCPE (carboxy-terminal fragment of pro-collagen C-terminal proteinase enhancer protein) 227
CWR22 31, 32, 35, 371, 381
cyclin dependent kinases (CDKs) 31, 112, 113, 115, 117
CDK2 112, 115
CDK4 112–115
cyclins 112, 179
Cyclin D 38, 112–114, 370
Cyclin E 112

cyclin G 348
cyclooxygenase-2 (COX-2) 51, 75, 77
Cyclooxygenases (COX)/prostaglandin H-synthase 88
cyproterone acetate 285, 286, 296
CYPs 89, 100, 101
cysteine protease inhibitors (CPI) 231, 232, 233
cysteine-rich secretory protein 3 (CRISP3) 50
cytochrome P450 89, 95
cytokeratins 132, 360, 383
cytokine production 69, 255, 344
cytokines 39, 40, 71, 90, 172, 198, 221, 222, 238, 253, 255, 339, 340, 360, 362, 365, 366, 369, 378
cytomegalovirus (CMV) 341, 344
cytoskeleton 171–173, 201, 203, 222
cytotoxic T-lymphocytes 156, 360, 378

Daxx 46
de-adenylating nuclease (DAN) 50
decorin 225
dehydroepiandrosterone 295
dendritic cells 321, 339, 378
desmoglein 70
desmoplasia 225
desmosomes 66
dexamethasone 263, 312, 315
DHA, see docosahexaenoic acid
dietary fats 95–97
diethylstilbesterol (DES) 7, 285
differential display (DD) 29, 45, 46, 348
differential injection sites 144
digital rectal exam 11, 382
dihomogamma linolenic acid (DGLA) 65–67, 71, 77
dihydrotestosterone (DHT) 284, 286, 295, 296
Dishevelled 176–178
DNA fragmentation 99
docetaxel 309, 312, 314–318, 320, 321, 362, 370, 371, 374, 375, 377
docosahexaenoic acid (DHA) 65, 70, 71, 73, 74, 77
dose-fractionation 323, 324
doxorubicin 316, 321, 328, 349, 371
Drg-1 74
DU-145 26, 74, 144, 149, 153, 154, 158, 159, 162, 184, 203, 204, 363
DU-145 MN1 cells 153
Dunning prostate carcinoma 119
Dunning R-3327 rat prostatic adenocarcinoma 129, 130, 135, 144, 320

Dunning rat model 129, 320, 321
Duplin 175, 178, 179

E2F 46, 112
E2F4 46
E-cadherin 22, 30, 35, 45, 70, 94, 128–132, 137, 171–174, 182–187, 202, 204–207, 357
ectopic transplantation 145
ED-B domain 225
EGF 74
EGFR, see epidermal growth factor receptor
eicosanoids 65, 66, 69, 75, 87–89
12-HETE 65, 66
13-HODE 65
eicosapentaenoic acid (EPA) 65, 67, 73, 74, 77
elastin 225
embryogenesis 201
EMMPRIN 226
encephalomyocarditis virus (IRES) 160, 345
endoglin 136, 373
endothelial binding 254
endothelial cells 27, 71, 72, 128, 135, 136, 138, 182, 202, 210, 224, 255, 341, 373
endothelin receptor antagonists 320, 321
endothelin-1 253, 255
endothelium 70, 71, 201, 254, 255
entactin 222
EORTC 285, 318
EPA, see eicosapentaenoic acid
epidermal growth factor 98, 173, 284
epidermal growth factor receptor (EGFR) 154, 155, 367, 372–374
epigenetic alteration 25
epirubicin 312, 316, 319
epithelial/mesenchymal transition 32, 51, 128, 187, 374
epithelial-to-mesenchymal transformation 226, 357
epoxide hydrolase 348
epoxyeicosa- tetraenoic acids (EpTrEs) 89
erythropoetin (EPO) 260, 261
E-selectin 71
essential fatty acid deficiency (EFA D) 66, 70
Essential Fatty Acids 63–66
estradiol 93, 96, 186, 311
estramustine 287, 288, 311, 312, 316–320, 328, 377
estrogens 8, 96, 283, 285, 286, 301, 310–312
etidronate 266–269
etoposide 312, 385
external beam radiotherapy 322, 325, 326, 372

extracellular matrix (ECM) 22, 28, 39, 40, 69–71, 94, 201–205, 221, 207, 222, 225–227, 233, 234, 236–239, 364
ezrin-ridixin-moesin family 71

FAK 70, 116
familial adenomatous polyposis (FAP) 176
FAP (separase) 226
farnesyl pyrophosphate synthase 269
farnesyl-pyrophosphates 269
fatty acid desaturates (FAD) 68, 78
F-box proteins 115, 175, 177
feminization 285
fibroblast growth factors 155, 255, 284, 311, 373
fibroblasts 130, 151, 174, 198, 201, 208, 224, 225, 255
fibronectin 28, 35, 70, 179, 205, 222, 225, 231, 234–236
FISH 37, 38, 153
flutamide 286, 291–293, 296, 298–300, 312
fra-1 179
Frizzled 177, 178

galectin-1 225
gamma glutamyl transpeptidase 89
gamma linolenic acid (GLA) 65–67, 74–7, 209
ganciclovir (GCV) 157, 337, 341–343, 347, 348, 350, 378
gap junctions 255
GCV, see ganciclovir
gelatin 235, 237
gene therapy 143, 155, 309, 337–343, 345, 346, 348–350, 360, 378, 380, 384
genome wide expression screens 23
geranylgeranylpyrophosphates 269
glandular kallikrein (hK2) 233, 235, 236
Gleason grade 9, 14, 42, 135, 229, 230, 362
Gleason grading system 6
Gleason score 6, 7, 12, 13, 15–17, 42, 45, 185, 227–229, 233, 236, 237, 290, 291, 343, 363, 367, 374
Gleevec (STI-571, or imatinib mesylate) 369, 374
GM-CSF gene modified cancer cell vaccination 339
goserelin 287, 288, 290–293, 298
G-protein linked receptors 98
Grb2 201
green fluorescent protein (GFP) 32, 133, 134, 143, 147, 151, 152, 160–162, 368
Groucho 178, 179
GSK-3ß (glycogen synthase kinase-3ß) 172, 173, 175–178, 180–182, 184, 187

GTPase-activating protein (GAP) 201
GTP-binding proteins 269
gynaecomastia 283

haematuria 322
haemoglobin 260, 262, 310, 313
Ha-ras 94
heat shock protein 90 (hsp90) 374, 376
Heat shock proteins 113
hemibody irradiation (HBI) 324
hemidesmosomes 224
heparan sulfate 146, 205, 222–225
heparan sulfate proteoglycan 146, 205, 222, 224
heparin 199, 225, 320
hepatoblastomas (HB) 180, 181
hepatocellular carcinomas (HCC) 180, 181
hepatocyte growth factor activator inhibitor (HAI) 237
hepatocyte growth factor/scatter factor (HGF/SF) 172, 197–199
hepatocyte growth-factor (HGF)-converting enzyme 199
hepatopoietin A 198
hepsin 33, 45, 221, 237
HER-2/neu 362
Herpes Simplex Virus (HSV) thymidine kinase (tk) gene 157, 341, 378
heterocyclic amines 100
hevin 39, 226
HGF 51, 181–184, 197–211, 367
highly unsaturated fatty acids (HUFA) 64
histologic differentiation 6
histomorphometric studies 256
Histone deacetylase (HDAC) 113, 178, 357
hK10 (NES1) 236
hK11 (hippostasin/PRSS20) 236, 237
hK4 (prostase) 236
hK6 (neurosin) 236
HMG box transcription factors 179
hormone response elements (HRE) 284
hormone-independent prostate cancer 310
hot flushes 285, 286, 290
HPV18 26
H-ras 32
HRPC 261, 262, 264, 272, 273, 314, 316, 318–321
HSV-tk 157, 337, 341–343, 347, 348, 350, 378
HT-15 cells 99
HT-29 cells 99
Human Genome Program 27
HUVEC 349
huWAP2 237
hyaluronidases (hyal-1) 152

402

hydrocortisone 312–315
hydroxprogesterone acetate 286
hydroxyeicosatetranoic acids (HETEs) 65, 66, 75, 89
hydroxyproline 267
hypercalcaemia 87, 261, 262, 268, 269

ibandronate 266, 267, 269, 272, 273
ICAM-1 22, 71
IGFs 98, 235, 270, 361
IkappaBalpha 152
IL-10 153, 154
IL-8 152, 153, 155
immune surveillance 99
immunoglobulin superfamily 70
immunoglobulins 49
immunohistochemistry 148, 185, 186, 227, 234
immunomodulatory gene therapy 339–341, 346, 378, 380
immunophilin fkbp 51 74
impotence 283, 285, 286, 290
In Situ Gene Therapy 337, 340, 342
incadronate 266, 267, 269
indomethacin 69, 92, 93, 98, 100
injurin 199, 200
iNOS 155, 347
insulin growth factor-1 284, 361
insulin-like growth factor binding protein-3 (IGFBP-3) 235
integrins 22, 30, 70, 154, 202, 203, 222, 229, 253, 255
interferon 312, 316
interferon-beta 155
Interleukin-12 (IL-12) 156, 337, 343–348, 350, 380
intermittent androgen deprivation (IAD) 284, 299–302
intermittent hormone therapy 287
intermittent therapy 287, 299
isoprenoid lipids 269

JF2S 155

KAI1 29, 34
Kaiso 174
kallikreins (hK) 221, 233–237
kallistatin 237
keratinocytes 98, 119, 182, 205, 366
ketoconazole 328
KLF6 117
kringle domains 199, 210

lactate dehydrogenase 47, 310
lamellipodia 28
lamina densa 222, 223
lamina rara 222, 224
laminin 22, 47, 70, 135, 138, 146, 222–225, 231, 234, 235
latent prostatic cancer 111, 128, 191, 356
leokotrienes 65, 69, 89, 100
leutenising hormone releasing hormone (LHRH)
leutrotrines 65, 89
Leydig tumor cells 268
Libido 285–287, 290, 300
linear accelerators 322
linoleic acid (LA) 64–66, 68, 69, 71–74, 77
liposomes 339
lipoxygenases (LOX) 66, 75, 88, 89, 99, 153, 361
LNCaP 25, 31, 34, 442, 94, 115, 144, 145, 147, 148, 150–152, 158, 186, 237, 362, 370, 372, 375
LNCapFGC 147, 183, 184, 202, 204, 206
LNCaP-GFP cells 183, 202, 204, 206
LNCaP-LN3 148, 152
LNCaP-Pro5 148, 152
loss of heterozygosity (LOH) 24, 31, 37, 42, 114, 116
low density lipoprotein receptor (LDLr) 75
luteinising hormone releasing hormone agonist 318
lymphoedema 322
lymphokines 100
lysosome membrane-associated proteins (LAMP) 230
lysosomes 204, 230–232

macroarrays 48
macrophage colony stimulating factor (M-CSF) 257
macrophages 69, 100, 156, 229, 321, 339, 344, 347, 349, 364, 365
MAP kinase (MAPK) 67, 366
MAPK kinase 4 29, 34
marrow failure 253, 254, 260
maspin 30, 40, 45, 71, 221, 237
mass-spectrometry 47, 49
matrigel 27, 133, 144, 146, 202, 206
matrilysin 162, 205–207, 226
matrilysin (MMP-7) 205
matrix metalloproteinase (MMP) 22, 132, 138, 205, 207, 226, 227, 239, 359, 364–366
matrix metalloproteinase-7 (MMP-7) 179, 226, 229, 230, 205, 207
MMP-1 205, 229

MMP-14 205
MMP-2 132, 133, 154, 225, 227–229, 238, 359, 376
MMP-3 205, 207
MMP-9 152, 153, 205, 228, 229, 366
maximal androgen blockade 273
MC3T3 E1 cells 98
MCF-7 69, 207
McGill-Melzack Pain Questionnaire 313
MDCK cells 210
MDCKts.srcCl2 207
MDM2 348
mdr-1 155
Medical Research Council 272, 291, 294, 295, 369, 370
medroxyprogesterone acetate 286
MEF 349
Melanoma 28, 29, 35, 128, 132, 136, 138, 268, 359
Membrane-type serine protease 1 (MT-SP1, Matriptase) 237, 238
mesenchymal transformation 187, 207, 226
mesodermal cell lineages 255
mesothelioma 205
metastasis activators 23, 25
metastasis suppressor genes 24, 29
metastasis suppressors 23, 24, 26, 29, 42, 348
mevalonate 269, 270
microarray analysis 29, 32, 255, 338, 359
micrometastases 147, 155, 255, 338, 359
microsatellites 42
microtubule assembly 311
minodronate 268, 269
mitomycin C 318
mitoxantrone 272, 312–319, 371
mixed function monooxygenase 92
MNNG-HOS 201
Moloney Sarcoma Virus 100
monocyte chemotactic protein-3 (MCP-3) 179
monocyte/neutrophil elastase inhibitor (MNEI) 237
morphogenesis 72, 187, 201, 227, 239
motogen 198, 201, 202, 204, 210, 211
multiple xenograft variants 26
myofibroblastic cells 208
myofibroblasts 225

N-[4,5-nitro-2-furyl]-2-thiazole] formamide 100
National Cancer Institute (NCI) 10, 382
natural killer (NK) cells 100, 156, 157, 341, 344, 347, 348, 380

N-benzyl-N-hydroxy-5-phenylpentamide (BHPP) 153
NC-37 344
neo-adjuvant 283, 284, 289, 291–293, 342
neo-adjuvant hormone therapy 283, 287, 288
neridronate 269
neuroendocrine cells 31, 236, 358, 385
neuron-specific enolase 229
nexin 234
NF-kappaB/relA 152
NFkb 257
NIH 3T3 201
Nilutamide 286, 287, 296, 298, 300
nitric oxide synthase 155, 156
NK4 115, 203, 209, 210
NKX 3.1 31, 35, 39
Nkx3.1 31, 35, 39
NLK (NEMO-like kinase) 175, 178, 179
N-methyl-N'-nitrosoguanidine 201
nomograms 17
Non-steroidal anti inflammatory drugs (NSAIDs) 92–95, 97–100,
non-steroidal antiandrogens (NSAA). 283
NS-398 92, 94

oleic acid (OA) 74
olpadronate 267, 269
oncogenes 24, 29–31, 52, 94, 116, 154, 174, 180, 199, 201, 363, 374, 382
orchidectomy 267, 273, 284–287, 291, 293, 294, 296, 298, 301, 318
orchiectomy 7
ornithine decarboxylase (ODC) 74, 98, 118–120
orthotopic injection 145–148, 156, 157
orthotopic models 147, 150, 153, 155, 349, 367, 373
orthotopic tumors 145, 148, 156, 157, 343, 344, 346, 347, 380
orthotopic-implantation (SOI) 143, 145–147, 149, 150, 152–154, 158, 159, 162, 368
osteoblastic reaction 325
osteoblasts 40, 98, 253, 255, 257, 258, 260, 261, 270
osteoclast 253, 255, 257, 258, 260, 261, 267, 269, 271, 273, 368, 369
osteogenic sarcoma 201
osteopontin 226
osteoporosis 267, 269, 273, 274, 302
osteoprotegerin 39, 257
ovarian carcinoma 128, 136

p120^{cas} 173, 174
p120^{ctn} 186
P16/INK4A/MTS/CDKN2 115
p185neu-T 154
p21 117, 349
p27 KIP1 31, 114
p300/CBP histone acetyltransferase (HAT) 179
p53 29, 34 67, 117, 156, 157, 348, 349, 371
paclitaxel 270, 312, 369, 373, 374
pamidronate 253, 266–268, 271–274
paraplegia 264
parathyroid hormone 40, 253, 267
pathologic grade 6, 10, 11
pathological fracture 253, 254, 260, 262, 263, 271–273
paxillin 70
PC-3 25, 29, 31, 42, 73, 74, 144, 145, 147–149, 151, 153–155, 157–162, 182, 184, 237, 363, 370, 371, 376
PC-3 cells 25, 31, 116, 117, 144, 145, 148, 151, 154, 157, 160–162, 182, 184, 237, 363, 371
PC-3 ML 153, 154
PC-3M 147, 148, 150, 152, 154–156
PC-3M-LN4 148, 152, 153, 373
PC-3M-Pro4 148, 152
PC-3P 14 153
pepsinogen II 236
perineural invasion 76, 363
peripheral blood stem cell support 326, 342
peroxidase 91, 100
peroxides 67
peroxisome-proliferator activated receptors (PPAR) 69, 75–78
Peroxy radicals 101
Phenylacetates 75
Phophatidylcholine 73
phorbol 12,13-dibutyrate 345
phorbol-12-myristate-13-acetate 207
phosphatidylinositol 3-kinase (PI3K) 32, 201, 366, 371
phospholipase-C-γ (PLC-γ) 201
phospholipids 88, 89, 97
phosphorous-32 (^{32}P) 324
phosphorylation 47, 70, 99, 112, 114, 172–174, 176–178, 180, 182
PI-3 kinase 116
pim-1 33
PLA2 89
plakoglobin 129, 171, 173, 174
plasminogen activator inhibitor-type 1 (PAI-1) 71, 221, 234
plasminogen activators 39, 71, 117, 199, 221, 226, 234, 236

plasminogen preactivation peptide (PAP) 199
polyamines 98, 111, 117–120
spermidine 118, 119
spermine 118
Polyunsaturated fatty acids (PUFAs) 63, 64, 66, 67, 69, 70, 72, 75–77, 89, 97, 361
Pontin52 175, 179
PP2A 176, 178
pp$^{60c-src}$ 201
PPARδ 69, 75, 77, 179
prednisolone 312, 315, 316, 318–321, 370
prenylation 269
probasin 30, 162
procollagen I 226
progesterone 8
promotor methylation 112
prostaglandins 65, 69, 72, 75, 87–89
  PGE2 66, 75, 89, 93, 94, 96–102
  PGF2 89, 96, 98
  PGG2 66, 88, 89
  PGI2 89, 99
  synthesis 87, 88, 90, 92, 96–102
prostasin 237
prostate cancer incidence 97
Prostate Cancer Trialist Collaborative Group (PCTCG) 296, 297
Prostate Expression database 50
prostate, female 385
prostate specific antigen (PSA, hK3) 1, 11, 113, 127, 127, 147, 152, 186, 208, 285, 309, 355, 383
prostate specific membrane antigen (PSMA) 49, 158, 371
Prostate stem-cell antigen (PSCA) 39, 157
prostatic acid phosphatase 12, 48, 321, 385
prostatic intraepithelial neoplasia (PIN) 31, 208, 222, 226, 227, 230, 237, 363
proteasome pathway 374, 375
protein kinase C (PKC) 74
proteoglycans 146, 205, 222–225, 231
proteomics 21, 23, 46–48
proteosome 175–177, 187
PS-341 375
PSA 1, 2, 6, 7, 11–13, 17, 48, 49, 74, 113, 127, 147, 148, 158, 159, 186, 208, 233–236, 285, 287, 289, 290, 300, 301, 309–317, 319–321, 326, 338, 342, 343, 345, 355, 362, 365, 372, 373, 378, 379, 381–383, 385
PSA doubling time 301, 342
PSMA, see prostate specific membrane antigen
PTEN 31, 32, 34, 35, 45, 111, 116, 363
PTEN - PI3-K/Akt pathway 116
PTEN/MMAC1 16, 120

PTH-rP 258
PZ-HPV-7 184

R-3327–5 144
Rab 269
Rac 269
radiation fields 322
radiation therapy 322, 341, 342, 371, 372, 377
radical prostatectomy 2, 7, 10, 12, 185, 283, 287, 289, 290, 337, 338, 342, 345, 356, 357, 363
radiotherapy 12, 253, 262, 263, 265, 283, 290–293, 309, 322–326, 343, 345, 370, 372, 376, 384
RANK ligand 253, 257, 258
Ras 29, 32, 34, 94, 201, 269
Rat Dunning tumor 29
RC-121 321
Receptor tyrosine kinases (RTK) 173, 201, 210
RECK (reversion-inducing cysteine-rich protein with Kazal motiffs) 227
red bone marrow 254, 261
Reptin52 178, 179
reticular lamina 222
Retinoblastoma (Rb) protein 112, 116
retinoic acid (RA) 39, 69, 209
RGD binding 226
Rhenium-186-Hydroxyethylene diphosphonate (^{186}Re-HEDP) 324–327
Rho 29, 35, 269
RhoC 28, 29
ribonuclease protection assay 135
risedronate 267, 269
RM-9 145, 156, 343, 344, 346, 347
Rous Sarcoma Virus (RSV) 173, 341
RTOG 291, 293, 324
RT-PCR 45, 49, 94, 151, 185, 255, 359
RTVP-1 (related to testes-specific, vespid and pathogenesis proteins) 337, 348–350

S100P 32, 33, 35
Samarium-153 (^{153}Sm) 324, 325, 327, 328
SAMP repeats 176
SC-58125 99
scatter factor (SF) 172, 182–184, 197–211
SCF^{SKP2} 115
SCID 144, 151
SCID mice 26, 31, 145, 152–154, 157, 162, 381
SELDI 47, 49
Serial Analysis of gene expression (SAGE) 46
SAGE tagging 43
serine protease 199, 221, 233, 234, 236–239, 358, 365

serine proteinase inhibitors (serpins) 40, 71, 221, 234, 236, 237
serpin 71, 221, 234, 236, 237
sex-hormone binding globulin (SHBG) 285
SGN-15
sialic acid 225, 381
Single Nucleotide Polymorphisms (SNP's) 42
SMAD 2, 32
somatostatin analogues 321
somatostatin receptors 321
SOS 201
spinal cord compression 253, 254, 260, 262, 264, 286, 322
spontaneous bone metastasis model 145, 151
squamous cell carcinomas 100, 182
src 39, 173, 174, 201, 207
stefin (cystatin) 231
Stilboestrol 311, 312
strontium-89 (89Sr) 324–326, 328
superoxides 67, 99
suramin 311, 312, 314, 315
Surveillance, Epidemiology and End Results (SEER) 10
SV40 30, 162

T antigen 30, 31, 162
T cell proliferation 100
T cells 22, 156, 157, 175, 179, 321, 339, 342–344, 346–348, 360, 364, 366, 372, 378, 380
T45D 69
Tag 30, 44, 46, 162
TATA-box binding protein (TBP) 179
taxanes 311, 319, 372
T-cell activation 156, 348
T-cells 22, 100, 175, 321, 339, 342, 346, 348, 372
TCF/LEF-1 (T cell factor/lymphoid enhancer factor-1) 175, 178
tenascin 225, 226, 239
Testosterone 93, 96, 253, 284–286, 301, 310
TFPI-2 (tissue factor pathway inhibitor-2) 227
TGF beta (TGFβ) 30, 32, 35, 40, 51, 117, 154, 155, 202, 235, 255, 270, 373
TGF-β1 154, 155, 202, 373
Th1 339, 350
Th2 339, 366
thalidomide 316, 320
thrombin receptor 136
thrombospondin 227, 229
thrombospondin-1 205
thromboxanes 88, 89

thymosin β4 28, 35
TIE-1 136
TIE-2 136
tiludronate 268, 269
Tissue Inhibitors of Metalloproteinases (TIMP's) 22, 154, 162, 205, 207, 221, 227, 229
TIMP-1 154
tissue-type plasminogen activator (tPA) 71, 199
TLE (transducin-like enhancer-of-split) 179
TMPRSS2 237, 358, 359
topoisomerase II 311
total-human-genome probe 159
TRAMP mice 162
TRAMP model 30, 31, 162
transcription factors 39, 41, 112, 113, 117, 152, 174, 178–180, 187, 362
transferrin 117, 368
transglutaminase (TGases) 365, 366
transrectal ultrasonography (TRUS) 145, 146
transurethral resection of the prostate (TURP) 11
trastuzumab (Herceptin) 362
Triton X-100 183, 202
tropomyosin-β 47
trypsinogen 236
tumor cell plasticity 127, 128, 137, 139
tumor volume 5, 6, 10–13, 146, 287, 289, 338
tyrosine kinases 173, 201, 210, 362, 373, 376

ubiquitin 115, 118–120, 175, 177, 374, 375
ubiquitin ligase 115, 175, 177
ureteric obstruction 322
urokinase 30, 39, 71, 117, 199, 205, 234–238
urokinase receptor (uPAR) 234, 235

urokinase-type plasminogen activator (uPA) 39, 71, 74, 117, 199
urothelium 185

valacyclovir 341, 343
vascular endothelial (VE)-cadherin 72, 207
vascular endothelial growth factor (VEGF) 136, 152, 320, 372, 373
vasculogenic mimicry 127, 128, 132, 134–138, 364
VCAM-1 71
versican 225
Veterans Administration Co-operative Urological Research Group (VAGURG) 6, 285, 294
villin 49
vimentin 51, 132, 360, 376
vinblastine 312, 316, 328
vinca alkaloids 311
vinculin 172, 173
vinorelbine 312
vitronectin 70
von Willebrand factor 49

Walker 256 carcinoma cells 268
watchful waiting 9, 10, 14, 290, 294, 356
Wg receptor 177
whole genome analysis 23
Wnt 171, 173, 175–179, 181, 184, 187, 383

xenobiotics 91, 92, 100

ZD1839 373
zoledronate 266–269, 272, 273, 369
zymogens 226